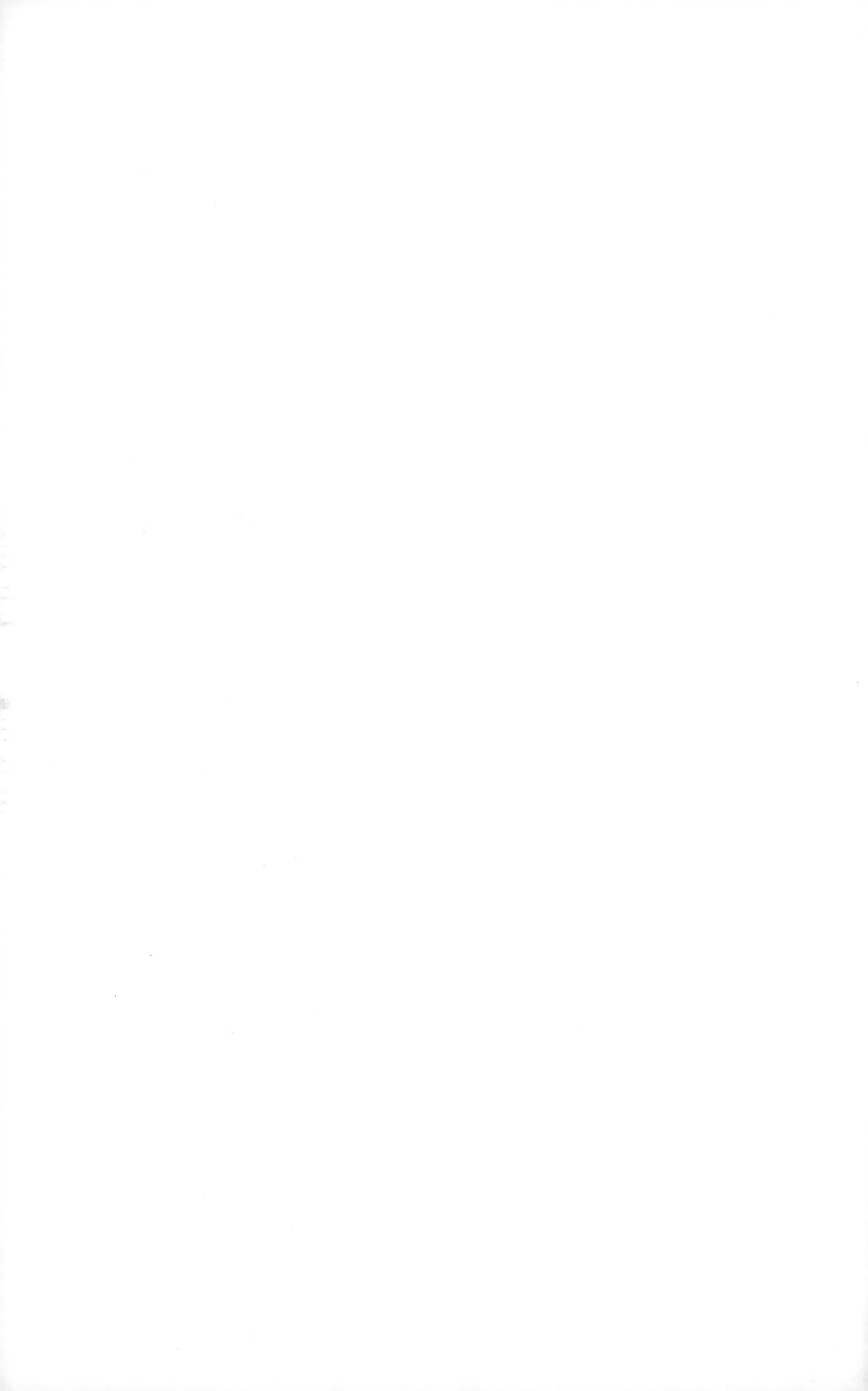

DYNAMICS OF ROMANTIC LOVE

Dynamics of Romantic Love

Attachment, Caregiving, and Sex

Edited by
MARIO MIKULINCER
GAIL S. GOODMAN

THE GUILFORD PRESS
New York London

A Division of Guilford Publications, Inc.
72 Spring Street, New York, NY 10012
www.guilford.com

Printed in the United States of America

This book is printed on acid-free paper.

Last digit is print number: 9 8 7 6 5 4 3 2 1

Library of Congress Cataloging-in-Publication Data

Dynamics of romantic love : attachment, caregiving, and sex / edited by Mario Mikulincer, Gail S. Goodman.
p. cm.
Includes bibliographical references and index.
ISBN-10 1-59385-270-3 ISBN-13 978-1-59385-270-2 (cloth)
1. Love. 2. Attachment behavior. 3. Sex. I. Mikulincer, Mario. II. Goodman, Gail S.
BF575.L8D96 2006
152.4′1—dc22

2005031503

About the Editors

Mario Mikulincer, PhD, obtained his doctorate in psychology from Bar-Ilan University, Ramat Gan, Israel, in 1985, and has been Professor of Psychology there since 1992. Between 1995 and 1999, Dr. Mikulincer acted as the Chair of the Psychology Department and today he serves as the Chair of Interdisciplinary Studies. He has published more than 220 articles and book chapters and one book, *Human Learned Helplessness: A Coping Perspective* (1994). Dr. Mikulincer's research interests include attachment styles in adulthood, terror management theory, personality processes in interpersonal relationships, evolutionary psychology, and trauma and posttraumatic processes. He currently serves on the editorial boards of several academic journals and as associate editor of *Personal Relationships* and the *Journal of Personality and Social Psychology.* In 2004 he received the EMET Prize in Social Science, sponsored by the A. M. N. Foundation for the Advancement of Science, Art, and Culture in Israel, awarded by Prime Minister Ariel Sharon, for Dr. Mikulincer's contributions to psychology.

Gail S. Goodman, PhD, obtained her doctorate in developmental psychology from the University of California, Los Angeles, in 1977, and conducted postdoctoral research at the University of Denver and the Université René Descartes in Paris, France. She is Professor of Psychology and Director of the Center for Public Policy Research at the University of California, Davis, and Professor of Forensic Psychology at the University of Oslo, Norway. Her research focuses on memory development, including attachment and memory, and forensic developmental psychology. Dr. Goodman has served as president of two divisions (Division 37, Child, Youth, and Family Services; and Division 41, Psychology and Law) and one section (Child Maltreatment) of the American Psychological Association. She has received many awards for her research, including two Distinguished Contributions awards in 2005 from the American Psychological Association (the Distinguished Contributions to Research in Public Policy Award and the Distinguished Professional Contributions to Applied Research Award).

Contributors

Colleen J. Allison, MA, Department of Psychology, Simon Fraser University, Burnaby, British Columbia, Canada

Arthur Aron, PhD, Department of Psychology, State University of New York at Stony Brook, Stony Brook, New York

Elaine N. Aron, PhD, Department of Psychology, State University of New York at Stony Brook, Stony Brook, New York

Kim Bartholomew, PhD, Department of Psychology, Simon Fraser University, Burnaby, British Columbia, Canada

Ellen Berscheid, PhD, Department of Psychology, University of Minnesota, Minneapolis, Minnesota

Claudia Chloe Brumbaugh, MA, Department of Psychology, University of Illinois, Urbana–Champaign, Illinois

Mary Campa, MA, Department of Human Development, Cornell University, Ithaca, New York

Lorne Campbell, PhD, Department of Psychology, University of Western Ontario, London, Ontario, Canada

Nancy L. Collins, PhD, Department of Psychology, University of California, Santa Barbara, California

M. Lynne Cooper, PhD, Department of Psychological Sciences, University of Missouri, Columbia, Missouri

Deborah Davis, PhD, Department of Psychology, University of Nevada, Reno, Nevada

Lisa M. Diamond, PhD, Department of Psychology, University of Utah, Salt Lake City, Utah

Brooke C. Feeney, PhD, Department of Psychology, Carnegie Mellon University, Pittsburgh, Pennsylvania

Máire B. Ford, MA, Department of Psychology, University of California, Santa Barbara, California

R. Chris Fraley, PhD, Department of Psychology, University of Illinois, Urbana–Champaign, Illinois

Omri Gillath, PhD, Department of Psychology, University of California, Davis, California

Gail S. Goodman, PhD, Department of Psychology, University of California, Davis, California

AnaMarie C. Guichard, MA, Department of Psychology, University of California, Santa Barbara, California

Nurit Gur-Yaish, MA, Department of Human Development, Cornell University, Ithaca, New York

Cindy Hazan, PhD, Department of Human Development, Cornell University, Ithaca, New York

Ejay L. Jack, BS, Department of Psychology, Pennsylvania State University, University Park, Pennsylvania

Kristen M. Kelly, PhD, Department of Psychology, Pennsylvania State University, University Park, Pennsylvania

Ash Levitt, BA, Department of Psychological Sciences, University of Missouri, Columbia, Missouri

Kenneth N. Levy, PhD, Department of Psychology, Pennsylvania State University, University Park, Pennsylvania

Lada Micheas, MS, Department of Psychological Sciences, University of Missouri, Columbia, Missouri

Mario Mikulincer, PhD, Department of Psychology, Bar-Ilan University, Ramat Gan, Israel

Mark Pioli, PhD, Department of Psychological Sciences, University of Missouri, Columbia, Missouri

Harry T. Reis, PhD, Department of Clinical and Social Sciences in Psychology, University of Rochester, Rochester, New York

Dory A. Schachner, MA, Department of Psychology, University of California, Davis, California

Phillip R. Shaver, PhD, Department of Psychology, University of California, Davis, California

Jeffry A. Simpson, PhD, Department of Psychology, University of Minnesota, Minneapolis, Minnesota

Keren Slav, MA, Department of Psychology, Bar-Ilan University, Ramat Gan, Israel

Amelia E. Talley, MA, Department of Psychological Sciences, University of Missouri, Columbia, Missouri

Yanna J. Weisberg, MA, Department of Psychology, University of Minnesota, Minneapolis, Minnesota

Preface

This book grew out of a conference that was held in September 2004 to celebrate Phillip Shaver's 60th birthday and his receipt of the honorary title "Distinguished Professor of Psychology" at the University of California, Davis. As explained in Chapter 1, Phil had requested such a conference instead of conventional birthday and congratulations gifts. Because he and many of his colleagues and former students thought it was time in any case to review the status of the research field that he and Cindy Hazan had initiated with their 1987 article, "Romantic Love Conceptualized as an Attachment Process," we contacted people in the field to see if they would be willing to present their work at such a conference and turn their talks into polished book chapters.

As you can see by skimming the table of contents, an amazing group of scholars accepted the invitation. The 2 days of talks, reunions among old friends, discussion-filled meal sessions, and a lovely outdoor dinner party provided many opportunities for creative contributors to the study of adult attachment and close relationships to compare ideas; have their work appreciated, discussed, and critiqued; and consider how the study of adult attachment has developed over the past 18 years and might develop further. The goal was to evaluate and expand on Cindy and Phil's early ideas about how romantic love typically involves a combination of three behavioral systems discussed by John Bowlby in his trilogy on attachment theory: attachment, caregiving, and sex.

The three behavioral systems provided the core organizational framework for the book. Preceding the three major sections on the behavioral systems are introductory chapters by us, the editors, that lay out the issues to be discussed and provide both a lighthearted commentary and a serious psychobiography of the guest of honor, Phil Shaver. At the end of the book, several authors comment on the attachment theory of romantic love, constructively criticize it, and supplement it with other important perspectives. In a final chapter, Phil comments on the previous chapters and the field they represent, noting questions, conundrums, and possibilities for future theoretical and empirical work.

All but two of the conference speakers, Jude Cassidy and Lee Kirkpatrick, turned their talks into chapters, so the book provides a stimulating, detailed, and accurate picture of most of what was presented and discussed. Jude Cassidy is in the process of writing a much more extensive version of her talk than a book chapter could contain, and Lee Kirkpatrick published a book in 2005, with The Guilford Press, that presents his perspective on *Attachment, Evolution, and the Psychology of Religion*, so even those two excellent contributions to the conference, for which we are very grateful, are or will be available to interested readers.

We also wish to thank everyone who made the conference and the preparation of this book both possible and enjoyable. We are extremely grateful to all of the speakers and the contributors to the book. They flew to California for the celebratory conference and largely did so at their own expense. Even so, the meetings, the hotel rooms, and the meals were expensive, so we are thankful for the help we received in paying for them. About half of the costs were generously covered by the Dean of Social Sciences at UC Davis, Steven Sheffrin. He also generously opened the conference. A matching grant was provided by The Guilford Press, whose editor-in-chief, Seymour Weingarten, not only approved the grant but flew to California to attend the conference.

The arrangements for the conference were made by psychology department staff members, including Brenda Ruth, the department manager, Barbara Scoggins, and Tracey Pereida. Many of the on-site details and inevitable emergencies were handled by Omri Gillath, a postdoctoral fellow who was managing Phil's laboratory at the time. He provided invaluable assistance, and always with good humor. We owe him special thanks. Josi Cosca, the psychology department's technical expert, was also crucially helpful. Phil's undergraduate advisor, Karl Scheibe, flew in as a surprise guest—adding a wonderful touch to the festivities. Itzi Alonso-Arbiol, a young faculty member from the University of the Basque Country in Spain who had worked with Phil on several research projects, flew all the way from Spain for the event. Phil's longtime friends from UC Santa Barbara, Jim Blascovich and Brenda Major, also showed up to surprise and delight Phil. Several people gave touching and funny commentaries about Phil and his career, with each sharing a special anecdote or angle that was entertaining for the rest of us to hear. Many of the doctoral students in psychology at UC Davis provided rides for the guests to and from the airport and restaurants; they also helped make the talk sessions, breaks, and meals lively.

The chapter authors were a pleasure for us to work with, in our role as editors. They produced excellent first drafts and yet were willing to make small adjustments to allow the chapters to interlock and become more than a sum of separate parts. All of them went beyond their previously published work to create a forward-looking volume that will be a real asset to the field. Our aim was to create a book that would be truly valuable even aside from its goal of celebrating Phil Shaver's life and career. We believe we have succeeded, and we look forward to the book having an important impact on the field.

Finally, we would like to thank Phil. He also read and commented on every chapter, contributed to some of the chapters more extensively, and took all of the joking and ribbing he received at the conference in the same friendly and loving spirit with which it was imbued. By including the one special chapter in this book about Phil's life, we hope, without disrupting the experience of anyone who wishes simply to read the rest of the book as a coherent scientific volume, to give current and future researchers and students a sense of Phil himself and the origins of his interest in attachment theory. Too often, students get the impression that scientific ideas and projects arise from some abstract, crystalline realm to which they do not have access. But the work summarized in this book grew partly out of the life experiences of people like Phil who were willing to combine personal observations and perspectives with seminal theorizing and research by other investigators. As is often the case in personality, social, developmental, and clinical psychology, the researchers who study romantic love, attachment (secure and insecure), caregiving, and sex are to some extent studying and expressing themselves, just as novelists, playwrights, and filmmakers do. It's a credit to Phil that he is willing to allow readers of this book to peek behind the formal persona, behind a name in the scientific literature, to learn something about the interplay between science and life.

MARIO MIKULINCER
GAIL S. GOODMAN

Contents

Part I

Introduction

1

Attachment to Attachment Theory

A Personal Perspective on an Attachment Researcher

GAIL S. GOODMAN

The idea for the conference that turned into this book arose when I asked my husband, Phil Shaver, what he would like for his 60th birthday (September 7, 2004). To my surprise, Phil said he would like a combination birthday party and small conference on the application of attachment theory to romantic love, something he and his erstwhile doctoral student Cindy Hazan (now a faculty member at Cornell University and coauthor of Chapter 3 of this volume) had first proposed when Phil and I were faculty members at the University of Denver in the 1980s.

During his 60th year, Phil had attended more than one memorial service for deceased friends and relatives; helped his then 84-year-old mother, Frances Shaver, recover from a stroke; processed the paperwork (in his role as department chair) for some of his colleagues' retirements; and received the honorary title "Distinguished Professor" from the University of California, Davis. All of this happened only a year after Phil had almost gone blind in one eye before an MRI scan revealed a large pituitary tumor that was crushing his left optic nerve, a scary situation that required something akin to brain surgery. All of these events, coming in such close succession, caused Phil to say in a perhaps mockingly humorous tone, "I think I'd like to have a retirement party and a memorial service right now, while I'm still alive and able to enjoy it." After Phil's friend and research partner Mario Mikulincer and I began planning the conference/party, Phil took to calling it the "Phil is an old guy conference," which was not its official name. (The conference had the same title as this book.)

Although I have used attachment theory and some of Phil's measures in my own research on parental attachment styles and children's memory for traumatic experiences (e.g., Goodman, Quas, Batterman-Faunce, Riddlesberger, & Kuhn, 1994, 1997), which might have been the subject of my chapter in this book, I decided to devote the space to a sketch of Phil's life that may help future students and scholars understand how he and his interest in attachment theory came about. It should stimulate hope and courage in students who have little idea how to develop a career, including those who have been told by their mentors to do it in the conventional ways. As you'll see, Phil followed his own personal interests and combined personal with scientific concerns, and I think this partially explains how he managed to develop new ideas and studies year after year and to work long hours without losing interest or enthusiasm.

This chapter-length venture into psychobiography—a field developed to a substantial degree by two of Phil's and my colleagues at UC Davis, Alan Elms (1994; Elms & Heller, 2005) and Dean Simonton (2002)—is my first. It gave me an excuse to sort through a large drawer of old photographs that Phil and I usually have no time to examine. I retain in this chapter some of the informality, lightness, and attempt at humor that characterized my presentation of this psychobiography at the "Phil is an old guy conference." My presentation, which I meant to be both funny and serious, was part of a series of presentations by friends of Phil's in which, for example, Harry Reis showed old photographs from our years at the University of Denver (where Harry spent a sabbatical year and met his wife, Ellen) and Art Aron showed both real and humorously counterfeited e-mail messages from Phil in which Phil explained, month after month, year after year, why his reviews for the *Journal of Personality and Social Psychology* were late. (I'm still not sure whether one of the last messages Art displayed, in which Phil supposedly said, "I'm really, really sorry, but my daughters ate the manuscript," was true or invented by Art for this special occasion.)

The aim of psychobiography is to apply psychological theories and research to the lives of particular individuals. In the case of Elms's and Simonton's work, the target individuals have included writers, psychologists, musicians, and political figures, to name just a few of the target categories. Elms and Heller (2005) recently relied on attachment theory to explain certain features of Elvis Presley's personality and his relationships with women, including his mother. I wanted to see whether attachment theory could help explain Phil Shaver's development. Those of us at the conference know Phil to be a gregarious, charming, nurturant, scholarly, talkative, warm, witty, readaholic–workaholic alpha male. Was he always that way? What shaped this unusual man?

It all started when Frances Magdalene Quinn and Robert (Bob) Richard Shaver, Phil's parents, met at a roller skating rink in Iowa City, Iowa, just before World War II. (See photograph 1.) Fran grew up on a farm, as a religious Catholic (which she remains to this day), and was working in Iowa City as a hairstylist following graduation from a rural high school. Her father used to take Phil to the "Westerns" (i.e., cowboy movies) after he retired, when Phil was in early elementary school. He generously gave Phil his large collection of Indian arrowheads and tomahawk heads, dug up during decades of plowing fields on his Iowa farm. Bob's Protestant (English and German) family barely made it through the Great Depression, but by the time Phil was born, his grandfather (Bob's father) was running a small feed store out of his garage in a rural Iowa town of 300 people. He was a creative and gregarious person, like Phil, who was locally famous for inventing a cattle-feed mixture called Shaver's No-Bloat!

Phil used to go with his grandfather to customers' farms to deliver bags of feed and No-Bloat, and on those trips he learned a lot about Amish people, many of whom had horses and buggies in their driveways but forbidden radios and early television sets hidden behind special drapes in their houses. A few also had taboo cars in their barns, but always in black or dark blue or purple shades, as if a car might be okay with the Lord if it looked as similar as possible to a buggy. These were early hints to Phil that people's public behavior and their inner desires and conflicts were not always congruent, a useful realization for someone who would go on to develop an interest in psychodynamic theories.

In short, although Phil wasn't born into a financially privileged family, he was always surrounded by a sociable, supportive, fun-loving, and interesting group of extended family members. Despite her and her husband's generally traditional ideas about parenting and child rearing, Fran once told me that Phil's dad was "quite the mother hen." I knew Bob late in his life (near that fateful age of 65), when he was very kind to both Phil and me, and especially so to his young granddaughter, whom he telephoned on the day he died to say he loved her. While Fran was out grocery shopping, Bob died at home alone with a small bottle of nitroglycerine in his hand, prescribed to prevent a heart attack. He may have known he was suffering what might be, and was, a final, fatal heart attack. He used his last breaths to call his granddaughter and tell her he loved her instead of dialing 911. These are hints, I believe, about the combination of psychological and familial qualities that influenced the future Distinguished Professor Shaver's development.

Because World War II started while Bob and Fran were courting, they decided to get married when he enlisted in the Navy. (Bob's picture in photograph 1 was taken at that time.) They had a romantic but also worrisome

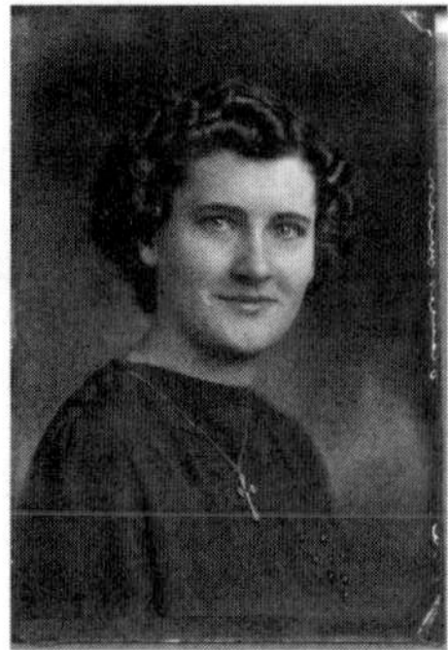

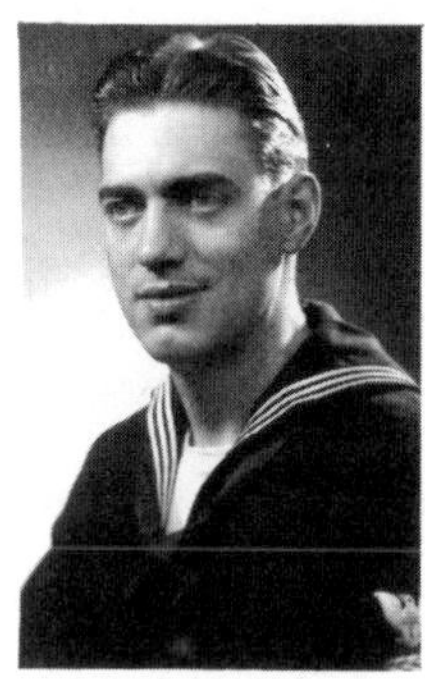

Photograph 1. Frances Quinn and Robert Shaver, before Phil Shaver was born.

few weeks at the University of Wisconsin in Madison, where Bob attended radio school before being shipped to Iceland and then to France. (Phil still thinks of the Madison campus as a romantic place, which makes it interesting that he and several of his professional friends attended the first "close relationships" conference in Madison in 1982, when the relationship research field was just getting under way and Phil was beginning to study romantic love.) Phil was conceived in Philadelphia (City of Brotherly Love), when Bob came home for a short leave and Fran took a train to the East Coast to be with him. After that, Fran was at home with baby Phil (photograph 2), who was named after a Civil War captain in the Shaver line, and she and one of her work colleagues lavished attention on him. The upside of this situation was, I believe, an early foundation of secure attachment to his mother, a greater than usual oedipal contest with his father, and a general

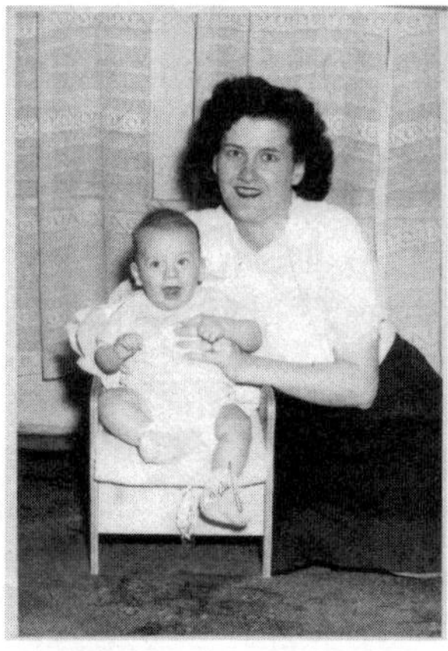

Photograph 2. Phil and Fran.

favoritism toward or comfort with women, which made it easy for him, like me, to favor having female children. (As I write, our only children, twin daughters, are 9 years old.)

When Phil underwent a 2-year, 4-day-a-week psychoanalysis years later, while he was teaching at Columbia and New York Universities during the 1970s, he kept dreaming about being a little boy and walking in a park with two women, each holding one of his hands. Because this image seemed to be linked in his free associations with a lingering tendency to get involved in a committed relationship with one woman while keeping another "in the wings," in case anything went awry with the primary relationship, Phil eventually called his mother long distance and asked what she thought the recurrent "two women" dreams and his dual-relationship strategy might mean. She said, "I think it refers to what actually happened. My coworker and I, both with husbands away in the military, really did hold your hands and walk with you in the park on weekends. And when I was busy or at work, she took care of you." This kind of accurate and enduring memory strengthened Phil's belief that early childhood experiences have lasting effects on relationship patterns, and it also kept him interested in psychodynamic approaches to psychology, as indicated by some of the papers he and Mario Mikulincer have written in recent years (e.g., Berant, Mikulincer, Shaver, & Segal, 2005; Shaver & Mikulincer, 2005).

Phil and I have had many debates during our decades together about the relative roles of environment and genes in personality development, with him remaining open to the possibility of a strong genetic contribution. He tends to think his Irish genes, as expressed in his mother's highly verbal and extroverted behavior, made him a talkative, fast-writing extrovert. When I look at photograph 3, I have to admit that his exhibitionistic tendencies were evident very early. But I would put much more weight on the fact that his mother spent a lot of time doting on him and talking with him.

When Phil's father returned from the war, he eventually went to work for what was then the Civil Aeronautics Administration (now the Federal

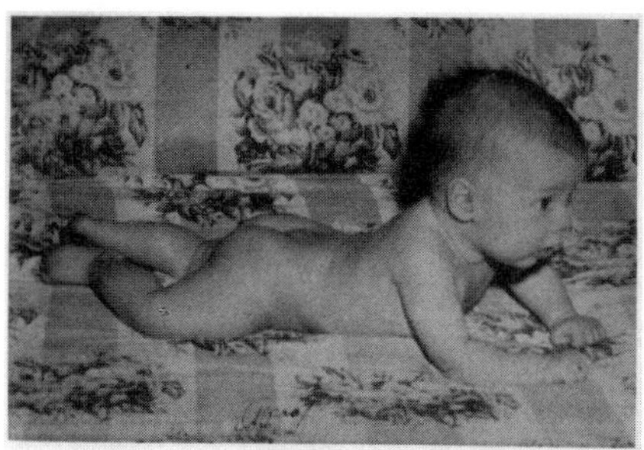

Photograph 3. Phil as an infant.

Aviation Administration). To make up for lost time and move up the government pay scale quickly, Bob bid on and accepted jobs in many different places. Phil's family therefore moved frequently during his childhood, causing him to live, at different times, in Iowa City; Redwing, Minnesota; Lincoln, Nebraska; Russell, Kansas; and eventually Cedar Rapids, Iowa, where Phil attended both junior high and high school. One important constant during most of those years, besides his parents, was his younger brother Craig (see photograph 4). It's my hypothesis that this important association with his then little brother, who was very upset by the frequent moves and couldn't understand the reasons for instability and change, helped to create in Phil a wonderful lifelong trait—nurturing others (see Chapters 7–9 in this volume, which deal with what attachment theorists call the "caregiving behavioral system"). Phil also noticed early on that the frequent moves caused Craig to vigorously follow his mother around the house, including up and down two flights of stairs, lest he find himself alone in novel surroundings (an issue addressed in Ainsworth's famous Strange Situation laboratory procedure; Ainsworth, Blehar, Waters, & Wall, 1978).

The constant moving to new cities and schools may have helped Phil develop his amazing ability to make friends quickly, enter new groups seamlessly, and become a group's leader. He was repeatedly elected to the presidency of this and that at every level of school. He was, for example, president of his high school student council and of his college fraternity. He has been the head of personality–social psychology programs at four different universities and chair of the UC Davis psychology department twice. He has been executive officer of the Society of Experimental Social Psychology. In these roles, as I believe his colleagues would agree, he is more oriented toward what Erikson (1950, 1974) called "generativity" (creatively helping

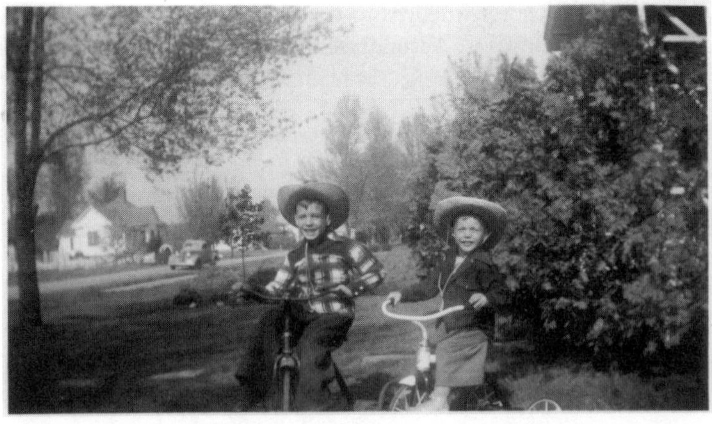

Photograph 4. Phil and his brother Craig.

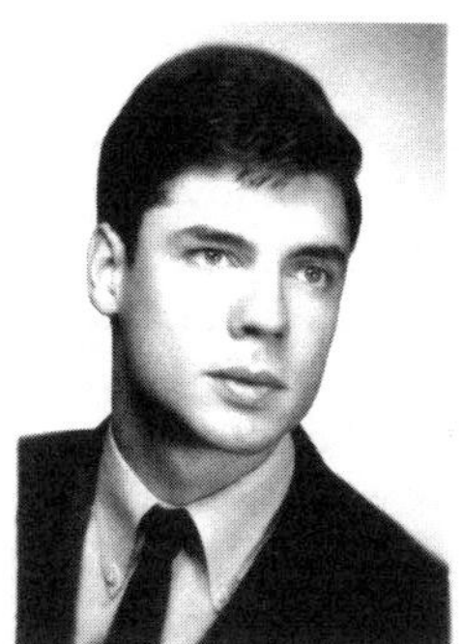

Photograph 5. Phil during his senior year in high school.

others, including social organizations and institutions) than toward power. This makes it easy for people to trust him and remain open to his vision.

Perhaps because of his secure attachment history and native intelligence, Phil was always at the top of his class academically. But as his high school graduation photograph (photograph 5) indicates, he was probably near the top of his class in looks, too. As a National Merit Scholar and valedictorian of his high school class, he could have had his pick of excellent universities, but he had little help in choosing one. It was Wesleyan University, a small liberal arts college in Connecticut, which had the foresight to send a recruiter to Iowa and actively seek Phil out. Phil's parents wanted him to stay near home, but fortunately the skilled Wesleyan recruiter convinced Phil's parents that, with all the scholarship funds they and the Merit Scholarship program would give Phil, it would be cheaper for him to go to school in Connecticut than in Iowa.

It was at Wesleyan that Phil took his first psychology class, taught partly by Dr. Karl Scheibe, a social psychologist who had recently received his PhD at Berkeley (and who attended the "Phil is an old guy conference" as an unannounced surprise guest—a delightful touch). That early class and Dr. Scheibe's subsequent support and mentoring led Phil to become a social psychologist. Phil had his first two papers accepted for publication as an undergraduate, with considerable help from Dr. Scheibe and a classmate, Sam Carrier (later president of Oberlin College)—one on a novel use of the Stroop color-naming task (Scheibe, Shaver, & Carrier, 1967), subsequently used in several studies by Mario Mikulincer and Phil, and one on "transformation of social identity" (Shaver & Scheibe, 1967), a recurring theme in Dr. Scheibe's subsequent work (see, e.g., his 2000 book, *The Drama of Everyday Life*).

With Karl's help, Phil was accepted by graduate programs at Berkeley, Duke, Harvard, Michigan, Minnesota, and Texas. He decided to attend the University of Michigan, which at that time had one of the largest and most prestigious social psychology programs in the country. Phil ended up working with Robert Zajonc, John Robinson, Jack French, Sidney Cobb, and Melvin Manis, as well as such fellow students as Carol Tavris, Peter Archibald, Robert Athanasiou, Philip Brickman, and Stanley Gaines, with all of whom he published articles and books during and just after graduate school. Before he was even sure what he wanted to do when he grew up, and while still getting used to the idea that he had survived a brush with malignant melanoma (which required two surgeries at the University of Michigan Hospital), he was offered jobs at Cornell and Columbia. (Phil and his family, including his younger brothers, Craig and Kevin, are shown around this time in photograph 6.) He accepted the job at Columbia and then quickly proposed and completed a doctoral dissertation (not the typical order of events in academia, then or now).

Phil hadn't decided before that point what he wanted to work on, but he nevertheless completed a dissertation in 6 months. It dealt with spatial imagery in problem solving, a topic that in Phil's mind settled an old score with one of his otherwise much-loved undergraduate mentors, Dick DeBold, who had assured Phil that psychology was way beyond such introspective concepts as mental imagery. Phil knew that he himself solved problems using mental imagery, so he decided that *behaviorism* was misguided, not he—a typical case of his mixing personal observations and intuitions with science. The dissertation was later supplemented and published (Shaver,

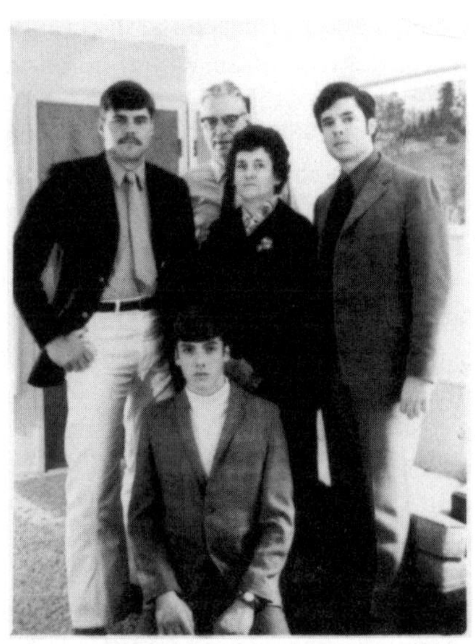

Photograph 6. The Shavers in the 1960s: Craig, Bob, Fran, Phil, and (in front) Kevin.

Pierson, & Lang, 1975), a tiny skirmish in the now-famous "cognitive revolution" in psychology.

Phil began his assistant professorship at Columbia University in 1971. He was exposed there to another group of highly creative and influential social psychologists, including Stanley Schachter, Richard Christie, Robert Krauss, and Jonathan Freedman. He did innovative jury selection research with Christie and published an influential article in *Psychology Today* titled "Recipe for a Jury: Jury Selection for the Harrisburg Conspiracy Trial" (Schulman, Shaver, Colman, Emrich, & Christie, 1973). That article was a foundational document in the field of social scientific jury selection. Phil and Jonathan Freedman also did innovative survey research on life satisfaction and happiness, which Freedman (1978) went on to develop into a popular and influential book.

During this time, Phil and his student collaborators published a number of influential articles about social facilitation, self-awareness, and fear of success, all related to interests he developed while at Michigan. In one of those papers, he and Valerie Geller (Geller & Shaver, 1976) used the Stroop color-naming procedure that he had previously used in his first study with Karl Scheibe at Wesleyan, a technique that subsequently became increasingly popular in studies of social cognition. Phil also collaborated with a young faculty colleague in the religion department, Wayne Proudfoot (now a full professor at Columbia), and together they applied Schachter's emotion theory to the study of religious experiences (Proudfoot & Shaver, 1975). Their article became one in a continuing series of psychology of religion articles by Phil and various coauthors (e.g., Kirkpatrick & Shaver, 1990, 1992; Spilka, Shaver, & Kirkpatrick, 1985), some of which have been reprinted in anthologies on the psychology of religion (for example, the one edited by Spilka & McIntosh, 1997). Lee Kirkpatrick, who spoke at the "Old Phil" conference, has continued to develop ideas he and Phil hatched together, as can be seen in Lee's thoughtful 2005 book, *Attachment, Evolution, and the Psychology of Religion.*

Phil taught personality psychology to a large number of undergraduates during his years at Columbia, and because so many of them had either been in psychoanalysis themselves or had parents or relatives who were psychoanalysts, Phil accepted an offer from the Columbia Psychoanalytic Institute for faculty members to undergo a 2-year analysis, on an "ability to pay" basis, with a medical resident who needed a final case study in order to achieve certification. At that time, Phil's assistant professor salary was around $15,000 a year, so his "ability to pay" was minimal. He thus received both psychotherapy and an important kind of professional training for a very low price (unless you factor in all of the cab rides from West 116th Street to East 96th Street and back; for some reason, even novice psychoanalysts in those days felt it necessary to have an office on the east side of Central Park).

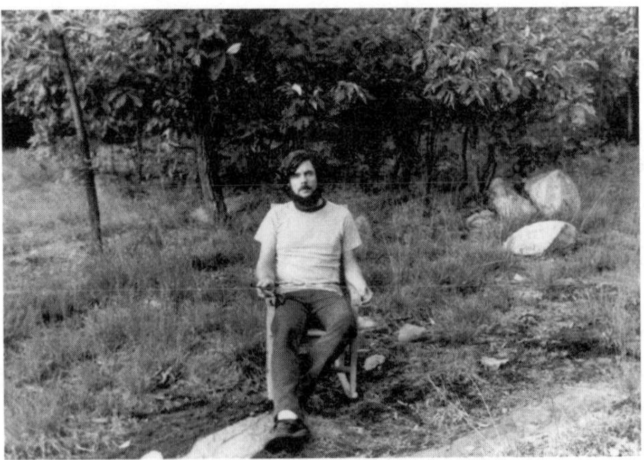

Photograph 7. Phil in 1972, during the anti-war movement.

This was the time of the Vietnam War, when antiwar social psychologists, like many students, sported long hair and beards. (See photograph 7, which shows Phil with a beard and long hair.) Phil had long-term romantic attachments, during graduate school and his assistant and associate professor years, with other talented young psychologists, including Carol Tavris, Susan Saegert, Diane Fenner, Cathy Pullis, and Tracey Revenson (all of whom are now accomplished researchers, writers, and professionals with whom Phil still maintains contact), but these attachments did not result in marriage, perhaps causing Phil—more than most men in their late 20s and early 30s—to become interested in the psychology of love, relationships, loneliness, and loss. To make matters worse, while he was in psychoanalysis, his younger brother Craig (then only 28) was diagnosed with testicular carcinoma (possibly an effect of chemicals encountered while Craig served in the Navy during the Vietnam War or of a drug, DES, taken by Fran during her childbearing years to prevent miscarriage).

Fortunately, when Phil's psychoanalyst, a physician, first learned of Craig's illness, he said, "I'd like to step outside the role of psychoanalyst for this session and explain to you why Craig is not likely to survive, and why you might want to turn your attention to dealing with his illness and likely death." Even though Phil learned and changed a great deal during his analysis, that one nonanalytic counseling session may have been the most important of all the turning points in the 2-year process. He decided to move for the summer to Minneapolis, where Craig lived and was being treated, and where Ellen Berscheid (famous relationship-research pioneer and author of Chapter 16 in this volume) allowed Phil to use an office at the University of Minnesota and stay at her home until he found an apartment. (He was also befriended by Mark Snyder, a faculty member at Minnesota, and Jeff

Simpson, a graduate student at the time but now a professor at Minnesota and one of the leading researchers studying adult attachment; see Chapter 9, this volume.)

Within a few months, Craig was dead, leaving Craig's young wife, Phil's younger brother Kevin, Phil's parents, and Phil himself devastated. Phil has always been extremely grateful to Ellen for her exceptional kindness during that period, another case of attachment-sustaining caregiving and compassion.

Being present when and just before Craig died, Phil noticed that Craig had what is called a "near-death" experience, which later caused Phil to read everything he could find about such experiences and even to review some of the literature professionally (Shaver, 1986). He wrote a brief note to *Psychology Today* magazine, which was published, suggesting how the reality or delusional quality of such experiences might be determined empirically by putting unexpected messages on the topsides of emergency room light fixtures. If a person really left his or her body during a near-death experience and looked down from the ceiling, as is often described, the person should be able to tell later (after being resuscitated) what was written on the lights. Today, researchers are actually conducting such studies, with, so far, no convincing evidence for sight without a body (although the book by Ring & Cooper, 1999, is certainly thought-provoking and has led to interesting lunch discussions between Phil and Ken Ring, who is retired and living in the San Francisco Bay area).

Phil returned to New York (he was on the faculty at NYU by that time, having been offered early tenure there along with the opportunity to direct their doctoral program in personality and social psychology) and tried to interest his graduate students in all of the books he was reading about loss and grief. He wanted to shift his research activities from self-awareness theory and fear of success, the topics he had mainly been studying (in addition to jury selection) up to that time, to grief. But not surprisingly, his young graduate students attributed this intense and, to them, morbid interest to Phil's own temporary grief; and with one exception they refused to go along with his newfound fascination with loss. The one exception was Carin Rubenstein, who negotiated a compromise with Phil according to which they would focus on loneliness (a salient concern for young adults) rather than grief. Phil agreed, and their work, which resulted in several coauthored articles and chapters and culminated in a 1982 book, *In Search of Intimacy* (Rubenstein & Shaver, 1982), helped shape the emerging field of close relationship research, which (as mentioned earlier) was launched with a landmark conference in Madison, Wisconsin, that same year. Reading about and researching loneliness is what first brought Phil into contact with John Bowlby's writings about attachment and loss, which had been applied to loneliness by Robert Weiss in 1974. Phil met Weiss in the late 1970s at an NIMH-sponsored conference on loneliness research, hosted by Anne Peplau and Dan Perlman, an important conference for both Phil and the emerging field of close relationship research.

In 1979, while working on what would become his and Rubenstein's 1982 book, Phil came to the University of Denver during a sabbatical leave from NYU. I was a postdoctoral fellow at the time. After Phil gave a "Hello, I'm the new visitor" colloquium on loneliness research, I did something I had never done before: Despite the fact that I was seeing someone else, I actually asked Phil out! I must say, this turned out to be a very smart move on my part. Totally unbeknownst to me, it was a time in Phil's life when he was longing for a new, deeper, more secure attachment. And it was certainly a time in my own life when I needed someone like Phil. I didn't realize then just how unusual and talented he is. The depth of his knowledge, and of his morality and kindness, still amaze me almost daily.

Aside from many other kindnesses he showed me, he offered me the sort of security that Bowlby and Ainsworth viewed as important for exploration. This allowed me to better focus my research attention on what had deeply interested me for some time—children in the legal system. I edited a special issue of the *Journal of Social Issues* on child eyewitness testimony (Goodman, 1984), a monograph that set the stage for what has since become an entire field, one that has sustained my interest and energy for more than 20 years (e.g., Goodman, 2005; Goodman et al., 1992; Goodman et al., 2003).

I think I returned Phil's support and provision of a "secure base for exploration" (an important concept in attachment theory), because he, with Cindy Hazan's considerable input and creativity, began to switch his interests away from loneliness and toward what lonely young adults (like he and I, before we met) longed for, *romantic love*, which we happily celebrated all the way from Jackson Hole, Wyoming, through the Grand Canyon, to the beaches of California. (This is a great way, incidentally, to spend parts of a sabbatical year or a postdoctoral fellowship!) Cindy and Phil began to realize that if love was what lonely adults were longing for, and if, as Cindy and Phil had noticed, people who were chronically vulnerable to loneliness were quite similar psychodynamically to the two main kinds of insecure babies discussed by Ainsworth et al. (1978) in their classic book on the Strange Situation, then there might be types of romantic love, eventually called "attachment styles" (Levy & Davis, 1988), that were similar to the patterns of infant–parent attachment described by Ainsworth. This idea, first broached in a paper by Cindy in one of Phil's graduate seminars at the University of Denver (and elaborated in this volume; see Chapter 3) and supplemented by their idea (e.g., Shaver, Hazan, & Bradshaw, 1988) that romantic love seemed to involve not only the attachment system but also the caregiving and sexual systems, became the foundation of the work summarized and creatively extended in this volume.

Not surprisingly, Phil's friends were quick to notice that, whereas he had studied loneliness following his brother's death, he began to study attachment, caregiving, and sex around the time he met me. I'm certainly happy to take some of the credit! (Seriously, this interweaving of personal preoccupations with creative research is something that has served both Phil and me well during our careers, and we recommend it to students, many of whom are told by their mentors that science shouldn't be personal.) During those years, Phil was regularly involved in a discussion group with Harry Reis, when Harry came to Denver during a sabbatical leave from the University of Rochester, and Phil's colleagues Howard Markman and Wyndol Furman. They and several postdocs and students jokingly called their group RUG (Relationship Understanding Group), and at the "Phil is an old guy" conference, Harry Reis showed pictures of what the group members looked like back then, wearing their special RUG T-shirts (see photograph 8).

Because I included Phil's high school graduation picture and mentioned that he was quite attractive for a valedictorian, I will also mention in passing that during the years in Denver, when he was writing about attachment, caregiving, and sex, he was selected by *Denver Magazine* as "one of the sexiest men in Denver over 40." A picture from that magazine is shown here as photograph 9. You can see that by this time Phil's hair and mustache were beginning to turn gray, but someone in one of his classes must nevertheless have nominated him as youthful and sexy. He was a popular teacher, that's for sure, and maybe sexiness was one of the reasons, along with his intellectual breadth, enthusiasm, and gregariousness.

Cindy and Phil's early work on romantic attachment mushroomed into one of the largest chunks of the now quite well-accepted field of close rela-

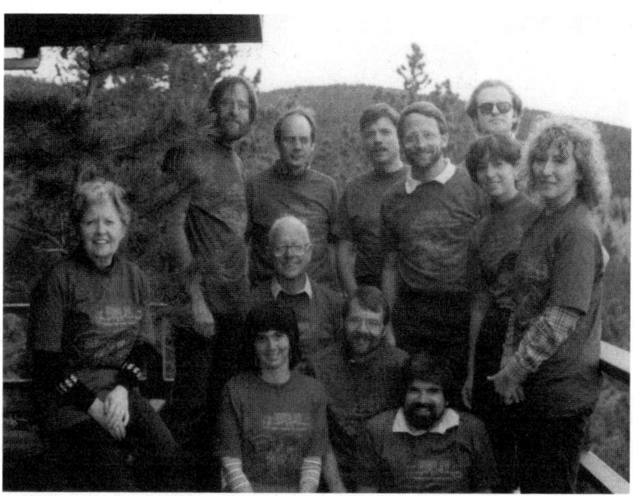

Photograph 8. The Relationship Understanding Group (RUG) in the early 1980s.

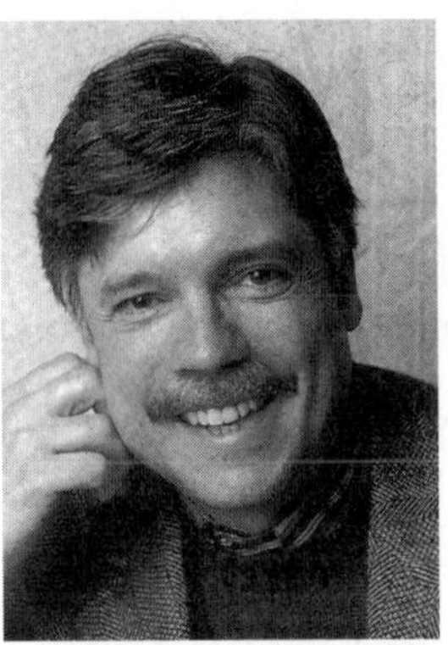

Photograph 9. Phil in *Denver Magazine*, 1986.

tionship research. It was expanded during those early years in Denver by doctoral students including Duane Buhrmester, Vicki Helgeson, Lee Kirkpatrick, Mary Klinnert, and Donald Sharpsteen, who, like Cindy, are now all tenured university professors or accomplished clinical researchers in their own right. The measures Cindy and Phil created have been expanded and translated into many languages. (I am deliberately skipping over other important research and writing Phil did during those years on emotions and emotion knowledge with Kurt Fischer, Judy Schwartz, Don Kirson, and Cary O'Connor because it is less directly relevant to this volume.)

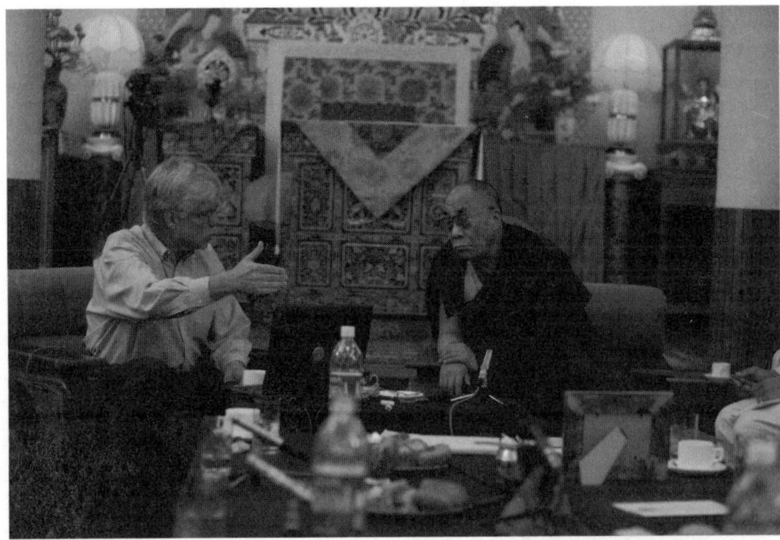

Photograph 10. Phil explaining attachment theory to the Dalai Lama, Dharamsala, India, 2004.

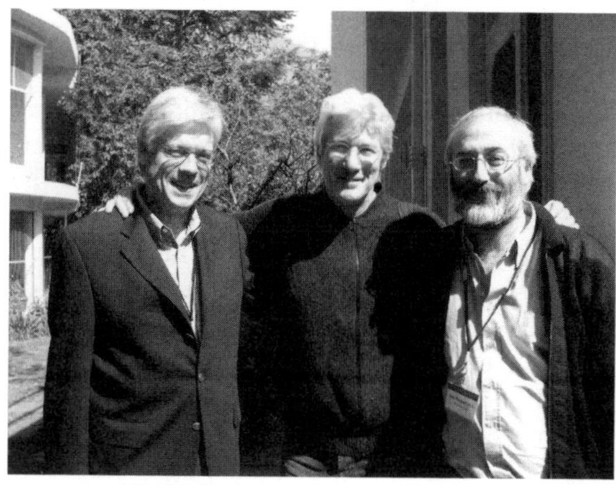

Photograph 11. Phil with Richard Gere and Mario Mikulincer, in Dharamsala, 2004.

One of the first people to follow up Phil and his students' work on attachment was Mario Mikulincer, coeditor of this book. His creative 1990 *Journal of Personality and Social Psychology* article on attachment styles and death anxiety (Mikulincer, Florian, & Tolmacz, 1990) provided the seed that has since developed into his and Phil's extremely productive collaboration. They have expanded the early work on romantic relationships to include other kinds of relationships and have expanded the number of behavioral systems under consideration beyond attachment, caregiving, and sex (e.g., Mikulincer & Shaver, 2003, 2006).

I will mention as one example of their creative collaboration the work that Mario and Phil have been doing with Omri Gillath on the facilitation of empathy, compassion, gratitude, and forgiveness (forms of caregiving) by experimentally manipulated boosts in attachment security (see the summary in Gillath, Shaver, & Mikulincer, 2005, and Chapter 8, this volume, by Mikulincer, Shaver, & Slav). This work led to Phil and Mario being invited to discuss their research with the Dalai Lama at his residence in Dharamsala, India, in October 2004, a development in their lives and work that was completely unexpected (see photograph 10, showing the now fully gray-haired Phil explaining his research to His Holiness the Dalai Lama, and photograph 11, showing Phil, Mario Mikculincer, and the actor Richard Gere, who also attended the meeting with the Dalai Lama). This is just one example of how Phil and Mario's friendship has resulted in new levels of creative scientific exploration, another example of attachment theory applied to real life.

As many people in the relationship field know, Phil loves to work collaboratively and has been extremely fortunate over the years to have talented students and professional colleagues, not only in whatever psychology department he was residing in at a particular time but from all over the country and other parts of the world, as indicated by the contributors to this volume. He has emotional ties to many smart and lovable people. We left the University of Denver in 1988 for a 4-year sojourn at the State University of New York at Buffalo, where Phil worked creatively with Bette Bottoms, Kelly Brennan, Linda Kunce, Ken Levy (coauthor, with his wife, Kristen Kelly, and Ejay Jack of Chapter 6 of this volume), Daria Papalia, Julie Rothbard, and Marie Tidwell, to name a few students with whom Phil coauthored papers. He also wrote collaborative papers with Jim Blascovich (a distinguished colleague at Buffalo who, along with his well-known social psychologist wife, Brenda Major, appeared as mystery guests at the "Phil is an old guy" conference), Lynne Cooper (another colleague at Buffalo and coauthor of Chapter 10 of this volume), and Harry Reis (a faculty member at the nearby University of Rochester and author of Chapter 15 of this volume). Except for the pervasive clouds and snow, Phil enjoyed his years at SUNY Buffalo, working with these inspiring students and colleagues.

After we moved from Buffalo to California, a move made mainly to bring me back to my native state and closer to my sister, Tina Goodman Brown, and my mother, Ruth Goodman, who was suffering from Alzheimer's disease, Phil had many other talented doctoral students, postdocs, and collaborators at UC Davis and other institutions, including Catherine Clark, Robin Edelstein, Chris Fraley (coauthor of Chapter 4 of this volume), Omri Gillath and Dory Schachner (coauthors of Chapter 13), Hillary Morgan, Caroline Tancredy, Nancy Collins (coauthor of Chapters 7 and

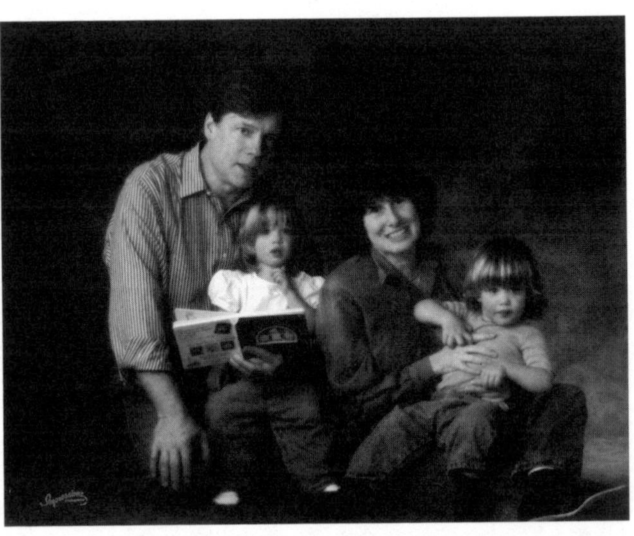

Photograph 12. Phil, Lauren, Gail, and Danielle.

10), Erik Noftle, Josh Hart, Rachel Nitzburg, and Jessica Tracy. He also published with faculty colleagues, including Rick Robins and Silvia Bunge, the latter of whom ushered Phil into the exciting new world of neuroimaging research (e.g., Gillath, Bunge, Shaver, Wendelken, & Mikulincer, 2005). His long professional friendship with Deborah Davis, a faculty member at the nearby University of Nevada, Reno, blossomed into collaborative research (e.g., Davis, Shaver, & Vernon, 2003, 2004), which is creatively extended in Chapter 12 of this volume. His work, which began via e-mail, with Itzi Alonso-Arbiol of the University of the Basque Country in Spain, has also produced collaborative papers, and we were delighted to have Itzi attend the conference. These professional relationships and friendships continue as I write.

I turn now to my final topic: Phil's caring relationships with our daughters, Lauren and Danielle (see photograph 12). They were born prematurely, Lauren weighing only 2 pounds 2 ounces, and Danielle only slightly more at 2 pounds 7 ounces. Phil spent hours in the intensive care nursery, rocking and playing with the tiny little girls, and they developed very secure attachments to him. He is, like his father, quite the mother hen. He is so nurturing, funny, personable, smart, comforting, and engaging with the girls that I'm sure he's influencing them to grow up to do great things, just as he has done. They are already showing clever senses of humor and clear signs of writing talent, very similar to his. This is a concrete example of the intergenerational transmission of attachment patterns, just as our 26-year-long relationship is an example of the effects of attachment security on relationship stability and professional creativity. It takes a great deal of good will and cooperation to allow two determined workaholics to carry on intense careers while sharing responsibility for two energetic daughters. Working 60 to 80 hours a week, Phil still takes time to get the girls ready for school every morning, and he takes them and their classmates on field trips to farms and art museums and grades homework papers for their teachers. He has read thousands of stories to the girls and accompanied them and me on many trips and adventures in the United States and abroad.

I hope this admittedly personal journey through time and photographs shows you how attachment theory as applied to romantic love was influenced by Phil's personal history and how the theory is useful for doing psychobiography. Phil began as a smiling baby boy in Iowa some 60 years ago, and through many unpredictable twists and turns, ups and downs, and transformations in interests he became a scholar of great distinction, a local and international leader in his field, a highly regarded teacher and mentor, a loving husband, and a caring, nurturant father. He has helped many people in their lives and careers, myself very much included.

In closing, I would like to do in writing what I did orally at what I, in contrast to Phil, called the "Phil is a young-at-heart guy conference"—thank Phil for all he has done for so many of us, and with great love and admiration dedicate this book to him. I wish him a long life with many more happy birthdays, and I look forward to seeing what he and the authors of this book discover in future years about the psychology of close relationships.

REFERENCES

Ainsworth, M. D. S., Blehar, M. C., Waters, E., & Wall, S. (1978). *Patterns of attachment: A psychological study of the Strange Situation.* Hillsdale, NJ: Erlbaum.

Berant, E., Mikulincer, M., Shaver, P. R., & Segal, Y. (2005). Rorschach correlates of self-reported attachment dimensions: Dynamic manifestations of hyperactivating and deactivating strategies. *Journal of Personality Assessment, 84,* 70–81.

Davis, D., Shaver, P. R., & Vernon, M. L. (2003). Physical, emotional, and behavioral reactions to breaking up: The roles of gender, age, emotional involvement, and attachment style. *Personality and Social Psychology Bulletin, 29,* 871–884.

Elms, A. C. (1994). *Uncovering lives: The uneasy alliance of biography and psychology.* New York: Oxford University Press.

Elms, A. C., & Heller, B. (2005). Twelve ways to say "lonesome": Assessing error and control in the music of Elvis Presley. In W. T. Schultz (Ed.), *Handbook of psychobiography* (pp. 142–157). New York: Oxford University Press.

Erikson, E. H. (1950). *Childhood and society.* New York: Norton.

Erikson, E. H. (1974). *Dimensions of a new identity.* New York: Norton.

Freedman, J. L. (1978). *Happy people: What happiness is, who has it, and why.* New York: Harcourt.

Geller, V., & Shaver, P. R. (1976). Cognitive consequences of self-awareness. *Journal of Experimental Social Psychology, 12,* 99–108.

Gillath, O., Bunge, S. A., Shaver, P. R., Wendelken, C., & Mikulincer, M. (2005). Attachment-style differences in the ability to suppress negative thoughts: Exploring the neural correlates. *NeuroImage, 28,* 835–847.

Gillath, O., Shaver, P. R., & Mikulincer, M. (2005). An attachment-theoretical approach to compassion and altruism. In P. Gilbert (Ed.), *Compassion: Conceptualizations, research, and use in psychotherapy* (pp. 121–147). London: Brunner-Routledge.

Goodman, G. S. (1984). The child witness: Conclusions and future directions for research and legal practice. *Journal of Social Issues, 40*(2), 157–175.

Goodman, G. S. (2005). Wailing babies in her wake. *American Psychologist, 60,* 872–881.

Goodman, G. S., Ghetti, S., Quas, J. A., Edelstein, R., Alexander, K. W., Redlich, A. D., et al. (2003). A prospective study of memory for child sexual abuse: New findings relevant to the repressed-memory controversy. *Psychological Science, 14,* 113–118.

Goodman, G. S., Quas, J. A., Batterman-Faunce, J. M., Riddlesberger, M. M., & Kuhn, J. (1994). Predictors of accurate and inaccurate memories of traumatic events experienced in childhood. *Consciousness and Cognition: An International Journal, 3,* 269–294.

Goodman, G. S., Quas, J. A., Batterman-Faunce, J. M., Riddlesberger, M. M., &

Kuhn, J. (1997). Children's reactions to and memory for a stressful event: Influences of age, anatomical dolls, knowledge, and parental attachment. *Applied Developmental Science, 1*(2), 54–75.

Goodman, G. S., Taub, E. P., Jones, D. P. H., England, P., Port, L. K., Rudy, L., et al. (1992). Testifying in criminal court: Effects on child sexual abuse victims. *Monographs of the Society for Research in Child Development, 57*(5, Serial No. 229).

Kirkpatrick, L. A. (2005). *Attachment, evolution, and the psychology of religion.* New York: Guilford Press.

Kirkpatrick, L. A., & Shaver, P. R. (1990). Attachment theory and religion: Childhood attachments, religious beliefs, and conversion. *Journal for the Scientific Study of Religion, 29*, 315–334.

Kirkpatrick, L. A., & Shaver, P. R. (1992). An attachment-theoretical approach to romantic love and religious belief. *Personality and Social Psychology Bulletin, 18*, 266–275.

Levy, M. B., & Davis, K. E. (1988). Lovestyles and attachment styles compared: Their relations to each other and to various relationship characteristics. *Journal of Social and Personal Relationships, 5*, 439–471.

Mikulincer, M., Florian, V., & Tolmacz, R. (1990). Attachment styles and fear of death: A case of affect regulation. *Journal of Personality and Social Psychology, 58*, 273–280.

Mikulincer, M., & Shaver, P. R. (2003). The attachment behavioral system in adulthood: Activation, psychodynamics, and interpersonal processes. In M. P. Zanna (Ed.), *Advances in experimental social psychology* (Vol. 35, pp. 53–152). New York: Academic Press.

Mikulincer, M., & Shaver, P. R. (2006). The behavioral systems construct: A useful tool for building an integrative model of the social mind. In P. A. M. van Lange (Ed.), *Bridging social psychology: Benefits of transdisciplinary approaches.* Mahwah, NJ: Erlbaum.

Proudfoot, W., & Shaver, P. R. (1975). Attribution theory and the psychology of religion. *Journal for the Scientific Study of Religion, 14*, 317–330.

Ring, K., & Cooper, S. (1999). *Mindsight: Near-death and out-of-body experiences in the blind.* Palo Alto, CA: William James Center for Consciousness Studies.

Rubenstein, C., & Shaver, P. R. (1982). *In search of intimacy.* New York: Delacorte.

Scheibe, K. E. (2000). *The drama of everyday life.* Cambridge, MA: Harvard University Press.

Scheibe, K. E., Shaver, P. R., & Carrier, S. C. (1967). Color association values and response interference on variants of the Stroop test. *Acta Psychologica, 26*, 286–295.

Schulman, J., Shaver, P. R., Colman, R., Emrich, B., & Christie, R. (1973). Recipe for a jury: Jury selection for the Harrisburg conspiracy trial. *Psychology Today, 6*, 37–44, 77–84.

Shaver, P. R. (1986). Consciousness without the body [Review essay based on *Heading toward omega* by K. Ring and *Flight of mind: A psychological study of the out-of-body experience* by H. J. Irwin]. *Contemporary Psychology, 31*, 645–647.

Shaver, P. R., Hazan, C., & Bradshaw, D. (1988). Love as attachment: The integration of three behavioral systems. In R. J. Sternberg & M. Barnes (Eds.), *The psychology of love* (pp. 68–99). New Haven, CT: Yale University Press.

Shaver, P. R., & Mikulincer, M. (2005). Attachment theory and research: Resurrection of the psychodynamic approach to personality. *Journal of Research in Personality*, *39*, 22–45.

Shaver, P. R., Pierson, L., & Lang, S. (1975). Converging evidence for the functional significance of imagery in problem solving. *Cognition*, *3*, 359–375.

Shaver, P. R., & Scheibe, K. E. (1967). Transformation of social identity. *Journal of Psychology*, *66*, 19–37.

Simonton, D. K. (2002). *Great psychologists and their times: Scientific insights into psychology's history*. Washington, DC: American Psychological Association.

Spilka, B., & McIntosh, D. N. (Eds.). (1997). *The psychology of religion: Theoretical approaches*. Boulder, CO: Westview Press.

Spilka, B., Shaver, P. R., & Kirkpatrick, L. (1985). A general attribution theory for the psychology of religion. *Journal for the Scientific Study of Religion*, *24*, 1–20.

Weiss, R. S. (1974). *Loneliness: The experience of emotional and social isolation*. Cambridge, MA: MIT Press.

2

Attachment, Caregiving, and Sex within Romantic Relationships

A Behavioral Systems Perspective

MARIO MIKULINCER

What is love? Countless answers have been offered by philosophers, theologians, creative writers, and—in recent times—psychiatrists and psychologists. In the late 1980s, Shaver and his coauthors (Hazan & Shaver, 1987; Shaver & Hazan, 1988; Shaver, Hazan, & Bradshaw, 1988) suggested extending Bowlby's (1969/1982, 1973, 1979, 1980) attachment theory, which was designed to characterize human infants' love for and attachment to their caregivers, to create a framework for studying romantic love and adult couple relationships. The core assumption was that romantic relationships—or pair bonds, as evolutionary psychologists call them—involve a combination of three innate behavioral systems described by Bowlby (1969/1982): attachment, caregiving, and sex. Each of these behavioral systems has its own evolutionary functions, and although the systems affect each other in various ways, they are conceptualized as distinct. Viewed from this theoretical perspective, love is a dynamic state involving both partners' needs and capacities for attachment, caregiving, and sex. The profound joy and affection, self-protective anxiety, numbing boredom, corrosive anger, lustful passion, uncontrollable jealousy, and intense sorrow experienced in romantic relationships are reflections of the central importance of these behavioral systems in a person's emotional life.

BEHAVIORAL SYSTEMS DEFINED

In explaining the motivational bases of human behavior and personality development, Bowlby (1969/1982) borrowed from ethology the concept of *behavioral system*, a species-universal neural program that organizes an individual's behavior in ways that increase the likelihood of survival and reproductive success in the face of environmental demands. Each such system governs the choice, activation, and termination of behavioral sequences so as to produce a predictable and functional change in the person–environment relationship. Each behavioral system involves a set of contextual activating triggers; a set of interchangeable, functionally equivalent behaviors that constitute the *primary strategy* of the system for attaining its particular goal state; and a specific set goal (a state of the person–environment relationship that terminates the system's activation). Because each behavioral system was evolutionarily "designed" to increase the likelihood of survival and adaptation to environmental demands, its optimal functioning has important implications for social adjustment, mental health, and quality of life.

Bowlby (1969/1982) also assumed that behavioral systems include "ontogenetically learned" components that reflect a person's particular history of behavioral-system activation in particular kinds of contexts. Although behavioral systems are innate neural structures, which presumably operate mainly at a subcortical level and in a mechanistic manner, their ability to achieve the desired set goal depends on the extent to which the individual can correct and adjust the primary strategy of the system in response to contextual affordances and demands. Therefore, Bowlby (1969/1982) assumed that, to make goal attainment more likely, each behavioral system also includes cognitive-behavioral mechanisms, such as monitoring and appraising the effectiveness of behaviors enacted in a particular context, which allow flexible, goal-corrected adjustment of the primary strategy whenever necessary to put it back on the track of goal attainment. Borrowing from more recent feedback-control theories (e.g., Carver & Scheier, 1981, 1990), we can say that Bowlby's view of behavioral system functioning involves self-regulatory feedback loops that shape the course of the system's primary strategy and help a person decide whether to persist in or disengage from this strategy after discovering that it is unsuccessful in a given context.

Over time, after operating repeatedly in similar environments, a person's behavioral systems become molded by social encounters so that the neural/behavioral capacities fit better with important relationship partners and other relational constraints. According to Bowlby (1973), the residues of such experiences are stored as mental representations of person–environment transactions (*working models of self and others*), which organize memories of behavioral system functioning and guide future attempts to attain the system's set goal. These representations, which operate partly unconsciously but also partly at the level of conscious thoughts and intentions, become part of a behavioral system's programming and are sources of both individual differences and within-person continuity in the system's functioning.

In the realm of romantic relationships, Shaver and his coauthors (Hazan & Shaver, 1987; Shaver & Hazan, 1988; Shaver et al., 1988) argued that optimal functioning of the attachment, caregiving, and sexual systems facilitates the formation and maintenance of stable and mutually satisfactory affectional bonds, whereas malfunctioning of these systems creates relational tensions, conflicts, dissatisfaction, and instability and often leads to relationship breakup. Shaver and Hazan (1988) also proposed that a person's working models explain individual variations in relational goals, beliefs, emotions, and behaviors. Beyond this individual-difference perspective, Shaver et al. (1988) suggested that relational, interactional factors also contribute to the functioning of the various behavioral systems (e.g., signals of a partner's waning interest) and that the dynamic interplay of different behavioral systems within a relationship can be important for understanding relational processes and outcomes.

Because Hazan and Shaver's (1987) germinal study on romantic attachment focused mainly on the conceptualization and assessment of individual differences in attachment, researchers subsequently conducted many studies focused on these individual differences without paying much attention to either the underlying dynamics of the attachment behavioral system itself or to the other behavioral systems—sex and caregiving—involved in romantic love. More recently this imbalance has begun to be corrected, and more studies have employed a combination of self-report measures of adult attachment orientations with powerful laboratory techniques borrowed from cognitive psychology (e.g., semantic priming) in order to study the underlying dynamics of the attachment system (e.g., Baldwin, Fehr, Keedian, Seidel, & Thomson, 1993; Fraley & Shaver, 1997; Mikulincer, 1998). Moreover, several studies have been conducted that examine relations between the attachment and caregiving systems and between the attachment and sexual systems (e.g., Collins & Feeney, 2000; Kunce & Shaver, 1994; Schachner & Shaver, 2004). In the following sections, I present a very brief overview of what we have learned so far and what we can learn from this book about the interplay of the attachment, caregiving, and sexual systems within romantic relationships.

ATTACHMENT PROCESSES IN COUPLE RELATIONSHIPS

According to Bowlby (1969/1982), the presumed biological function of the attachment system is to protect a person (especially during infancy and early childhood) from danger by assuring that he or she maintains proximity to caring and supportive others (who are called *attachment figures* in the theory). In Bowlby's (1969/1982) view, the need to seek out and maintain proximity to attachment figures (what he called "stronger and wiser" caregivers) evolved in relation to the prolonged helplessness and complete dependence of human infants, who are unable to defend themselves from predators and other dangers. Bowlby (1969/1982, 1980, 1988) assumed that although the attachment system is most frequently activated during infancy, it continues to function throughout life, as indicated by adults' needs for proximity and support and their prolonged emotional reactions to the loss of attachment figures.

During infancy, primary caregivers (usually one or both parents, but also grandparents, older siblings, day-care workers, and so on) are likely to serve attachment functions. In adulthood, romantic partners become the most important attachment figures, such that proximity maintenance to these partners in times of need becomes a crucial source of support, comfort, and reassurance (e.g., Fraley & Davis, 1997; Hazan & Zeifman, 1999). However, not every romantic partner becomes a major attachment figure. In fact, the transformation of a romantic partner into an attachment figure is a gradual process that depends on the extent to which the person functions as (1) a target for proximity seeking; (2) a source of protection, comfort, support, and relief in times of need (*safe haven*); and (3) a *secure base*, encouraging the individual to pursue his or her goals in a safe relational context (e.g., Ainsworth, 1991; Hazan & Shaver, 1994; Hazan & Zeifman, 1999). These three functions are mainly found in long-lasting, highly committed romantic relationships.

Bowlby (1969/1982) also specified the set goal of the attachment system and described the typical cycle of attachment-system activation and deactivation. The goal of the system is a sense of protection or security (called by Sroufe & Waters, 1977, *felt security*), which normally terminates the system's activation. This goal is made particularly salient by encounters with actual or symbolic threats and by appraising an attachment figure as not sufficiently near, interested, or responsive. In such cases, the attachment system is activated and the individual is driven to seek and reestablish actual or symbolic proximity to an external or internalized attachment figure. When the set goal of security is attained, proximity bids are terminated, and the individual calmly returns to other, nonattachment activities.

In infants, attachment-system activation includes nonverbal expressions of neediness and desire for proximity, such as crying and pleading, as well as active behaviors aimed at reestablishing and maintaining proximity, such as moving toward the caregiver and clinging (Ainsworth, Blehar, Waters, & Wall, 1978). In adulthood, the primary attachment strategy does not necessarily entail actual proximity-seeking behaviors. Instead, felt security can be attained by the activation of soothing, comforting mental representations of relationship partners who regularly provide care and protection or even self-representations associated with these partners (Mikulincer & Shaver, 2004). These cognitive representations help people deal successfully with threats and allow them to continue pursuing nonattachment goals without having to interrupt these activities to engage in actual proximity bids.

Bowlby (1979) viewed the smooth functioning of the attachment system as necessary for the formation of satisfactory close relationships. Every interaction in which a relationship partner is helpful in alleviating distress and restoring felt security reaffirms the adaptive advantage of closeness and strengthens affectional bonds with a particular partner. In this way, people gradually consolidate a relationship-specific sense of attachment security (the belief that a particular romantic partner will be available and supportive in times of need). Although this sense can be biased by a person's generic working models of attachment relationships, it can also be affected by a partner's actual supportive behaviors and become a potent regulator of relational cognitions and behaviors and a major contributor to relationship quality. From an emotion-regulation perspective, the attachment system acts as a dynamic, homeostatic mechanism that can contribute to or interfere with emotional equanimity. Within a relational context, the smooth functioning of this system is crucial for deescalating relational tensions and conflicts, maintaining a positive affective tone, and encouraging relationship stability.

Attachment theorists and researchers (e.g., Cassidy & Kobak, 1988; Main, 1990; Mikulincer & Shaver, 2003) have extensively documented the negative consequences of attachment-system dysfunctions that can occur during interactions in which bids for proximity or support or the mental activation of internalized attachment figures fail to provide a sense of protection and security. In such cases, the distress that activated the system is compounded by serious doubts and fears about the feasibility of attaining a sense of security: "Is the world a safe place or not? Can I trust my relationship partner in times of need or not? Do I have the resources necessary to bring my partner close to me?" These worries about self and relationship partners can keep the attachment system in a continually activated state, cause a person's mind to be preoccupied with threats and the need for protection, and drastically interfere with the functioning of other behavioral systems.

Negative attachment interactions indicate that the primary attachment strategy, proximity and support seeking, is failing to accomplish its set goal. As a result, the operating parameters of the attachment system have to be adjusted, and certain *secondary attachment strategies* are likely to be adopted. Attachment theorists (e.g., Cassidy & Kobak, 1988; Main, 1990; Shaver & Mikulincer, 2002) have emphasized two such secondary strategies: *hyperactivation* and *deactivation* of the attachment system. Hyperactivating strategies (which Bowlby, 1969/1982, called *protest*) are "fight" responses to the frustration of attachment needs; they involve strong activation of the attachment system aimed at demanding or coercing the attachment figure's love and support. The main goal of these strategies is to get an attachment figure, viewed as unreliable or insufficiently available and responsive, to pay attention and provide protection or support. This goal can be achieved by maintaining the attachment system in a chronically activated state until an attachment figure is perceived to be adequately available and responsive. Such hyperactivation involves exaggeration of appraisals of danger and of signs of attachment-figure unavailability; intensification of demands for attention, affection, and assistance; clinging and controlling actions toward a relationship partner; and overdependence on the partner as a source of protection (Shaver & Mikulincer, 2002). From an outside observer's perspective, it is easy to see why this strategy interferes with good communication, emotional tranquility, and mature personal development.

In contrast, deactivating strategies include inhibition of proximity seeking and cultivation of what Bowlby (1980) called "compulsive self-reliance" and "detachment." The primary goal of these strategies is to keep the attachment system turned off or down-regulated to avoid the frustration and distress of attachment-figure unavailability (Shaver & Mikulincer, 2002). These strategies require denial of attachment needs; avoidance of intimacy and dependence in relationships; and maximization of cognitive, emotional, and physical distance from others. They also involve the dismissal of threat- and attachment-related cues and suppression of threat- and attachment-related thoughts and emotions that might cause unwanted activation of the attachment system (Shaver & Mikulincer, 2002).

Attachment theory in general, and Hazan and Shaver's (1987) application of the theory to the realm of romantic love in particular, have been unusual in stimulating a huge body of empirical research that examines whether and how individual differences in attachment-system functioning affect the quality of romantic relationships (see J. Feeney, 1999; Shaver & Hazan, 1993; and Shaver & Mikulincer, in press, for extensive reviews). Initially, Hazan and Shaver (1987) created a simple three-category (secure, anxious, avoidant) measure of what has come to be called "attachment style"—the habitual pattern of relational expectations, emotions, and behaviors that results from a particular history of attachment experiences. However, subsequent studies (e.g., Bartholomew & Horowitz, 1991; Brennan, Clark, & Shaver, 1998) indicated that attachment styles are more appropriately conceptualized as regions in a continuous two-dimensional space. The first dimension, attachment *avoidance*, reflects the extent to which a person distrusts relationship partners' goodwill, deactivates the attachment system, and strives to maintain behavioral independence and emotional distance from partners. The second dimension, attachment *anxiety*, reflects the degree to which a person worries that a partner will not be available in times of need and engages in hyperactivating strategies. People who score low on both dimensions are said to be secure or securely attached. The two dimensions can be measured with reliable and valid self-report scales, such as the Experience in Close Relationships scale (ECR; Brennan et al., 1998).

Attachment research in personality and social psychology has been successful in generating a large body of theory-consistent findings showing that attachment insecurities defined in terms of the anxiety and avoidance dimensions are associated with low levels of relationship stability, satisfaction, and adjustment in both dating and married couples (see Mikulincer, Florian, Cowan, & Cowan, 2002; Shaver & Mikulincer, in press, for extensive reviews). For example, Davila, Karney, and Bradbury (1999) collected data every 6 months for 3 years from newlywed couples and found that changes in husbands' and wives' reports of attachment orientations predicted concurrent changes in both partners' reports of marital satisfaction. Studies have also linked attachment insecurities with less relationship intimacy, affection, trust, and commitment (e.g., Collins & Read, 1990; Shaver & Brennan, 1992; Simpson, 1990), as well as with relationship-destructive patterns of emotional reactions to partner behaviors and maladaptive strategies of conflict resolution (e.g., Rholes, Simpson, & Orina, 1999; Scharfe & Bartholomew, 1995). There is also extensive evidence showing that attachment-related anxiety and avoidance are both associated with negative expectations about a partner's behavior (e.g., Baldwin et al., 1993; Mikulincer & Arad, 1999) and relationship-damaging explanations of a partner's negative behaviors (e.g., Collins, 1996; Mikulincer, 1998).

Recent adult attachment studies have also found that availability, responsiveness, and supportiveness of a romantic partner in times of need—which are the crucial contextual factors that facilitate optimal functioning of the attachment system—have important beneficial relational outcomes and attenuate the harmful effects of chronic attachment insecurities (e.g., Feeney, 2002; Rholes, Simpson, Campbell, & Grich, 2001). Research has also revealed that a relationship-specific sense of attachment security is a potent regulator of interpersonal cognitions and behaviors within a particular relationship. For example, Kobak and Hazan (1991) found that partners with a relatively strong relationship-specific sense of security were less rejecting and more supportive during a problem-solving interaction. More important, Cozzarelli, Hoekstra, and Bylsma (2000) and Cowan and Cowan (2002) found that reports of secure attachment within a specific romantic relationship were more powerful predictors of satisfaction with that relationship than reports of global attachment security.

Part II of this book deals with the implications of variations in attachment-system functioning for the dynamics of romantic love. The chapters in this section present up-to-date theoretical ideas and empirical evidence concerning attachment processes and their implications for explaining normative aspects of couple relationships, as well as more maladaptive aspects (e.g., abusive dynamics, jealousy). Cindy Hazan, Nurit Gur-Yaish, and Mary Campa present recent findings on the behavioral, cognitive, and affectional "markers" of attachment at different stages of romantic relationship development. Chris Fraley and Claudia Brumbaugh propose a comparative-phylogenetic explanation of the functions of the attachment behavioral system in romantic relationships. Kim Bartholomew and Colleen Allison review evidence from a recent study of attachment dynamics observed in couples characterized by male violence. Finally, Ken Levy, Kristen Kelly, and Ejay Jack present new findings on the associations between attachment anxiety and avoidance and variations in the experience of romantic jealousy due to a partner's emotional or sexual infidelity.

INTERPLAY BETWEEN THE CAREGIVING AND ATTACHMENT SYSTEMS

In an early article expounding what they unabashedly called a "biased overview of the study of love," Shaver and Hazan (1988) explained that the caregiving behavioral system is also extremely important to the dynamics of romantic love. According to Bowlby (1969/1982), the caregiving system was crafted by evolution to provide protection and support to others who were either chronically dependent or temporarily in need. Although this system presumably evolved because it increased the inclusive fitness of individuals by making it more likely that children and other family members with whom an individual shared genes would survive and reproduce (Hamilton, 1964), its functioning in any present case is often truly altruistically aimed at alleviating distress and benefiting others who are suffering or needy (Gillath, Shaver, & Mikulincer, 2005).

"Caregiving" refers to a broad array of behaviors that complement another person's attachment behaviors or signals of need. The set goal of such behaviors is reduction of others' suffering (which Bowlby, 1969/1982, called providing a "safe haven") or fostering their growth and development (which Bowlby, 1969/1982, viewed as providing a "secure base" for exploration). The key mechanism for achieving these goals is the adoption of what Batson (1991) called an empathic attitude toward others' suffering—taking the perspective of the distressed person in order to sensitively and effectively help him or her reduce distress. The caregiving system is focused on another's welfare and therefore directs attention to the other's distress rather than to one's own emotional state. In its prototypical form, in the parent–child relationship, the set goal of the *child's attachment system* (proximity that fosters protection, reduces distress, increases safety, and establishes a secure base) is also the aim of the *parent's caregiving system*. Extending this conceptualization to the realm of romantic relationships, one partner's caregiving system is automatically activated by the other partner's attachment behaviors or signals of need, and its aim is to alter the needy partner's condition until signs of increased safety, well-being, and security are evident.

The smooth functioning of the caregiving system in romantic relationships has important implications for relationship satisfaction and stability. Evidence is rapidly accumulating that relational episodes in which an individual sensitively attends and empathically responds to a romantic partner's attachment behaviors and signals of need lead to positive emotional reactions in both the needy person (feelings of being loved and esteemed, feelings of gratitude, feelings of attachment security) and the caregiver (feelings of competence and generativity), as well as heightened relationship satisfaction (e.g., Collins & Feeney, 2000; Feeney, 2004; Feeney & Collins, 2003). In contrast, dysfunctions of the caregiving system—failure to respond empathically to a partner's needs and help the partner effectively to alleviate distress—is a major source of relational tensions and conflicts and can produce a host of relationship-damaging worries, negative attitudes, and destructive behaviors. Specifically, such dysfunctions can increase the needy person's relationship-specific attachment insecurities and heighten the caregiver's doubts about his or her interpersonal skills and love for the partner or, alternatively, can encourage distancing from the partner whenever he or she displays signs of vulnerability or distress.

Dysfunctions of the caregiving system can also trigger either hyperactivation or deactivation of this system. In the case of caregiving, hyperactivating strategies are intrusive, effortful, sometimes awkward attempts to convince oneself and one's partner that one can be an effective caregiver. These goals can be achieved by exaggerating appraisals of others' signals of need, adopting a hypervigilant attitude toward others' distress, and focusing on others' needs to the neglect of one's own. Unfortunately, this hyperactivation of the system is accompanied by heightened personal distress, doubts about one's efficacy as a caregiver, and controlling behavior aimed at coercing others to accept one's caregiving bids, which in turn result in rejection by the partner, increased relational distress, and acceleration of dysfunctional "caregiving" responses. On the other hand, deactivating strategies result in inhibition of empathy, compassion, and effective caregiving combined with increased interpersonal distance precisely when a partner seeks proximity. More specifically, a deactivated caregiving system results in less sensitivity and responsiveness to others' needs, dismissal or downplaying of others' distress, suppression of thoughts related to others' needs and vulnerability, and inhibition of sympathy and compassion.

Although no research instrument has been explicitly constructed to assess hyperactivation and deactivation of the caregiving system, an item analysis of the existing self-report measures of caregiving responses reveals that they tap various aspects of these dysfunctions. For example, Davis's (1983) Interpersonal Reactivity Index includes an Empathic Concern subscale that taps variations (mostly on the low end) of the deactivating dimension (e.g., "I often have tender, concerned feelings for people less fortunate than me") and a Personal Distress subscale that taps the self-focused aspects of the hyperactivating dimension (e.g., "Being in a tense emotional situation scares me"). Kunce and Shaver's (1994) measure of caregiving within romantic relationships includes items gauging distance from a suffering partner and lack of sensitivity to signals of need (e.g., "I sometimes push my partner away even though s/he seems to need me," "I sometimes miss the subtle signs that show how my partner is feeling"), as well as items tapping anxious, compulsive caregiving (e.g., "I tend to get overinvolved in my partner's problems and difficulties"). Items related to hyperactivation of the caregiving system can also be found in Helgeson's (1993) Unmitigated Communion Scale (e.g., "I worry about how other people get along without me when I am not there") and Jack and Dill's (1992) Silencing of Self Scale (e.g., "Caring means putting the other person's needs in front of my own"). However, the field still lacks a reliable and valid measure that, like the ECR scale in the attachment domain, is explicitly designed to assess global caregiving orientations along the deactivation and hyperactivation dimensions.

Following Bowlby's (1969/1982) reasoning about the interplay of the various behavioral systems, Shaver and Hazan (1988) proposed hypotheses about how attachment orientations might bias the functioning of the caregiving system. According to Bowlby (1969/1982), because of a person's urgent need to protect him- or herself from imminent threats, activation of the attachment system inhibits activation of other behavioral systems and interferes with nonattachment activities, including caregiving. Under conditions of threat, adults generally turn to others for support rather than thinking first about providing support to others. Only when they feel reasonably secure can people easily direct attention to others' needs and provide sensitive support. Possessing greater attachment security allows people to provide more effective care for others, because the sense of security is related to optimistic beliefs about distress management and feelings of self-efficacy when coping with distress.

Reasoning along these lines, Shaver and Hazan (1988) hypothesized that securely attached people would comfortably and effectively provide care to a needy partner, whereas insecure people would have difficulty providing sensitive, responsive care within romantic relationships. Furthermore, although both anxious and avoidant people are conceptualized as insecure, Shaver and Hazan (1988) hypothesized that they would exhibit different problems in caregiving. Specifically, avoidant people, who chronically attempt to distance themselves from partners, as well as from emotional signals of neediness and suffering, should be less able or willing to provide care and therefore should exhibit less compassion toward a needy partner. Anxious people, who seek to maximize closeness to a relationship partner, suffer from chronic frustration of their need for security and tend to be easily distressed in a self-focused way; they should react to others' suffering with personal distress, resulting in insensitive, intrusive, and ineffective care. In other words, whereas deactivation of the attachment system (avoidance) facilitates deactivation of the caregiving system, hyperactivation of the attachment system (anxiety) is associated with hyperactivation of the caregiving system.

In an initial test of these hypotheses, Kunce and Shaver (1994) examined caregiving orientations within romantic relationships and found that secure adults were indeed more sensitive to their partner's needs, reported more cooperative caregiving, and described themselves as more likely to provide emotional support than insecure individuals; and their romantic partners agreed with this assessment. Moreover, whereas avoidant people attempted to maintain distance from a needy partner, anxious people reported high levels of overinvolvement with their partner's problems and a pattern of compulsive, intrusive caregiving. These findings have been replicated using other self-report scales (e.g., Carnelley, Pietromonaco, & Jaffe, 1996; Feeney, 1996; Feeney & Hohaus, 2001).

The link between attachment security and sensitive caregiving has been further documented in observational studies by Feeney and Collins (2001), Simpson, Rholes, and Nelligan (1992), and Simpson, Rholes, Orina, and Grich (2002), who videotaped dating couples while one partner waited to endure a stressful task. Overall, as compared with insecure participants, those high in attachment security spontaneously offered more comfort to their distressed dating partner. Moreover, participants who were relatively secure and whose dating partners sought more support provided more support, whereas secure participants whose partners sought less support provided less. In contrast, more avoidant participants provided less support regardless of how much support their partner actually sought. In a related study, Collins and Feeney (2000) videotaped dating couples while one member disclosed a personal problem to his or her partner; they found that higher attachment anxiety was associated with provision of less instrumental support and more negative caregiving responses toward the distressed partner.

Part III of this book concerns the dynamic interplay of attachment and caregiving within romantic relationships. Nancy Collins and her coauthors deal with normative processes and individual differences in caregiving effectiveness and explain attachment-style differences in willingness and ability to provide responsive care to partners in times of need. Jeff Simpson, Lorne Campbell, and Yanna Weisberg present data from a recent diary study examining associations between attachment anxiety, perceptions of relationship-based conflict and support, and assessments of relationship quality. Mario Mikulincer, Phillip Shaver, and Keren Slav extend the boundaries of the attachment–caregiving connection and review recent evidence on the relations between attachment orientations, the prosocial virtues of gratitude and forgiveness, and the quality of romantic relationships.

ATTACHMENT, SEX, AND LOVE

The dynamics of romantic love cannot be understood without taking into account the activation and functioning of the sexual behavioral system (Berscheid, 1984; Shaver & Hazan, 1988). From an evolutionary perspective, the major function of the sexual system is to pass one's genes to the next generation by having sexual intercourse with an opposite-sex partner. However, sexual intercourse and impregnation are effortful, goal-oriented activities that demand coordination of two partners' motives and responses. Accordingly, in the course of human evolution, selection pressures have produced subordinate functional behaviors and psychological mechanisms that solve particular adaptive problems associated with reproduction and reproductive success (Buss & Kenrick, 1998). These behaviors and mechanisms are the primary strategies of the sexual behavioral system.

The set goal of this system is to impregnate an opposite-sex partner in order to pass one's genes to the next generation. The key mechanisms for achieving this set goal are to approach a potential fertile partner, persuade him or her to have sex, and engage in genital intercourse. That is, the primary strategies of the sexual system consist of bringing fertile partners together to have sex by heightening sensitivity to signals of fertility in opposite-sex partners, increasing one's attractiveness as a potential sexual partner, and using effective persuasive techniques to seduce a potential partner. From this perspective, sexual attraction is a motivating force that drives individuals to look for either short-term or long-term mating opportunities with a potential sexual partner (Buss, 1999; Fisher, Aron, Mashek, Li, & Brown, 2002). Because sexual attraction and attachment are discrete and functionally independent emotion-motivation systems (e.g., Diamond, 2003; Fisher et al., 2002), sexual relations often occur without affectional bonds, and affectional bonding between adults is not always accompanied by sexual desire. Still, the formation of a romantic relationship is frequently initiated by infatuation (Hazan & Zeifman, 1994), as well as sexual attraction (e.g., Berscheid, 1984; Sprecher & Regan, 1998). That is, successful human mating is likely to begin with sexual desire and attraction, and the feelings associated with attraction are powerful components of romantic love.

Beyond its tremendous importance in the initial stages of romantic love, the sexual system plays an important role in the consolidation and maintenance of satisfactory, long-lasting romantic relationships. There is growing empirical evidence that sexual interactions in which both partners gratify their sexual needs foster many positive emotional reactions (love, excitement, vitality, gratitude, and relaxation) and contribute to relationship satisfaction and stability (see Sprecher & Cate, 2004, for an extensive review). In contrast, dysfunctions of the sexual system are major sources of relational conflict that can raise doubts about being loved and loving a partner, heighten worries and concerns about one's relationship, increase one's interest in alternative sexual partners, and ultimately erode the affectional bond and destroy the relationship (e.g., Hassebrauck & Fehr, 2002; Sprecher & Cate, 2004).

Dysfunctions of the sexual behavioral system, like dysfunctions of the other systems, can be conceptualized in terms of hyperactivating and deactivating strategies. Hyperactivating strategies involve effortful, mentally preoccupying, sometimes intrusive, and even coercive attempts to persuade a partner to have sex. In the process, a person can overemphasize the importance of sexual activities within a relationship, exaggerate appraisals of a partner's sexual needs, and adopt a hypervigilance toward a partner's signals of sexual arousal, attraction, and rejection. This chronic sexual-system activation is accompanied by heightened anxieties and worries about one's sexual attractiveness, the extent to which one is able to gratify one's partner, and the partner's responses to one's sexual appeals. These anxieties and worries may provoke intrusive or aggressive responses aimed at coercing the partner to have sex, which in turn can lead to rejection and an exacerbation of sexual system dysfunction.

In contrast, deactivating strategies are characterized either by inhibition of sexual desire and an erotophobic or avoidant attitude toward sex or by a superficial approach to sex that divorces it from other considerations, such as kindness or intimacy. Deactivating sexual strategies can involve dismissal of sexual needs, distancing from or disparaging a partner when he or she expresses interest in sex, suppression of sex-related thoughts and fantasies, repression of sex-related memories, and inhibition of sexual arousal and orgasmic joy. They can also, paradoxically, promote sexual promiscuity driven by narcissism or self-advertisement without an intense sexual drive or even much enjoyment of sex per se (Schachner & Shaver, 2004).

As in the caregiving domain, no research instrument has been explicitly designed to assess hyperactivation and deactivation of the sexual behavioral system. However, we can gain important insights from more general scales designed to assess sexual attitudes and behaviors. For example, the erotophobia–erotophilia scale (Fisher, Byrne, White, & Kelley, 1988) assesses the tendency to respond to sexual stimuli in approach or avoidance terms, and this comes close to attachment theorists' understanding of the deactivation dimension (e.g., "I feel no pleasure during sexual fantasies"). The Revised Mosher Guilt Inventory (Mosher, 1988), the Sex Anxiety Inventory (Janda & O'Grady, 1980), and the Experience of Heterosexual Intercourse scale (Birnbaum & Laser-Brandt, 2002) assess some of the worry aspects of sexual-system hyperactivation (e.g., "Bothersome thoughts disturb my concentration during sexual intercourse").

In their attempt to interleave or integrate the attachment, caregiving, and sexual systems as aspects of romantic love, Shaver and Hazan (1988) offered explicit hypotheses concerning the relations between attachment and sex. Securely attached people were hypothesized to strive for mutual intimacy and pleasure during sexual activities, to enjoy sex, and to be attentive and responsive to partners' sexual needs. These are all signs of the smooth functioning of the sexual system. In contrast, anxiously attached people, who are focused on seeking protection and security, were expected to have trouble attending without desperation to their partner's sexual needs and preferences. They were expected to find it difficult to attain the relatively calm and secure state of mind that is helpful in fostering mutual sexual satisfaction (Shaver & Hazan, 1988). Avoidant attachment was also expected to interfere with or distort the sexual system. Whereas attachment avoidance favors emotional distance, mutual exploration of sexual pleasures with a lover risks movement toward psychological intimacy and vulnerability. This heightened closeness might cause avoidant people to feel especially uncomfortable during sexual intercourse.

Evidence is now emerging that shows that attachment processes shape sexual motives, experiences, and behaviors. For example, Tracy, Shaver, Albino, and Cooper (2003) found that securely attached adolescents engaged in sex primarily to show love for their partners and that they experienced fewer negative emotions and more positive and passionate emotions during sexual activity than their insecurely attached peers. Similarly, in adulthood, securely attached individuals have a more positive sexual self-schema (Cyranowski & Andersen, 1998), get pleasure from expressing affection and sexual interest through touch (Brennan, Wu, & Loev, 1998), and enjoy exploring sexuality freely within the context of affectionate long-term relationships (Hazan & Zeifman, 1994).

There is also evidence that adolescents who score high on attachment avoidance report relatively low sexual drive, are less likely to have and enjoy sex, and are motivated by self-enhancement and public reputation rather than by concern for their partners. They say they have sex, for example, so that they can say they have lost their virginity (Tracy et al., 2003) or brag about it to peers (Schachner & Shaver, 2004). Avoidant adults dismiss sex-related motives such as promoting emotional closeness or giving pleasure to a partner and instead seem to engage in sex so as to manipulate or control their partners, protect themselves from partners' negative affect, or achieve other nonromantic goals, such as reducing stress or increasing their prestige among peers (Davis, Shaver, & Vernon, 2004; Schachner & Shaver, 2004). Anxiously attached adolescents have been found to engage in sex primarily to avoid abandonment and hold onto a partner through sexual acquiescence, even when particular sexual acts are otherwise unwanted (Tracy et al., 2003). In adulthood, attachment-anxious individuals tend to use sex as a means for achieving emotional intimacy and reassurance, eliciting a partner's caregiving behaviors, and defusing a partner's anger (Davis et al., 2004; Schachner & Shaver, 2004). However, unfulfilled relational expectations and worries about partner's affection often lead to anxious individuals' sexual dissatisfaction (Brennan et al., 1998).

Part IV of this book deals with connections between attachment and sex. Lynne Cooper and her colleagues discuss a longitudinal study of the developmental trajectories of attachment orientation, sexual attitudes and behaviors, and relational processes from adolescence to young adulthood. Lisa Diamond presents a new conceptualization of the distinction between attachment and sexuality within the realm of *same-sex* romantic relationships and elaborates on the contribution of attachment theory to understanding the nature and development of various kinds of sexual attraction. Deborah Davis reviews recent findings from Internet surveys investigating the associations between attachment orientations and sexual motives, preferences, and behaviors, as well as experimental studies examining the effects of attachment-security primes on sexual responses. Omri Gillath and Dory Schachner describe recent studies of sex-related goals and strategies.

ATTACHMENT THEORY AND OTHER PERSPECTIVES ON ROMANTIC LOVE

Bowlby's (1969/1982) behavioral systems theory and Shaver and Hazan's (1988) approach to romantic love evolved from the confluence of diverse conceptual frameworks, such as evolutionary psychology, psychoanalysis, interdependence theory, research on social cognition, and humanistic psychology. Bowlby's (1969/1982) notion of behavioral systems was borrowed from his day's evolutionary psychology. His ideas about the transformation of attachment experiences into working models of self and others, the defensive nature of insecure working models, and the crucial role that working models play in maintaining stability of attachment orientations fit with the basic principles of modern psychoanalysis (e.g., Westen, 1998). Bowlby's (1973) idea that a relationship partner's responses to one's own attachment behaviors can change the operating parameters of the attachment system fits with interdependence theories of social behavior (e.g., Holmes & Cameron, 2005). The role Bowlby (1973) assigned to working models in explaining a person's relational expectations, emotions, and social behaviors fits with contemporary social cognition research (e.g., Baldwin, 2005). Moreover, the view that attachment security is an important human strength or resource that fosters mental health meshes with humanistic and "positive" psychological approaches that emphasize human strengths, virtues, and optimal development (e.g., Rogers, 1961; Seligman, 2002).

This does not mean that Bowlby's (1969/1982) theory can simply be equated with the other conceptual frameworks. For example, whereas contemporary psychoanalysis still views mental representations of self and others in adulthood as mental residues of childhood experiences, Bowlby (1988) believed that the developmental trajectory of working models is not simple and that these mental representations in adulthood are not exclusively based on early experiences. Rather, they can be updated throughout life and can be affected by a broad array of contextual factors, such as current interactions with a relationship partner who has his or her own patterns of behavioral-system functioning (Mikulincer & Shaver, 2003).

Unlike contemporary interdependence theories, Bowlby's (1969/1982) theory is not exclusively relational. Working models of self and others do not exclusively reflect the ways in which a person and his or her partner actually behave in a given interaction. Rather, they can be biased by defensive processes related to hyperactivating or deactivating attachment strategies (Bowlby, 1980). Furthermore, behavioral-system activation in adulthood can occur intrapsychically without any overt expression in interpersonal behavior and without demanding the intervention of an actual relationship partner (Mikulincer & Shaver, 2004). In other words, the seemingly perpetual tension between personality and social psychological approaches to social behavior and relationships is bridged in attachment theory, but it is always in danger of reasserting itself when researchers with one or the other perspective undertake attachment or relationship research. Moreover, working models of self and others cannot be simply equated with other kinds of social cognitions (Shaver, Collins, & Clark, 1996), even though it is natural for social cognition researchers to view them similarly. Attachment working models evolve not only from simple memories of actual experiences but also from dynamic processes of goal pursuit, emotion regulation, and psychological defense involved with wishes for proximity and security and fears of separation and helplessness.

There is also an important difference between Bowlby's (1969/1982) theory and humanistic or positive psychology: Whereas the positive, humanistic approaches focus mainly on growth-oriented, promotion-focused aspects of development and personality, Bowlby (1969/1982) emphasized both the prevention and the promotion aspects of human behavior. This dual focus is well illustrated in the functions of "safe haven" and "secure base" that qualify relationship partners as attachment figures. These figures need to protect a person from threats and calm his or her fears and conflicts. At the same time, they need to provide a "secure base" from which the person can explore the environment and engage in promotion-oriented activities. Bowlby (1969/1982) emphasized both the "dark" and the "bright" sides of human experience, which psychological researchers seem to have trouble capturing in a single theoretical framework. Bowlby showed how behavioral systems can deal with fears, frustrations, conflicts, and defenses while also fostering happiness, love, and growth.

Bowlby's rich conceptual framework is located at the intersection of psychoanalytic, relational, social cognition, and positive psychological approaches. The theory is unique in integrating different, perhaps even contradictory, views of human nature and maintaining a dialectical tension between opposites of four kinds: (1) the shaping and constraining influences of past experiences versus the influence of current contexts and experiences; (2) the intrapsychic nature of behavioral systems and working models versus the relational, interdependent nature of feelings, experiences, and social behaviors; (3) the goal-oriented, promotive, expansive, self-regulatory function of behavioral systems versus their defensive, protective, distress-regulating functions; and (4) the centrality of basic fears, conflicts, and prevention-focused motivational mechanisms, as well as promotion-focused motives and the capacity for growth and self-actualization.

Part V of this book deals with the interface between Bowlby's (1969/1982) behavioral systems theory and Shaver and Hazan's (1988) approach to romantic relationships on one hand and other conceptual perspectives of romantic love on the other hand. Arthur and Elaine Aron explore potential links between their self-expansion model of romantic love and attachment theory, with a special note on the Jungian "shadow" side of adult development. Harry Reis highlights the concept of "perceived partner responsiveness" and shows how it helps to integrate attachment theory and contemporary theories of intimacy. Ellen Berscheid discusses the nature of romantic love, attachment, caregiving, and sex across the seasons of a human life. Finally, Phil Shaver provides an integrative overview of the conceptual territory, with its current mysteries, controversies, and opportunities for further research and theory development.

CONCLUDING REMARKS

This book makes clear that Bowlby's behavioral system perspective and its use by romantic attachment researchers have been very fruitful over the past 20 years. I hope the ideas and findings presented in this book will stimulate other scholars to apply a behavioral system perspective to the study of love and that future research will be directed at the normative and individual-difference aspects of other behavioral systems discussed or hinted at by Bowlby, such as exploration, affiliation, and aggression/dominance. For each such system there are likely to be primary, functional behavioral strategies, as well as both hyperactivating and deactivating strategies that are often dysfunctional and damaging to both individuals and their social relationships. The attachment system was a good place for Bowlby to start, given his interest in infant and child development and the long-term effects of parental loss or "deprivation." The research discussed in this book has grown out of a heavy emphasis on attachment. What the field needs ultimately, however, is a more complete behavioral systems theory of personality and relationships, and this will require new research instruments, ideas, and creative studies. As always, when science works well, it is a pleasure both to see what has been accomplished in the study of love and what remains to be explored.

REFERENCES

Ainsworth, M. D. S. (1991). Attachment and other affectional bonds across the life cycle. In C. M. Parkes, J. Stevenson-Hinde, & P. Marris (Eds.), *Attachment across the life cycle* (pp. 33–51). New York: Routledge.

Ainsworth, M. D. S., Blehar, M. C., Waters, E., & Wall, S. (1978). *Patterns of attachment: A psychological study of the Strange Situation*. Hillsdale, NJ: Erlbaum.

Baldwin, M. W. (Ed.). (2005). *Interpersonal cognition*. New York: Guilford Press.

Baldwin, M. W., Fehr, B., Keedian, E., Seidel, M., & Thomson, D. W. (1993). An exploration of the relational schemata underlying attachment styles: Self-report and lexical decision approaches. *Personality and Social Psychology Bulletin, 19*, 746–754.

Bartholomew, K., & Horowitz, L. M. (1991). Attachment styles among young adults: A test of a four-category model. *Journal of Personality and Social Psychology, 61*, 226–244.

Batson, C. D. (1991). *The altruism question: Toward a social psychological answer.* Hillsdale, NJ: Erlbaum.

Berscheid, E. (1984). Interpersonal attraction. In G. Lindzey & E. Aronson (Eds.), *Handbook of social psychology* (Vol. 2, 3rd ed., pp. 413–484). Reading, MA: Addison-Wesley.

Birnbaum, G. E., & Laser-Brandt, D. (2002). Gender differences in the experience of heterosexual intercourse. *Canadian Journal of Human Sexuality, 11*, 143–158.

Bowlby, J. (1982). *Attachment and loss: Vol. 1. Attachment* (2nd ed.). New York: Basic Books. (Original edition published 1969)

Bowlby, J. (1973). *Attachment and loss: Vol. 2. Separation: Anxiety and anger.* New York: Basic Books.

Bowlby, J. (1979). *The making and breaking of affectional bonds*. London: Tavistock.

Bowlby, J. (1980). *Attachment and loss: Vol. 3. Loss: Sadness and depression*. New York: Basic Books.

Bowlby, J. (1988). *A secure base: Clinical applications of attachment theory.* London: Routledge.

Brennan, K. A., Clark, C. L., & Shaver, P. R. (1998). Self-report measurement of adult attachment: An integrative overview. In J. A. Simpson & W. S. Rholes (Eds.), *Attachment theory and close relationships* (pp. 46–76). New York: Guilford Press.

Brennan, K. A., Wu, S., & Loev, J. (1998). Adult romantic attachment and individual differences in attitudes toward physical contact in the context of adult romantic relationships. In J. A. Simpson & W. S. Rholes (Eds.), *Attachment theory and close relationships* (pp. 394–428). New York: Guilford Press.

Buss, D. M. (1999). *Evolutionary psychology: The new science of the mind.* Boston: Allyn & Bacon.

Buss, D. M., & Kenrick, D. T. (1998). Evolutionary social psychology. In D. T. Gilbert,

S. T. Fiske, & G. Lindzey (Eds.), *The handbook of social psychology* (Vol. 2, pp. 982–1026). New York: McGraw-Hill.

Carnelley, K. B., Pietromonaco, P. R., & Jaffe, K. (1996). Attachment, caregiving, and relationship functioning in couples: Effects of self and partner. *Personal Relationships, 3*, 257–277.

Carver, C. S., & Scheier, M. F. (1981). *Attention and self-regulation: A control-theory approach to human behavior.* New York: Springer-Verlag.

Carver, C. S., & Scheier, M. F. (1990). Origins and functions of positive and negative affect: A control-process view. *Psychological Review, 97*, 19–35.

Cassidy, J., & Kobak, R. R. (1988). Avoidance and its relationship with other defensive processes. In J. Belsky & T. Nezworski (Eds.), *Clinical implications of attachment* (pp. 300–323). Hillsdale, NJ: Erlbaum.

Collins, N. L. (1996). Working models of attachment: Implications for explanation, emotion, and behavior. *Journal of Personality and Social Psychology, 71*, 810–832.

Collins, N. L., & Feeney, B. C. (2000). A safe haven: An attachment theory perspective on support seeking and caregiving in intimate relationships. *Journal of Personality and Social Psychology, 78*, 1053–1073.

Collins, N. L., & Read, S. J. (1990). Adult attachment, working models, and relationship quality in dating couples. *Journal of Personality and Social Psychology, 58*, 644–663.

Cowan, P. A., & Cowan, C. P. (2002). What an intervention design reveals about how parents affect their children's academic achievement and behavior problems. In J. G. Borkowski, S. Ramey, & M. Bristol-Power (Eds.), *Parenting and the child's world: Influences on intellectual, academic, and social-emotional development* (pp. 75–98). Mahwah, NJ: Erlbaum.

Cozzarelli, C., Hoekstra, S. J., & Bylsma, W. H. (2000). General versus specific mental models of attachment: Are they associated with different outcomes? *Personality and Social Psychology Bulletin, 26*, 605–618.

Cyranowski, J. M., & Andersen, B. L. (1998). Schemas, sexuality, and romantic attachment. *Journal of Personality and Social Psychology, 74*, 1364–1379.

Davila, J., Karney, B. R., & Bradbury, T. N. (1999). Attachment change processes in the early years of marriage. *Journal of Personality and Social Psychology, 76*, 783–802.

Davis, D., Shaver, P. R., & Vernon, M. L. (2004). Attachment style and subjective motivations for sex. *Personality and Social Psychology Bulletin, 30*, 1076–1090.

Davis, M. H. (1983). Empathic concern and the muscular dystrophy telethon: Empathy as a multidimensional construct. *Personality and Social Psychology Bulletin, 9*, 223–229.

Diamond, L. M. (2003). What does sexual orientation orient? A biobehavioral model distinguishing romantic love and sexual desire. *Psychological Review, 110*, 173–192.

Feeney, B. C. (2004). A secure base: Responsive support of goal strivings and exploration in adult intimate relationships. *Journal of Personality and Social Psychology, 87*, 631–648.

Feeney, B. C., & Collins, N. L. (2001). Predictors of caregiving in adult intimate relationships: An attachment theoretical perspective. *Journal of Personality and Social Psychology, 80*, 972–994.

Feeney, B. C., & Collins, N. L. (2003). Motivations for caregiving in adult intimate relationships: Influence on caregiving behavior and relationship functioning. *Personality and Social Psychology Bulletin*, *29*, 950–968.

Feeney, J. A. (1996). Attachment, caregiving, and marital satisfaction. *Personal Relationships*, *3*, 401–416.

Feeney, J. A. (1999). Adult romantic attachment and couple relationships. In J. Cassidy & P. R. Shaver (Eds.), *Handbook of attachment: Theory, research, and clinical applications* (pp. 355–377). New York: Guilford Press.

Feeney, J. A. (2002). Attachment, marital interaction, and relationship satisfaction: A diary study. *Personal Relationships*, *9*, 39–55.

Feeney, J. A., & Hohaus, L. (2001). Attachment and spousal caregiving. *Personal Relationships*, *8*, 21–39.

Fisher, H. E., Aron, A., Mashek, D., Li, H., & Brown, L. L. (2002). Defining the brain systems of lust, romantic attraction, and attachment. *Archives of Sexual Behavior*, *31*, 413–419.

Fisher, W. A., Byrne, D., White, L. A., & Kelley, K. (1988). Erotophobia-erotophilia as a dimension of personality. *Journal of Sex Research*, *25*, 123–151.

Fraley, R. C., & Davis, K. E. (1997). Attachment formation and transfer in young adults' close friendships and romantic relationships. *Personal Relationships*, *4*, 131–144.

Fraley, R. C., & Shaver, P. R. (1997). Adult attachment and the suppression of unwanted thoughts. *Journal of Personality and Social Psychology*, *73*, 1080–1091.

Gillath, O., Shaver, P. R., & Mikulincer, M. (2005). An attachment-theoretical approach to compassion and altruism. In P. Gilbert (Ed.), *Compassion: Its nature and use in psychotherapy* (pp. 121–147). London: Brunner-Routledge.

Hamilton, W. D. (1964). The genetical evolution of social behavior. Parts I, II. *Journal of Theoretical Biology*, *7*, 1–52.

Hassebrauck, M., & Fehr, B. (2002). Dimensions of relationship quality. *Personal Relationships*, *9*, 253–270.

Hazan, C., & Shaver, P. R. (1987). Romantic love conceptualized as an attachment process. *Journal of Personality and Social Psychology*, *52*, 511–524.

Hazan, C., & Shaver, P. R. (1994). Attachment theory as an organizational framework for research on close relationships. *Psychological Inquiry*, *5*, 1–22.

Hazan, C., & Zeifman, D. (1994). Sex and the psychological tether. In K. Bartholomew & D. Perlman (Eds.), *Advances in personal relationships: Vol. 5. Attachment processes in adulthood* (pp. 151–177). London: Kingsley.

Hazan, C., & Zeifman, D. (1999). Pair-bonds as attachments: Evaluating the evidence. In J. Cassidy & P. R. Shaver (Eds.), *Handbook of attachment: Theory, research, and clinical applications* (pp. 336–354). New York: Guilford Press.

Helgeson, V. S. (1993). Implications of agency and communion for patient and spouse adjustment to a first coronary event. *Journal of Personality and Social Psychology*, *64*, 807–816.

Holmes, J. G., & Cameron, J. (2005). An integrative review of theories of interpersonal cognition: An interdependence theory perspective. In M. W. Baldwin (Ed.), *Interpersonal cognition* (pp. 415–447). New York: Guilford Press.

Jack, D. C., & Dill, D. (1992). The Silencing the Self Scale: Schemas of intimacy associated with depression in women. *Psychology of Women Quarterly*, *16*, 97–106.

Janda, L. H., & O'Grady, K. E. (1980). Development of a sex anxiety inventory. *Journal of Consulting and Clinical Psychology, 48*, 169–175.

Kobak, R. R., & Hazan, C. (1991). Attachment in marriage: Effects of security and accuracy of working models. *Journal of Personality and Social Psychology, 60*, 861–869.

Kunce, L. J., & Shaver, P. R. (1994). An attachment-theoretical approach to caregiving in romantic relationships. In K. Bartholomew & D. Perlman (Eds.), *Advances in personal relationships* (Vol. 5, pp. 205–237). London: Kingsley.

Main, M. (1990). Cross-cultural studies of attachment organization: Recent studies, changing methodologies, and the concept of conditional strategies. *Human Development, 33*, 48–61.

Mikulincer, M. (1998). Attachment working models and the sense of trust: An exploration of interaction goals and affect regulation. *Journal of Personality and Social Psychology, 74*, 1209–1224.

Mikulincer, M., & Arad, D. (1999). Attachment working models and cognitive openness in close relationships: A test of chronic and temporary accessibility effects. *Journal of Personality and Social Psychology, 77*, 710–725.

Mikulincer, M., Florian, V., Cowan, P. A., & Cowan, C. P. (2002). Attachment security in couple relationships: A systemic model and its implications for family dynamics. *Family Process, 41*, 405–434.

Mikulincer, M., & Shaver, P. R. (2003). The attachment behavioral system in adulthood: Activation, psychodynamics, and interpersonal processes. In M. P. Zanna (Ed.), *Advances in experimental social psychology* (Vol. 35, pp. 53–152). New York: Academic Press.

Mikulincer, M., & Shaver, P. R. (2004). Security-based self-representations in adulthood: Contents and processes. In W. S. Rholes & J. A. Simpson (Eds.), *Adult attachment: Theory, research, and clinical implications* (pp. 159–195). New York: Guilford Press.

Mosher, D. L. (1988). Revised Mosher Guilt Inventory. In C. M. Davis, W. C. Yarber, & R. S. L. Davis (Eds.), *Sexuality-related measures* (pp. 75–88). Lake Mills, IA: Davis.

Rholes, W. S., Simpson, J. A., Campbell, L., & Grich, J. (2001). Adult attachment and the transition to parenthood. *Journal of Personality and Social Psychology, 81*, 421–435.

Rholes, W. S., Simpson, J. A., & Orina, M. M. (1999). Attachment and anger in an anxiety-provoking situation. *Journal of Personality and Social Psychology, 76*, 940–957.

Rogers, C. R. (1961). *On becoming a person.* Boston: Houghton Mifflin.

Schachner, D. A., & Shaver, P. R. (2004). Attachment dimensions and motives for sex. *Personal Relationships, 11*, 179–195.

Scharfe, E., & Bartholomew, K. (1995). Accommodation and attachment representations in couples. *Journal of Social and Personal Relationships, 12*, 389–401.

Seligman, M. E. P. (2002). *Authentic happiness: Using the new positive psychology to realize your potential for lasting fulfillment.* New York: Free Press.

Shaver, P. R., & Brennan, K. A. (1992). Attachment styles and the "big five" personality traits: Their connections with each other and with romantic relationship outcomes. *Personality and Social Psychology Bulletin, 18*, 536–545.

Shaver, P. R., Collins, N., & Clark, C. L. (1996). Attachment styles and internal working models of self and relationship partners. In G. J. O. Fletcher & J. Fitness (Eds.), *Knowledge structures in close relationships: A social psychological approach* (pp. 25–61). Hillsdale, NJ: Erlbaum.

Shaver, P. R., & Hazan, C. (1988). A biased overview of the study of love. *Journal of Social and Personal Relationships*, *5*, 473–501.

Shaver, P. R., & Hazan, C. (1993). Adult romantic attachment: Theory and evidence. In D. Perlman & W. Jones (Eds.), *Advances in personal relationships* (Vol. 4, pp. 29–70). London: Kingsley.

Shaver, P. R., Hazan, C., & Bradshaw, D. (1988). Love as attachment: The integration of three behavioral systems. In R. J. Sternberg & M. Barnes (Eds.), *The psychology of love* (pp. 68–99). New Haven, CT: Yale University Press.

Shaver, P. R., & Mikulincer, M. (2002). Attachment-related psychodynamics. *Attachment and Human Development*, *4*, 133–161.

Shaver, P. R., & Mikulincer, M. (in press). Attachment theory, individual psychodynamics, and relationship functioning. In D. Perlman & A. Vangelisti (Eds.), *Handbook of personal relationships*. New York: Cambridge University Press.

Simpson, J. A. (1990). Influence of attachment styles on romantic relationships. *Journal of Personality and Social Psychology*, *59*, 971–980.

Simpson, J. A., Rholes, W. S., & Nelligan, J. S. (1992). Support seeking and support giving within couples in an anxiety-provoking situation: The role of attachment styles. *Journal of Personality and Social Psychology*, *62*, 434–446.

Simpson, J. A., Rholes, W. S., Orina, M. M., & Grich, J. (2002). Working models of attachment, support giving, and support seeking in a stressful situation. *Personality and Social Psychology Bulletin*, *28*, 598–608.

Sprecher, S., & Cate, R. M. (2004). Sexual satisfaction and sexual expression as predictors of relationship satisfaction and stability. In J. H. Harvey, A. Wenzel, & S. Sprecher (Eds.), *Handbook of sexuality in close relationships* (pp. 235–256). Mahwah, NJ: Erlbaum.

Sprecher, S., & Regan, P. C. (1998). Passionate and companionate love in courting and young married couples. *Sociological Inquiry*, *68*, 163–185.

Sroufe, L. A., & Waters, E. (1977). Attachment as an organizational construct. *Child Development*, *48*, 1184–1199.

Tracy, J. L., Shaver, P. R., Albino, A. W., & Cooper, M. L. (2003). Attachment styles and adolescent sexuality. In P. Florsheim (Ed.), *Adolescent romance and sexual behavior: Theory, research, and practical implications* (pp. 137–159). Mahwah, NJ: Erlbaum.

Westen, D. (1998). The scientific legacy of Sigmund Freud: Toward a psychodynamically informed psychological science. *Psychological Bulletin*, *124*, 252–283.

Part II

Basic Attachment Processes in Couple Relationships

3

What Is Adult Attachment?

CINDY HAZAN, MARY CAMPA,
and NURIT GUR-YAISH

The question posed by the title of this chapter may strike some readers as odd, coming nearly two decades after the field of adult romantic attachment was born. In less than 20 years, hundreds of studies on the topic have been published, along with many additional edited volumes and review papers. Surely by now we know the answer!

Our reasons for asking the question may be elucidated by reframing it: How do researchers who conduct studies of adult romantic attachment know—that is, what "markers" do they use to determine—whether study participants are attached to their romantic partners? In fact, this question has yet to be fully answered because, as a field, we have yet to fully address it.

In all areas of scientific inquiry the specific issues that occupy researchers at any given point in time often follow directly from the most recent developments and discoveries. Normative aspects of infant–caregiver attachment, such as the process by which they are established, were the primary focus of Bowlby's (1969/1982) original theory and subsequently the focus of early attachment research. But when Ainsworth and her colleagues (Ainsworth, Blehar, Waters, & Wall, 1978) published the results of their landmark study revealing "secure," "ambivalent," and "avoidant" patterns of infant attachment, the emphasis shifted to individual differences.

The field of adult romantic attachment grew more out of Ainsworth et al.'s research than out of Bowlby's theory. It was founded on self-report and interview measures designed to capture adult versions of the infant patterns (Bartholomew & Horowitz, 1991; Brennan & Shaver, 1995; Collins & Read, 1990; Hazan & Shaver, 1987; Levy & Davis, 1988; Simpson, 1990). Much has since been learned about the nature and correlates of adult attachment patterns or "styles" (see Feeney, 1999, for a review).

However, as a result of this near-exclusive focus on individual differences, relatively little progress has been made on the normative front. Increasingly, investigators in the fields of both infant and adult attachment (e.g., Berlin & Cassidy, 1999; Diamond, 2001; Fraley & Shaver, 2000; Hazan & Zeifman, 1994; Hazan, Gur-Yaish, & Campa, 2004; Kobak, 1999; Main, 1999; Marvin & Britner, 1999; Simpson & Rholes, 1998) are calling for more research on normative aspects of attachment. They (and we) have argued that attachment research thus far has not taken full advantage of all that Bowlby's deep and rich theory of human affectional bonding has to offer. Many basic issues remain entirely unexplored.

Our aim here is not to provide a definitive answer to the question raised in the title. In fact, we do not believe it *can* be answered satisfactorily from the empirical evidence currently available. Instead, we wish to make the case that the question itself is important and deserving of research attention. In our view, identifying markers of adult attachment is a crucial next step for the field. And we think the payoff in terms of theoretical advance could be significant.

The development of an attachment bond is presumed to result from the interaction of multiple intraindividual and interindividual processes operating at multiple levels over time. This includes the different levels at which attachment has already been studied—that is, behavior, cognition, emotion, and physiology. Thus, in addition to finding multilevel markers of attachment, it will be important to specify *what* the related processes are and *how* they change over time.

We begin with a brief theoretical background that focuses on Bowlby's definition of attachment and normative model of attachment formation. In the second section, we describe some of the research challenges of defining adult attachment in terms of markers and processes. In the third section, we offer additional thoughts on potential markers and processes as a way of suggesting possible areas and avenues for future research on adult attachment.

THEORETICAL BACKGROUND

Bowlby (1969/1982) defined attachment bonds in terms of four distinct but interrelated classes of behavior, all of which are regulated by an innate behavioral system: *proximity maintenance, safe haven, separation distress*, and *secure base*. These features of attachment and the dynamic functioning of the attachment system are most readily observable in the behavior of 12-month-olds in relation to their primary caregivers (typically mothers). The infant continuously monitors the caregiver's whereabouts and makes adjustments as necessary to maintain proximity, retreats to her as a haven of safety in the event of perceived threat, is actively resistant to and upset by separations from her, and uses her as a base of security from which to explore the environment. Although infants often direct one or more of these behaviors toward individuals to whom they are not attached, it is the selective orientation of all four behaviors toward a specific individual that defines attachment.

Bowlby (1969/1982) proposed four phases in the development of infant–caregiver attachments, which Ainsworth (1972) further elaborated and labeled as follows. In the *preattachment* phase (birth to 2 months of age), infants are inherently interested in and responsive to social interaction with virtually anyone. In the *attachment-in-the-making* phase (2–6 months), they begin to show preferences by, for example, smiling and vocalizing to and settling more quickly with some caregivers than others. In the *clear-cut attachment* phase (beginning at around 6 or 7 months), all of the behaviors that define attachment are selectively directed toward the primary caregiver. This is evident in the infant's efforts to maintain proximity (differential following), the use of this individual as a haven of safety (differential comfort seeking) and secure base (differential exploration), and reactions to separation (differential distress). In the fourth phase, *goal-corrected partnership* (after about 2 years), children have less urgent needs for physical proximity and are increasingly capable of negotiating with caregivers regarding separations and availability.

The separation-distress feature of attachment is particularly important for both theoretical and historical reasons. A major source of inspiration for attachment theory was reports during the 1940s and 1950s (e.g., Burlingham & Freud, 1944; Robertson, 1953) that infants and young children who are separated from primary caregivers for extended periods of time pass through a predictable sequence of reactions. At first, they actively resist by crying and searching in an attempt to regain contact. Eventually, agitation and anxiety are replaced by deeper and more pervasive signs of distress, including depressed mood, decreased appetite, and disturbed sleep. In time these symptoms subside, giving the appearance of full recovery. It is only when they are reunited with caregivers that otherwise invisible lingering effects of the separation show up in the form of emotional withdrawal or anger mixed with anxious clinging. This sequence of reactions is known as *protest*, *despair*, and *detachment*.

According to Bowlby (1979), romantic relationships or "pair bonds" are the prototype of attachment in adulthood. Nevertheless, adult attachments differ from infant–caregiver bonds in at least two important respects. First, they tend to be more reciprocal in the sense that partners alternately seek care from and provide care to each other. Second, such relationships are inherently sexual in nature. Thus adult attachments involve not only the attachment system but also the caregiving/parental and sexual/reproductive systems (Ainsworth, 1990; Hazan & Shaver, 1994; Shaver, Hazan, & Bradshaw, 1988).

The earliest reported evidence that pair bonds qualify as true attachments came from reports that adults grieving the death of a spouse exhibit a similar protest–despair–detachment sequence of reactions (Parkes, 1972; Weiss, 1975). Differential separation distress is still considered the standard marker of attachment in infancy (Ainsworth et al., 1978; Sroufe & Waters, 1977a).

RESEARCH CHALLENGES

At the Level of Behavior

In theory, if person A maintains proximity to person B, uses B as a haven of safety and base for exploration, and is distressed by separations from B, then person A is attached to person B. There are two major challenges that need be addressed if these behaviors are to be used as markers of adult attachment. Given that adults do not usually behave like babies, the first challenge is to operationally (re)define the behaviors in adult terms. The second is to determine the contexts in which the behaviors do and do not indicate the existence of an attachment bond.

Although many adult attachment studies have focused directly or indirectly on the behaviors that Bowlby proposed to define attachment, the vast majority have relied solely on self-reports as opposed to actual behavior. Two noteworthy exceptions are a laboratory-based experiment and a naturalistic observational study.

Simpson, Rholes, and Nelligan (1992) designed an experimental paradigm similar in several respects to the laboratory procedure developed by Ainsworth et al. (1978) to assess infant attachment. Female undergraduates were separated from their male romantic partners and then (falsely) led to expect a stressful experience. Subsequent reunions with partners were unobtrusively videotaped and later coded. The experimental manipulation was designed to elicit anxiety and attachment behavior, and in females with a "secure" attachment style it did. The more anxious they were, the more they sought contact with and comfort from their partners.

The Simpson et al. (1992) study is an excellent example of how attachment behaviors can be investigated in adulthood. In considering the specific behaviors the researchers observed—proximity seeking and safe haven—as potential markers of adult attachment, it is essential to take contextual and relational factors into account. The researchers engineered a context that should elicit attachment behavior. However, in situations that arouse anxiety, individuals of all ages have been shown to seek contact with and comfort from whoever is nearby, even relative strangers (Shaver & Klinnert, 1982). In theory, what sets attachment figures apart is that they are reliably preferred over other targets of distress alleviation.

Fraley and Shaver (1998) observed couples in an airport lobby awaiting either a joint trip on a departing flight or a separation entailed by one person departing while the other remained behind. In this study, the impending separation was expected to elicit anxiety and thereby trigger attachment behavior. In general, contact seeking (e.g., hugging, kissing, hand holding) was significantly higher in couples facing a separation than in those traveling together. The incidence of these behaviors also varied as a function of relationship length. Overt displays of attachment behavior were less common in longer term compared with shorter term couples.

The Fraley and Shaver (1998) study represents another creative approach to investigating attachment behavior in adults, and the results accord well with theoretical predictions that actual or anticipated separations from attachment figures activate proximity and comfort seeking. Further, the specific behaviors the researchers observed (e.g., kissing, hand holding) are not likely to be directed toward strangers. Such physical intimacy signals a special relationship, but it still may be insufficient evidence of attachment. Romantic partners tend to be most physically affectionate at the beginning of their relationships. Fraley and Shaver (1998) found that the longer the couples in their study had been together, the less they exhibited various proximity and contact maintenance behaviors. If one assumes that longer term couples are more likely than shorter term couples to be attached, the limitations of inferring attachment solely on the basis of such behaviors become clear.

Recall that separation reactions in infancy and childhood undergo qualitative change over time. The immediate (protest) response is anxiety, agitation, and heightened activity, whereas the later (despair) response is depression, lethargy, and diminished activity. In considering response to separation as a potential marker of adult attachment, it is important to distinguish between acute and slower developing reactions. It is also necessary to take into account how manifestations of separation distress change over the course of bond development. If children in the goal-corrected phase of attachment formation are able to tolerate short-term separations without undue upset, presumably adult partners can, also. It may require more than a few days of separation to elicit measurable distress in romantic couples.

Vormbrock's (1993) review of research on marital separations lasting weeks or months revealed that responses also differ depending on whether one leaves or is left behind. Reactions of homebound spouses included protest, despair, and detachment behaviors, but responses on the part of traveling spouses did not.

Individual differences or attachment styles complicate the picture even further. In the Simpson et al. (1992) experiment, the behavior of avoidant females was opposite that of secure females. Instead of turning to their partners when they were most anxious and thus in greatest need of support, they exhibited less proximity and comfort seeking the more anxious they were. This is reminiscent of the findings reported by Ainsworth et al. (1978) that avoidant infants are more likely to evade contact with caregivers under high- than under low-stress conditions. It is also consistent with results from Fraley and Shaver's (1998) airport study. Avoidant women sought more contact with their partners when the two were traveling together and less when a separation was imminent.

In summary, the challenges associated with using attachment behaviors as markers of adult attachment bonds include the facts that proximity and comfort seeking are sometimes directed toward strangers and occur more frequently in shorter term than longer term couples and that reactions to separation vary as a function of individual differences, relationship length, separation duration, and leaver versus left behind status.

At the Level of Physiology

Attachment theory specifies a broad range of ways that infants are affected by relationships with primary caregivers. What the theory underestimates, in the opinion of some, are the effects of attachment figures on infant physiology (Kraemer, 1992; Polan & Hofer, 1999; Reite & Capitano, 1985). Interest in this issue has grown in recent years, and there is now a large body of empirical work on the psychophysiology of infant–caregiver attachment (reviewed in Fox & Card, 1999). The main focus of this research has been individual differences, especially the effects of temperament and attachment organization on infant reactivity.

A few studies of adult attachment have incorporated physiological measures (e.g., Feeney & Kirkpatrick, 1996; Fraley & Shaver, 1997; Mikulincer, 1998), again with an emphasis on how attachment styles influence arousal under various conditions. In the field of health psychology, hundreds of studies have examined the physiological correlates of social interaction (reviewed in Uchino, Cacioppo, & Kiecolt-Glaser, 1996). Although many of the findings are relevant to attachment issues and questions, the studies were not designed explicitly to address them. Missing from the literature are systematic investigations of the physiological underpinnings of normative adult attachment (Diamond, 2001).

In contrast, animal researchers have made significant progress in identifying the neuroanatomical and neurobiological substrates of attachment in a variety of mammalian species (see Carter, Lederhendler, & Kirkpatrick,

1997, for a review). Several (e.g., Carter, 1998; Hofer, 1994; Reite & Boccia, 1994; Suomi, 1999) have explicitly discussed the implications of their findings for research on human attachment.

Prominent among them is Hofer, who, in a 1987 *Child Development* article, summarized his research on separation distress in rat pups. The work was motivated by the question of what, exactly, the pups missed about their mother during separations from her. To find out, Hofer and his colleagues designed a series of experiments in which they introduced specific features of the absent mother, one by one, and then measured the effect of each on the pups' distress. The studies revealed that each of the pups' distress symptoms was tied to a specific maternal feature. For example, in her absence, the pups became listless, but warming the cage to match her body temperature normalized their activity levels. Their heart rates returned to normal when gastric canulas were used to fill their stomachs with her milk. By imitating her grooming behavior with rhythmic stroking, sleep disturbances were corrected.

The major discovery was that each maternal feature alleviated a single distress symptom while having no effect on the others. Hofer (1987) interpreted the findings as evidence that specific features of the mother regulate the pups' physiological systems. In his view, the reason that the pups showed the constellation of symptoms that in human young and bereaved adults is called despair was because in the mother's absence all of these "hidden" regulators were also absent. The fact that extended separations cause behavioral and physiological disorganization is widely accepted as evidence that an attachment exists. The flip side, according to Hofer, is that attachment bonds are what keep these systems organized and regulated. In essence, he raised the intriguing possibility that across species and ages, physiological coregulation may be an inherent part and reliable marker of attachment.

Extrapolating findings from one species to another can be risky, but cross-species comparisons can also be an invaluable source of new ideas. In formulating attachment theory, Bowlby drew inspiration from Harlow's experiments on affectional bonding in rhesus monkeys and from research by Lorenz on imprinting behavior in goslings, both of which led him to postulate an innate system to regulate human attachment behavior.

It is relatively easy to accept that the physiology of helpless newborn rats is regulated by the mother who nurses, protects, and grooms them. But is this a plausible model of attachment in our species, especially beyond infancy? In fact, there is ample evidence for the social entrainment of biological rhythms in human adults. Biological systems have a 24-hour functional rhythm run by two pacemakers in the hypothalamus. These pacemakers require daily synchronization, and for every species there are specific aspects of the environment (*Zeitgebers*, from the German word for timekeepers) that entrain the rhythms. For example, insect timekeepers include such things as ambient temperature and light–dark cycles. A major *Zeitgeber* for humans is social interaction.

The field of chronobiology is replete with examples of this phenomenon. Vernikos-Danellis and Winget (1979, cited in Hofer, 1984) found that adults who are removed from their usual surroundings and housed in sensory-deprivation environments show circadian rhythm synchronization. Examples from other literatures include evidence of menstrual synchrony among coresident women (McClintock, 1971), earlier pubertal onset for girls sharing households with unrelated adult males (Moffitt, Caspi, Belsky, & Silva, 1992; Surbey, 1990), and more regular ovulation in women with steady male sexual partners (Veith, Buck, Getzlaf, Van Dalfsen, & Slade, 1983).

A different kind of coregulation is suggested by evidence (Carter, 1998; Carter et al., 1997; Hennessy, 1997) that, across mammalian species, bonds between infants and caregivers and between adult reproductive partners involve the same psychoneuroendocrine core: the hypothalamic–pituitary–adrenocortical (HPA) axis and the autonomic nervous system (ANS). The primary function of this core is to up-regulate system activity to prepare an organism to take action in potentially harmful situations and then down-regulate system activity to restore homeostasis after the threat has passed. Evidence that this physiological core is involved in attachment comes from both human and animal research.

In a sample of cohabiting and married couples, Gump, Polk, Kamarck, and Shiffman (2001) used blood pressure as an index of ANS activity. All participants wore ambulatory monitors during waking hours for 1 week. At least once per hour, blood pressure was recorded, and participants made diary entries to report what they were doing and feeling and whether anyone was with them at the time. Blood pressure was found to be significantly lower when partners were present than during one-on-one interactions with others or when alone. Although exchanges with partners were rated as more intimate, this did not mediate the association with blood pressure.

Mason and Mendoza (1998) have found evidence of physiological markers of attachment in titi monkeys. Specifically, HPA effects appear to be uniquely associated with attachment bonds. Titi mates maintain close proximity, often sitting shoulder-to-shoulder for hours with their long tails intertwined, and they show extreme distress and increased HPA activation when separated. In contrast, they do not display attachment behaviors toward their offspring, nor do they experience increased HPA activation when separated from them. Titi infants tend to be primarily attached to their fathers. Correspondingly, separations from fathers, but not mothers, are associated with increased HPA activation in the infants.

Carter (1998) has investigated physiological markers of attachment in prairie voles, another pair-bonding species. Prairie vole pairs simply housed in the same cage eventually become attached, but the process is speeded by sexual contact and stress. Carter's work focuses on the hormones oxytocin and vasopressin, which are closely associated with the parasympathetic branch of the ANS and have a down-regulating effect on arousal. Through a series of experiments, Carter et al. (1997) demonstrated that oxytocin and vasopressin play central roles in the formation of pair bonds. For example, prairie voles display proximity maintenance and separation distress in relation to mates, but these behaviors are precluded by the administration of an antagonist (see also Insel, 2000).

Based on their findings, Carter (1998) proposed a model of prairie vole attachment formation: It begins with sustained proximity, sexual contact, and/or stress, all of which trigger HPA activation and social approach. HPA activation signals the hypothalamus, which in turn signals the posterior pituitary to release oxytocin or vasopressin. The ensuing hormone-induced state of calm is thus experienced in the context of social contact. When contact and calming coincide with sufficient frequency or intensity, conditioning occurs. That is, a specific individual becomes associated with feelings of security.

In humans, oxytocin is best known for triggering labor in pregnant women and milk letdown in nursing mothers and is thought to foster infant bonding via a similar mechanism—a conditioned association between the mother and feelings of security (Uvnas-Moberg, 1994, 1998). Oxytocin release is not limited to infant–caregiver relationships. In fact, levels are highest in both men and women at the moment of sexual orgasm (Uvnas-Moberg, 1997). This suggests that the effects of intimate physical contact on adult attachment formation may also be hormonally mediated and involve a similar conditioning mechanism. Of course the challenge for researchers will be to distinguish between sex-related and attachment-related releases of oxytocin.

In summary, animal research on the neurobiology of pair bonding has resulted in normative models of mammalian attachment to mates that have tremendous potential for human application. In addition, research on the physiological effects of human social interaction offers clues and methods that should prove useful in the development of a normative model for our species. These literatures highlight two processes that appear to be good candidates for markers of romantic attachment, each of which involves a different type of coregulation.

One type is evident when individuals modulate each other's physiological arousal in specific situations. Most pertinent to attachment is the attenuation of arousal responses to threats and stressors. In considering this form of coregulation as a possible marker of adult attachment, at least two challenges must be addressed.

The first is that studies comparing the effectiveness of (presumed) attachment figures versus others in buffering stress reactivity have produced conflicting results. In the Gump et al. (2001) study, participants had significantly lower blood pressure in the presence of partners than in the presence of others or alone, but other studies (e.g., Fontana, Diegnan, Villeneuve, & Lepore, 1999) have found supportive strangers to be as effective as close friends in attenuating physiological responses to stress. Clearly, these inconsistencies will need to be resolved if physiological stress buffering is to be used as a marker of attachment.

The second challenge concerns the complicating effects of attachment style. In one study (Carpenter & Kirkpatrick, 1996), undergraduate females experienced a physiological stressor on two separate occasions, once in the presence of romantic partners and once alone. For secure women, the presence of a partner had no effect on physiological responses. In contrast, avoidant women had higher blood pressure with a partner present than when alone. Whether there are circumstances in which partner effects on physiological stress responses are reliable markers of attachment remains to be seen.

The other type of coregulation involves more generalized effects on multiple physiological systems of the sort that Hofer (1987) identified in rat pups. The primary challenge associated with using this kind of physiological coregulation as a marker of adult attachment is that our physiological systems, even in adulthood, remain "open" to a variety of social influences. Some may be indicative of attachment whereas others may not.

At the Level of Cognition

As individuals mature they become less dependent on the physical presence of attachment figures and increasingly reliant on mental representations of them. Some of the most exciting new work on adult attachment takes advantage of this normative shift to the level of representation by borrowing methods from the field of cognitive psychology.

Using a lexical decision task and cognitive priming paradigm, Mikulincer, Gillath, and Shaver (2002) tested the hypothesis that activating the attachment system via threat would increase the accessibility of mental representations of attachment figures. Study participants completed a shortened version (Fraley & Davis, 1997) of a self-report measure (WHOTO) created by Hazan and Zeifman (1994) that asks respondents to name the targets of the four behaviors that, according to Bowlby, define attachment. In addition, they provided names of close or known others not mentioned as targets of attachment behavior. Subsequently, on a computer screen, they were subliminally exposed to either a neutral ("hat") or threatening ("separation") prime word followed by the name of an attachment figure, close or known other, or a nonword. Their task was to indicate as quickly as possible, by a key stroke, whether the string of letters that appeared on the screen was a word or a nonword. The dependent measure was reaction time (RT).

The findings supported the main hypothesis: Following the threatening but not the neutral prime word, participants more quickly recognized as words the names of individuals they had listed as attachment figures. Importantly, this effect was observed across attachment styles. Regardless of how participants scored on measures of avoidance, ambivalence, or security, their RTs were shorter in response to attachment than to nonattachment figures.

Another cognitive method that shows promise for investigating adult attachment comes from the work of Andersen and colleagues (Andersen & Glassman, 1996; Andersen, Reznik, & Chen, 1997). Their research program is based on the clinical concept of transference, the idea that mental representations of important interpersonal relationships affect how information about a new person is processed. To explore this concept, they have developed a paradigm that incorporates idiographic methods into a nomothetic experimental design. For example, in a sentence-completion task, participants provide descriptions of individuals with whom they have a "significant" personal relationship. In a follow-up, weeks later, they are presented with descriptions of several new persons. The test set contains descriptions composed to resemble one significant other of each participant. Afterward, participants complete a standard recognition memory task consisting of sentences, some of which were taken from the descriptions they provided at Time 1, some of which were included in the test set at Time 2, and some that were included as fillers. Across a series of studies (reviewed in Andersen & Berk, 1998), the results support their transference hypotheses. One finding is that participants are more likely to falsely remember having seen an unpresented sentence if it was derived from a description of their significant other. Another is that they make more errors when unknown persons are described as having traits in common with their significant other.

In summary, these methods show great promise for identifying cognitive markers of adult attachment. But, again, there are challenges to be addressed.

One is the apparent inconsistency in findings across studies and methods, as well as inconsistencies between the findings and predictions derived from attachment theory. Bowlby (1969/1982) emphasized the distinction between attachment behaviors and attachment bonds. As previously noted, attachments are defined by the presence of four specific behaviors: proximity maintenance, safe haven, separation distress, and secure base. Importantly, some of these behaviors may, under certain circumstances, be directed toward nonattachment figures. Thus the presence of any one or two may or may not indicate the existence of an attachment bond. As also noted, separation distress is considered the standard marker of infant attachment because it is the one behavior that is selectively directed toward individuals who are presumed to be primary attachment figures. In other words, not all attachment behaviors are equally indicative of an attachment bond.

Hazan and Zeifman's (1994) WHOTO instrument asks respondents to name the individuals toward whom they direct proximity-seeking, safe-haven, separation-distress, and secure-base behaviors (e.g., the persons they most want to spend time with, turn to when upset, hate being away from, and count on to be available when needed). In a 1994 study, they administered the WHOTO to a sample of adults. On the proximity and safe-haven items, nearly all participants named a romantic partner or close friend. In contrast, for the separation-distress items, they tended to name either a romantic partner or parent. Among the participants who reported having a romantic partner at the time of the study, the difference in whether they named the partner or a parent on separation-distress items depended on the length of their romantic involvement. Over 80% of those whose romantic relationships met the definitional criteria for attachment (i.e., contained all four behavioral components) had been with their partners for 2 or more years, compared with 30% who had been with their partners for less than 2 years.

In analyses of the data from their cognitive priming study, Mikulincer et al. (2002) did not distinguish among items representing different types of attachment behavior. Individuals who were named on any item were considered attachment figures, and reaction times were averaged across them (for comparison with individuals not named on any items). Thus it is unclear whether every individual named would meet Bowlby's definition of an attachment figure, whether the priming effects would have been observed for all named persons if considered individually, or whether in adults separation distress is simply not a better marker of attachment than other behaviors.

In the Hazan and Zeifman (1994) study, which used all four criterion behaviors, parents and partners often qualified as attachment figures, whereas friends rarely did. However, this finding may have resulted from the method they used. Participants were asked to name just one individual (the "most important") on each item. In a study by Trinke and Bartholomew (1997), participants were allowed to name as many people as they wished, and friends were often included on the lists (as they were in the Mikulincer et al., 2002, study). Andersen and Berk (1998) also found that friends were frequently cited as "significant" others. Trinke and Bartholomew (1997) argued that although infants tend to have one *primary* attachment figure, they also typically have additional *secondary* attachment figures, and, therefore, the same could reasonably be expected of adults.

It seems reasonable to assume that the way people process social information will be influenced more by mental representations of individuals who are of greater (versus lesser) significance to them. But deciding when a particular cognitive effect indicates the existence of an attachment bond will require additional research. In this effort we should not be limited by theoretical notions of what types of relationships are more or less likely to qualify as attachments.

At the Level of Emotion

Emotions occupy a central place in attachment theory. "Many of the most intense emotions arise during the formation, the maintenance, the disruption, and the renewal of attachment relationships" (Bowlby, 1979, p. 130). In the first volume of his trilogy, Bowlby (1969/1982) emphasized the importance of physical proximity to attachment figures. In the second volume (Bowlby, 1973), he placed greater emphasis on the child's appraisal of attachment figure availability. Specifically, feelings of security or insecurity derive less from the physical presence or absence of particular individuals than from the sense of their availability or unavailability.

The proximal function of attachment bonds is to modulate individuals' emotional states in a manner that facilitates effective coping and exploratory engagement—that is, to reduce anxiety and induce security. The primary source of "felt security" (Sroufe & Waters, 1997a) is the perception that attachment figures are accessible and responsive; maintaining proximity to them is the primary strategy for achieving it. Accordingly, adult attachment researchers have viewed emotion regulation as a core feature of romantic relationships (e.g., Brennan & Shaver, 1995; Feeney, 1995; Simpson & Rholes, 1994).

Several findings described earlier are relevant here. In the Simpson et al. (1992) experiment, secure females whose behavior indicated anxiety sought contact with their partners, presumably for the purpose of anxiety reduction. In the Fraley and Shaver (1998) airport study, couples awaiting an anxiety-provoking separation sought contact with their partners, again for what is assumed to be the same reason. In the Gump et al. (2001) study, participants' blood pressure was lower during interactions with partners, an indication that contact with them had a calming, anxiety-reducing effect. All of these studies provide support for Bowlby's conceptualization of attachment bonds as serving an emotion regulation function. Note, however, that in each case emotions or internal feeling states were inferred from other indicators (see also Mikulincer, Hirschberger, Nachmias, and Gillath, 2001).

Emotions are inherently multilevel, multicomponent processes (Frijda & Mesquita, 1998). Most involve some degree of *cognitive* appraisal, though not necessarily deliberative or conscious. They also have a *physiological* component. Arousal is a common feature, though no clear link has been established between specific emotions and particular patterns of physiological response (Caccioppo, Klein, Berntson, & Hatfield, 1993). Additionally emotions have *behavioral* components, including facial expressions, as well as action tendencies (e.g., to run away in fear, strike out in anger).

In summary, research thus far suggests that potential emotional markers of adult attachment may be found in behavioral, cognitive, and physiological indicators. If so, then identifying emotional markers will present essentially the same challenges as identifying possible markers in these other realms. An additional challenge is posed by the frequent lack of correspondence across behavioral, cognitive, and physiological indicators of emotion, which makes it difficult to draw inferences about internal feeling states from any single level.

ADDITIONAL THOUGHTS ON FUTURE RESEARCH

We have argued thus far that adult attachment formation is a process that unfolds over time and occurs at multiple levels. Implicit in this argument is the recommendation that it be studied over time and at multiple levels. In our view, it is important to know not only what changes as adult attachment bonds are established but also how the changes come about. This will require the identification of attachment markers, as well as the underlying processes that ultimately result in attachment.

One potentially helpful starting point is to think about how new romances evolve into long-term pair bonds and the changes that occur along the way. Even casual observations of couples can reveal whether they are just getting to know each other, are in the throes of romantic infatuation, or have settled into comfortable coexistence. The good news for researchers is that these qualitative changes in the ways partners interact take place over a relatively short period of time. If they reflect attachment-related developments, as we believe they do, it may be possible to capture the process of adult attachment formation in short-term longitudinal studies.

Zeifman and Hazan (1997) proposed that, in the absence of a framework for studying adult attachment processes, Bowlby and Ainsworth's four-phase model of infant attachment formation could serve as a preliminary research guide. In what follows we use this model to speculate about the types of changes that may occur at various levels as adult attachments develop. Our main objective in doing so is to suggest potentially fruitful areas and avenues of research by highlighting possible attachment markers and processes.

At the Level of Behavior

To date, there have been no descriptive longitudinal studies of attachment behavior over the course of romantic relationship development. Zeifman and Hazan (1997) hypothesized that phases in the development of attachment bonds between romantic partners would involve a logical progression in the emergence of attachment-defining behaviors.

In a hypothetical pair, the process of attachment formation at the level of behavior might look something like this: In the preattachment phase, sexual attraction and/or romantic interest draws partners together into flirtatious and arousing interactions. During this phase an increase in selective proximity seeking takes place, but other forms of attachment behavior are not yet evident. If the two begin to fall in love, the stage is set for the attachment-in-the-making phase. During this phase, physical contact is at its highest. In addition, the partners begin to display various forms of safe-haven behavior, such as increased proximity and comfort seeking when anxious or stressed. Repeated instances of intimate physical and verbal exchanges that reduce arousal foster the development of an attachment bond. Partners come to be preferred over others as sources of comfort and anxiety alleviation. If the relationship survives the inevitable waning of romantic infatuation, they may find themselves in the phase of clear-cut attachment. They have habituated to and are thus no longer as aroused by each other's presence. They have sex less often and experience less urgent needs for physical contact, but each has become sufficiently reliant on the other that separations are now distressing. And they begin to use each other as bases of security. With growing confidence that the relationship will endure, they enter the final, goal-corrected phase. From the base of security that has been established, attention is redirected toward previously neglected friendships, work obligations, and so forth. There are fewer overt displays of attachment behavior, and interactions between partners take on a more mundane, less passionate quality.

Even if this hypothetical scenario captures the major qualitative changes in behavior that occur as a secure attachment is established, it neglects the question of how the behavior of insecure individuals or couples might differ. Are there attachment-style-free behaviors that one could confidently point to as markers of adult attachment?

Infant and child attachment researchers continue to caution against confusing *quality* of attachment with *strength* of attachment (Main, 1999). Insecure children are differently but no less attached than their secure counterparts. So what do they all have in common? It is that their attachment behaviors are primarily organized around a specific person. This person may or may not be reliably responsive, may or may not be effective in alleviating distress, may or may not be approached for contact comfort in threatening or stressful situations. But she or he is nonetheless the selective target toward whom attachment behaviors are directed and around whom they are organized.

Similar patterns of selective orientation and organization might also be found in adults, perhaps in style-adjusted, mean-level changes in attachment behavior over time. Avoidant adults would not be expected to share their concerns with or request a reassuring hug from partners as readily as secure adults would, but when anxious they may nonetheless show an increase in their own version of safe-haven behavior. Avoidant infants do not try to stay as far away from their attachment figures as possible but rather maintain a "safe" distance from them (Ainsworth et al., 1978). It is easy to imagine a comparable adult strategy of not overtly expressing anxiety or actively seeking comfort but instead engaging in more distal forms of approach (e.g., hanging around but not talking, calling but not disclosing, self-soothing in proximity to an attachment figure). If attachment behaviors are conceptualized and operationalized flexibly enough, they may reveal markers that supersede attachment style.

At the Level of Physiology

The hypothesis that romantic partners become attached at a physiological level has yet to be empirically tested, but there is evidence consistent with it. As Hofer (1984) pointed out, the cardiovascular, endocrine, and immunological changes that occur in adults grieving the loss of a long-term partner are similar to those found in rat pups during prolonged separations from their mothers. From his perspective, if the extended absence of attachment figures reliably leads to dysregulation in physiological systems, it implies that attachment figures play a major role in regulating these systems. Hofer's experiments have convincingly demonstrated that such coregulation occurs in rats. In a recent set of recommendations for future directions in attachment research, Main (1999) urged investigators to begin searching for hidden physiological regulators in humans.

In a hypothetical romantic pair, the process might unfold as follows: In the preattachment phase, partners would not show any signs of physiological coregulation beyond what has been observed among strangers. In the attachment-in-the-making phase, they would engage in the kinds of physically intimate and arousal-modulating exchanges known to foster the development of coregulation in multiple physiological systems, especially those related to distress. At some point, as a result of conditioning, they would begin to have unique effects on one another's acute stress reactions and chronic physiological functioning. These context-specific and more generalized effects could mark the onset of clear-cut attachment. In the goal-corrected phase, the effects may be further consolidated and less dependent on physical proximity or interaction.

Earlier we reviewed evidence of the effects of attachment style on physiology. In the Carpenter and Kirkpatrick (1996) study, avoidant women had higher blood pressure when their partners were present than absent, whereas secure women showed no difference. The findings are consistent with results from a study in which the heart rates of 1-year-olds were monitored during separations from and reunions with their mothers (Sroufe & Waters, 1977b). All infants, whether secure or insecure, appeared to be distressed by the separations, as indicated by heart rate acceleration. But there were striking individual differences in reactions to reunion. Secure infants' heart rates returned to preseparation levels after less than a minute of maternal contact. Avoidant infants, who by definition avoid contact when stressed, continued to show increased heart rate well into the reunion.

In light of these and related findings, is there any basis for thinking that coregulation of stress reactivity is a marker of adult attachment? There may be. In the Sroufe and Waters (1977b) study, avoidant infants were distressed in both their mother's absence and her presence. We suspect that these reactions would not have been observed in relation to individuals other than the mothers, nor would we expect the avoidant women in Carpenter and Kirkpatrick's (1996) study to show elevated blood pressure in the presence of individuals other than their partners. As for the question of whether there are normative attachment markers to be found in physiological stress reactivity, the answer may lie not in *how* partners regulate each other but rather in the fact that they *do*. In situations of high stress, whether a partner's presence has a soothing or additionally arousing effect may be less revealing of attachment status than whether he or she has a significant effect of any kind.

At the Level of Cognition

A cornerstone of attachment theory is the idea that attachment experiences are internalized. The inborn attachment system enhances survival not by regulating behavior in a fixed or rigid manner but rather in a way that is adapted to the local environment, and attachment representations are the mechanism by which such adaptation occurs. Nearly all of the adult research on "internal working models" of attachment has been designed to explore attachment style differences (see Pietromonaco & Feldman Barrett, 2000, for a review). Indeed, the terms "working models" and "attachment styles" are often used interchangeably.

From an individual-differences perspective, the contents of people's representations are of interest, such as whether others are perceived as rejecting or responsive. Of course, simply knowing whether an individual expects his or her partner to be rejecting or responsive is insufficient for determining whether he or she is attached to the partner. From a normative perspective, of greater interest is whether partner representations are selectively activated under relevant circumstances and whether they have selective processing effects.

Assuming that long-term partners have mental representations of each other that they did not have before they met, theoretically it should be possible to track the development of such representations. In the absence of research on this topic, we speculate as follows:

Partners may begin to construct mental representations of each other in the preattachment phase, but the nature of their interactions during the attachment-in-the-making phase is highly conducive to the formation of more extensive representations. Partners spend long periods in close physical proximity and intimate contact, which provides ample opportunities to get familiar with each other's faces, bodies, voices, and so forth, as well as each other's availability and responsiveness. At some point, partner representations begin to be activated in attachment-relevant (e.g., stressful, threatening) contexts and have specific effects on information processing (e.g., by being chronically accessible). The emergence of these effects marks the onset of clear-cut attachment. Partner representations may undergo further elaboration and/or organizational changes that would signal a goal-corrected phase, such as faster activation or more pervasive processing influence.

Mikulincer et al. (2002) found that attachment figures were called to mind more quickly following a threat prime than a neutral prime, and this result held across attachment styles. Had the researchers instead asked participants to report which persons they think of first when feeling threatened, the results may well have been different. The methods used by Andersen et al. (1997) and Mikulincer et al. (2002) may be useful for discovering basic cognitive markers of adult attachment precisely because they circumvent conscious processing. These methods could also be useful for addressing questions about the organization of attachment representations and, specifically, the unresolved issue of whether they are organized hierarchically. For example, one could test whether (following a threatening prime) individuals are reliably quicker to recognize the names of some attachment figures rather than others. And for the purpose of identifying potential cognitive markers of adult attachment, one could test whether reaction times to partner names change as relationships progress.

At the Level of Emotion

As Bowlby (1979) noted, emotions are central to attachment theory for two reasons—first, because the proximal function of the attachment system is to regulate emotions and, second, because the most intense emotions are experienced within the context of attachment relationships. Emotions must therefore also be central in attachment research. But as discussed previously, emotion research typically involves inferring internal feeling states from behavioral, cognitive, and/or physiological indices. Thus attempts to identify attachment markers and processes at the level of emotion will necessarily involve other levels of analysis. As for the hypothesized phases of adult attachment formation, we suspect that the changes in emotion, and specifically in partners' regulation of each other's emotions, will be reflected in changes occurring at the levels of behavior, cognition, and/or physiology as couples progress toward clear-cut attachment and beyond. Whether attachment occurs simultaneously at all levels is yet another matter for future research.

CONCLUSION

In 1987 Hazan and Shaver published an article titled "Romantic Love Conceptualized as an Attachment Process." The idea that romantic involvement fosters the development of adult attachment bonds was taken directly from Bowlby: "In terms of subjective experience, the formation of an adult attachment bond is described as falling in love" (1979, p. 69). It takes a minimum of 6 months for infants to become fully attached to their primary caregivers, and this is within a context of near-total dependency and (in most parts of the world) almost nonstop contact. Common sense suggests that it would take at least this long, if not longer, for adult partners to become attached.

Maybe the model of infant–caregiver bonding is not applicable to adult attachment formation. If that proves to be the case, specifying what is changing and how it is changing at each level—and finding those elusive markers—would nonetheless lead to a deeper understanding of exactly what adult attachment is.

To our knowledge, the only study to date that offers clear evidence of an adult attachment marker is the one published in 2002 by Mikulincer, Gillath, and Shaver. It may be informative to think about why their approach worked. The key, we think, is that they tapped into a process very much like the one that Aron and colleagues (Aron, Aron, & Norman, 2001; Aron, Norman, Aron, & Lewandowski, 2002; see Chapter 14, this volume) have been investigating—that is, the integration of another person into the self.

In many respects attachment figures are like everyone else in our social networks. We may seek proximity to them, turn to them for comfort when stressed, and even become entrained to their physiological rhythms. What distinguishes our attachment figures from everyone else is that, in a very literal sense, they reside inside of us. Their effects on us do not require their physical presence. We carry around mental images of them that we invoke when we need comforting. We go about our daily business more confidently because we know that they are cheering us on and ready to help if needed. Our emotional reactions are tempered by anticipating their embrace or reassuring words. Our physiological homeostasis is sustained beyond immediate interactions because our physiological systems have been conditioned to them.

The overarching challenge for adult attachment researchers is to figure out how romantic partners go from being completely separate (others) to being integral parts of each other's selves. It may not be easy or straightforward, but it will surely be stimulating!

REFERENCES

Ainsworth, M. D. S. (1972). Attachment and dependency: A comparison. In J. L. Gewirtz (Ed.), *Attachment and dependency* (pp. 97–137). Washington, DC: Winston.

Ainsworth, M. D. S. (1990). Some considerations regarding theory and assessment relevant to attachments beyond infancy. In M. T. Greenberg, D. Cicchetti, & E. M. Cummings (Eds.), *Attachment in the preschool years: Theory, research, and intervention* (pp. 463–488). Chicago: University of Chicago Press.

Ainsworth, M. D. S., Blehar, M. C., Waters, E., & Wall, S. (1978). *Patterns of attachment: A psychological study of the Strange Situation.* Hillsdale, NJ: Erlbaum.

Andersen, S. M., & Berk, M. S. (1998). The social-cognitive model of transference: Experiencing past relationships in the present. *Current Directions in Psychological Science*, 7, 109–115.

Andersen, S. M., & Glassman, N. S. (1996). Responding to significant others when they are not there: Effects on interpersonal inference, motivation, and affect. In R. M. Sorrentino & E. T. Higgins (Eds.), *Handbook of motivation and cognition: Vol. 3. The interpersonal context* (pp. 262–321). New York: Guilford Press.

Andersen, S. M., Reznik, I., & Chen, S. (1997). The self in relation to others: Motivational and cognitive underpinnings. In J. G. Snodgrass & R. L. Thompson (Eds.), The self across psychology: Self-recognition, self-awareness, and the self concept. *Annals of the New York Academy of Sciences, 818*, 233–275.

Aron, A., Aron, E., & Norman, C. (2001). Self-expansion model of motivation and cognition in close relationships and beyond. In G. Fletcher & M. Clark (Eds.), *Blackwell handbook of social psychology: Interpersonal processes* (pp. 478–502). Malden, MA: Blackwell.

Aron, A., Norman, C., Aron, E., & Lewandowski, G. (2002). Shared participation in self-expanding activities: Positive effects on experienced marital quality. In P. Noller & J. Feeney (Eds.), *Understanding marriage* (pp. 177–196). Cambridge, UK: Cambridge University Press.

Bartholomew, K., & Horowitz, L. M. (1991). Attachment styles among young adults: A test of a four-category model. *Journal of Personality and Social Psychology, 61*, 226–244.

Berlin, L. G., & Cassidy, J. (1999) Relations among relationships: Contributions from attachment theory and research. In J. Cassidy & P. R. Shaver (Eds.), *Handbook of attachment: Theory, research, and clinical applications* (pp. 688–712). New York: Guilford Press.

Bowlby, J. (1982). *Attachment and loss: Vol. 1. Attachment* (2nd ed.). New York: Basic Books. (Original edition published 1969)

Bowlby, J. (1973). *Attachment and loss: Vol. 2. Separation: Anxiety and anger.* New York: Basic Books.

Bowlby, J. (1979). *The making and breaking of affectional bonds.* London: Tavistock.

Brennan, K. A., & Shaver, P. R. (1995). Dimensions of adult attachment, affect regulation, and romantic relationship functioning. *Personality and Social Psychology Bulletin, 21*, 267–283.

Burlingham, D., & Freud, A. (1944). *Young children in wartime*. London: Allen & Unwin.

Cacioppo, J. T., Klein, D. J., Berntson, G. G., & Hatfield, E. (1993).The psychophysiology of emotion. In M. Lewis & J. M. Haviland-Jones (Eds.), *Handbook of emotions* (pp. 119–142). New York: Guilford Press.

Carpenter, E. M., & Kirkpatrick, L. A. (1996). Attachment style and presence of a romantic partner as moderators of psychophysiological responses to a stressful laboratory situation. *Personal Relationships, 3*, 351–367.

Carter, C. S. (1998). Neuroendocrine perspectives on social attachment and love. *Psychoneuroendocrinology, 23*, 779–818.

Carter, C. S., Lederhendler, I. I., & Kirkpatrick, B. (Eds.). (1997). *The integrative neurobiology of affiliation*. Cambridge, MA: MIT Press.

Collins, N. L., & Read, S. J. (1990). Adult attachment, working models, and relationship quality in dating couples. *Journal of Personality and Social Psychology, 58*, 644–663.

Diamond, L. M. (2001). Contributions of psychophysiology to research on adult attachment: Review and recommendations. *Personality and Social Psychology Review, 5*, 276–295.

Feeney, B. C., & Kirkpatrick, L. A. (1996). Effects of adult attachment and presence of romantic partners on physiological responses to stress. *Journal of Personality and Social Psychology, 70*, 255–270.

Feeney, J. A. (1995). Adult attachment and emotional control. *Personal Relationships, 2*, 143–159.

Feeney, J. A. (1999). Adult romantic attachment and couple relationships. In J. Cassidy & P. R. Shaver (Eds.), *Handbook of attachment: Theory, research, and clinical applications* (pp. 355–377). New York: Guilford Press.

Fontana, A. M., Diegnan, T., Villeneuve, A., & Lepore, S. J. (1999). Nonevaluative social support reduces cardiovascular reactivity in young women during acutely stressful performance situations. *Journal of Behavioral Medicine, 22*, 75–91.

Fox, N. A., & Card, J. A. (1999). Psychophysiological measures in the study of attachment. In J. Cassidy & P. R. Shaver (Eds.), *Handbook of attachment: Theory, research, and clinical applications* (pp. 226–245). New York: Guilford Press.

Fraley, R. C., & Davis, K. E. (1997). Attachment formation and transfer in young adults' close friendships and romantic relationships. *Personal Relationships, 4*, 131–144.

Fraley, R. C., & Shaver, P. R. (1997). Adult attachment and the suppression of unwanted thoughts. *Journal of Personality and Social Psychology, 73*, 1080–1091.

Fraley, R. C., & Shaver, P. R. (1998). Airport separations: A naturalistic study of adult attachment dynamics in separating couples. *Journal of Personality and Social Psychology, 75*, 1198–1212.

Fraley, R. C., & Shaver, P. R. (2000). Adult romantic attachment: Theoretical developments, emerging controversies, and unanswered questions. *Review of General Psychology, 4*, 132–154.

Frijda, N. H., & Mesquita, B. (1998). The analysis of emotions: Dimensions of variation. In M. F. Mascolo & S. Griffin (Eds.), *What develops in emotional develop-*

ment? Emotions, personality, and psychotherapy (pp. 273–295). New York: Plenum Press.

Gump, B. B., Polk, D. E., Kamarck, T. W., & Shiffman, S. M. (2001). Partner interactions are associated with reduced blood pressure in the natural environment: Ambulatory monitoring evidence from a healthy, multiethnic adult sample. *Psychosomatic Medicine, 63*, 423–433.

Hazan, C., Gur-Yaish, N., & Campa, M. (2004). What does it mean to be attached? In W. S. Rholes & J. A. Simpson (Eds.), *Adult attachment: Theory, research, and clinical implications* (pp. 55–85). New York: Guilford Press.

Hazan, C., & Shaver, P. (1987). Romantic love conceptualized as an attachment process. *Journal of Personality and Social Psychology, 52*, 511–524.

Hazan, C., & Shaver, P. R. (1994). Attachment as an organization framework for research on close relationships. *Psychological Inquiry, 5*, 1–22.

Hazan, C., & Zeifman, D. (1994). Sex and the psychological tether. In K. Bartholomew & D. Perlman (Eds.), *Advances in personal relationships: Vol. 5. Attachment processes in adulthood* (pp. 151–177) London: Kingsley.

Hennessy, M. B. (1997). Hypothalamic–pituitary–adrenal responses to brief social separation. *Neuroscience and Biobehavioral Reviews, 21*, 11–29.

Hofer, M. A. (1984). Relationships as regulators: A psychobiologic perspective on bereavement. *Psychosomatic Medicine, 46*, 183–197.

Hofer, M. A. (1987). Early social relationships: A psychobiologist's view. *Child Development, 58*, 633–647

Hofer, M. A. (1994). Hidden regulators in attachment, separation, and loss. In N. Fox (Ed.), The development of emotion regulation: Biological and behavioral considerations. *Monographs of the Society for Research in Child Development, 59*(2–3, Serial No. 240), 192–207.

Insel, T. R. (2000). Toward a neurobiology of attachment. *Review of General Psychology, 4*, 176–185.

Kobak, R. (1999). The emotional dynamics of disruptions in attachment relationships: Implications for theory, research, and clinical intervention. In J. Cassidy & P. R. Shaver (Eds.), *Handbook of attachment: Theory, research, and clinical applications* (pp. 21–43). New York: Guilford Press.

Kraemer, G. W. (1992). A psychobiological theory of attachment. *Behavioral and Brain Sciences, 15*, 493–541.

Levy, M. B., & Davis, K. E. (1988). Lovestyles and attachment styles compared: Their relations to each other and to various relationship characteristics. *Journal of Social and Personal Relationships, 5*, 439–471.

Main, M. (1999). Epilogue. Attachment theory: Eighteen points with suggestions for future studies. In J. Cassidy & P. R. Shaver (Eds.), *Handbook of attachment: Theory, research, and clinical applications* (pp. 845–887). New York: Guilford Press.

Marvin, R. S., & Britner, P. A. (1999). Normative development: The ontogeny of attachment. In J. Cassidy & P. R. Shaver (Eds.), *Handbook of attachment: Theory, research, and clinical applications* (pp. 44–67). New York: Guilford Press.

Mason, W. A., & Mendoza, S. P. (1998). Generic aspects of primate attachments: Parents, offspring and mates. *Psychoneuroendocrinology, 23*, 765–778.

McClintock, M. K. (1971). Menstrual synchrony and suppression. *Nature, 229*, 244–245.

Mikulincer, M. (1998). Adult attachment style and individual differences in functional versus dysfunctional experiences of anger. *Journal of Personality and Social Psychology, 74*, 513–524.

Mikulincer, M., Gillath, O., & Shaver, P. R. (2002). Activation of the attachment system in adulthood: Threat-related primes increase the accessibility of mental representations of attachment figures. *Journal of Personality and Social Psychology, 83*, 881–895.

Mikulincer, M., Hirschberger, G., Nachmias, O., & Gillath, O. (2001). The affective component of the secure base schema: Affective priming with representations of attachment security. *Journal of Personality and Social Psychology, 81*, 97–115.

Moffitt, T. E., Caspi, A., Belsky, J., & Silva, P. A. (1992). Childhood experience and the onset of menarche: A test of a sociobiological model. *Child Development, 63*, 47–58.

Parkes, C. M. (1972). *Bereavement studies of grief in adult life*. New York: International Universities Press.

Pietromonaco, P. R., & Feldman Barrett, L. (2000). The internal working models concept: What do we really know about the self in relation to others? *Review of General Psychology, 4*, 155–175.

Polan, H. J., & Hofer, M. A. (1999). Psychobiological origins of infant attachment and separation responses. In J. Cassidy & P. R. Shaver (Eds.), *Handbook of attachment: Theory, research, and clinical applications* (pp. 162–180). New York: Guilford Press.

Reite, M., & Boccia, M. L. (1994). Physiological aspects of adult attachment. In M. B. Sperling & W. H. Berman (Eds.), *Attachment in adults: Clinical and developmental perspectives* (pp. 98–127). New York: Guilford Press.

Reite, M., & Capitano, J. P. (1985). On the nature of social separation and social attachment. In M. Reite & T. Field (Eds.), *The psychobiology of attachment and separation* (pp. 3–49). New York: Academic Press.

Robertson, J. (1953). *A two-year-old goes to hospital* [Film]. London: Tavistock Child Development Research Unit.

Shaver, P. R., Hazan, C., & Bradshaw, D. (1988) Love as attachment: The integration of three behavioral systems. In R. J. Sternberg & M. L. Barnes (Eds.), *The psychology of love* (pp. 68–99). New Haven, CT: Yale University Press.

Shaver, P. R., & Klinnert, M. (1982). Schachter's theories of affiliation and emotions: Implications of developmental research. In L. Wheeler (Ed.), *Review of personality and social psychology* (Vol. 3, pp. 37–71). Beverly Hills, CA: Sage.

Simpson, J. A. (1990). Influence of attachment styles on romantic relationships. *Journal of Personality and Social Psychology, 59*, 971–980.

Simpson, J. A., & Rholes, W. S. (1994). Stress and secure base relationships in adulthood. In K. Bartholomew & D. Perlman (Eds.), *Advances in personal relationships: Vol. 5. Attachment processes in adulthood* (pp. 181–204). London: Kingsley.

Simpson, J. A., & Rholes, W. S. (1998). Attachment in adulthood. In J. A. Simpson & W. S. Rholes (Eds.), *Attachment theory and close relationships* (pp. 3–21). New York: Guilford Press.

Simpson, J. A., Rholes, W. S., & Nelligan, J. S. (1992). Support seeking and support giving within couples in an anxiety-provoking situation: The role of attachment styles. *Journal of Personality and Social Psychology, 62*, 434–446.

Sroufe, L. A., & Waters, E. (1977a). Attachment as an organizational construct. *Child Development, 48*, 1184–1199.

Sroufe, L. A., & Waters, E. (1977b). Heart rate as a convergent measure in clinical and developmental research. *Merrill Palmer Quarterly, 23*, 3–27.

Suomi, S. (1999). Attachment in rhesus monkeys. In J. Cassidy & P. R. Shaver (Eds.), *Handbook of attachment: Theory, research, and clinical applications* (pp. 181–197). New York: Guilford Press.

Surbey, M. K. (1990). Family composition, stress, and the timing of human menarche. In T. E. Ziegler & F. B. Bercovitch (Eds.), *Monographs in primatology: Vol. 13. Socioendocrinology of primate reproduction* (pp. 11–32). New York: Wiley-Liss.

Trinke, S. J., & Bartholomew, K. (1997). Hierarchies of attachment relationships in young adulthood. *Journal of Social and Personality Relationships, 14*, 603–625.

Uchino, B. N., Cacioppo, J. T., & Kiecolt-Glaser, J. K. (1996). The relationship between social support and physiological processes: A review with emphasis on underlying mechanisms and implications for health. *Psychological Bulletin, 119*, 488–531.

Uvnas-Moberg, K. (1994). Oxytocin and behaviour. *Annals of Medicine, 26*, 315–317.

Uvnas-Moberg, K. (1997). Physiological and endocrine effects of social contact. *Annals of the New York Academy of Sciences, 807*, 146–163.

Uvnas-Moberg, K. (1998). Oxytocin may mediate the benefits of positive social interaction and emotions. *Psychoneuroendocrinology, 23*, 819–835.

Veith, J. L., Buck, M., Getzlaf, S., Van Dalfsen, P., & Slade, S. (1983). Exposure to men influences the occurrence of ovulation in women. *Physiology and Behavior, 31*, 313–315.

Vormbrock, J. K. (1993). Attachment theory as applied to wartime and job-related marital separation. *Psychological Bulletin, 114*, 122–144.

Weiss, R. S. (1975). *Marital separation: Coping with the end of a marriage and the transition to being single again.* New York: Basic Books.

Zeifman, D., & Hazan, C. (1997). A process model of adult attachment formation. In S. Duck (Ed.), *Handbook of personal relationships* (2nd ed., pp. 179–195). Chichester, UK: Wiley.

4

The Evolution of Attachment in Romantic Relationships

CLAUDIA CHLOE BRUMBAUGH
and R. CHRIS FRALEY

In their landmark paper, Hazan and Shaver (1987) argued that romantic love is an attachment process—one involving the same motivational system (i.e., *the attachment behavioral system*) that gives rise to the bond that develops between infants and their primary caregivers. Over the past two decades, an extraordinary amount of research has been conducted on the role that the attachment system plays in the development, maintenance, and dissolution of romantic relationships (see Feeney, 1999; Hazan & Zeifman, 1999). Despite the empirical advances that have been made, a fundamental question remains: Why does the attachment system play *any* role in adult romantic relationships?

This question is particularly puzzling because, although most mammalian species exhibit some form of attachment in infancy, humans are one of the few that exhibit attachment in their romantic relationships. For example, bonobo chimpanzees do not forge close, emotional bonds with one another despite the fact that they share over 98% of their genes with humans (de Waal & Lanting, 1997; Sibley & Ahlquist, 1984). The fact that our relational behavior differs so much from that of our primate kin suggests that understanding why attachment exists in adult relationships is important not only for advancing adult attachment theory but also for better appreciating the place of love in the natural world.

In this chapter, we review several hypotheses concerning the evolution of love that have been discussed in the literature on attachment and close relationships and evaluate those hypotheses in light of comparative data on primates and within-species data on humans. It is critical that we present two qualifications and clarifications from the outset. First, throughout this chapter, we use the terms "adult attachment," "pair-bonds," and "love" interchangeably. We wish to state explicitly, however, that "romantic love" is a complex emotional state that reflects much more than the attachment that exists between two people (Bersheid, Chapter 16, this volume; Kirkpatrick, 1998). For example, the early stages of romantic love often involve lust, mutual fascination, and an idealization of one's partner—experiences that likely serve to bring two individuals together for just enough time to enable a viable sexual union. We believe, however, that the passionate aspects of love are driven by a different motivational system than the one that gives rise to feelings of attachment, companionship, and security (Diamond, 2003; Shaver, Hazan, & Bradshaw, 1988). Although we believe that sexual desire plays a critical role in romantic love, the evolutionary story behind desire, as rich and fascinating as it is, appears to be relatively straightforward (see Buss, 1994). What is not well understood from an evolutionary perspective is why two individuals would continue to feel emotionally bound to one another once they have reproduced successfully.

Second, we note that the concept of "attachment" is relatively nuanced and involves a number of distinctions that are not made in the literature we review. For most of our review we operationalize attachment relationships as *socially monogamous* ones—relationships that are characterized by mates' maintenance of proximity to one another and distress over physical separation. This conceptualization captures some of the key features of attachment relationships discussed by Bowlby (1969), such as proximity seeking and separation distress. However, it omits some key features, such as the use of the other as a safe haven in times of threat and the use of the other as a secure base from which to explore the world. Because these latter two features have rarely been considered in research on animal behavior, we focus on the first two as a workable, if limited, analogue to adult attachment.

In this chapter we explore the possible functions that romantic attachment may serve and, importantly, provide new empirical evidence that helps to elucidate the conditions under which attachment may have evolved, both within humans and in other species. We organize our discussion around three hypotheses concerning the evolution of love: the paternal-care hypothesis, the developmental-immaturity or neoteny hypothesis, and the concealed-ovulation hypothesis. Although scholars have debated the merits of these hypotheses for several decades, there are few signs that any progress has been made toward evaluating them. One reason for the lack of progress is that there are many challenges involved in trying to answer evolutionary questions. The study of evolution is a historical enterprise, and, as such, much of the data needed to evaluate evolutionary hypotheses are unavailable. Despite such challenges, we argue that the primary reason little progress has been made toward understanding the evolution of love is that existing data have rarely been used to evaluate evolutionary hypotheses *systematically.* Instead, evolutionary hypotheses tend to be treated as claims to be defended in a court of law. Hypotheses are often stated emphatically and, instead of being systematically evaluated, are buttressed only with evidence that is consistent with them.

In this chapter we seek to advance the discussion by evaluating each of these evolutionary hypotheses using data drawn from multiple species—species that, a priori, may or may not behave in ways that are consistent with theoretical expectations. We also focus on some of the factors that might give rise to variation in the experience of attachment within humans. We hope that this dual approach (i.e., one that focuses on both across- and within-species variations in attachment) will serve as a useful first step toward answering what we consider to be some of the most challenging questions in the field: Why does attachment exist in adult relationships? What functions does it serve? And how did attachment evolve over the course of evolutionary history? We begin with a brief overview of the role of attachment in infant–caregiver relationships.

THE FUNCTION OF ATTACHMENT BEHAVIOR

One of Bowlby's goals was to explain the nature of the bond that develops between children and their caregivers (Bowlby, 1969). Bowlby and his colleagues noticed that children who had been separated from their parents frequently expressed intense distress, often vigorously trying to regain their missing caregivers by crying, clinging, and searching (Bowlby, Robertson, & Rosenbluth, 1952; Heinicke & Westheimer, 1966). Bowlby (1969) argued that these *attachment behaviors* were regulated by an innate motivational system, the *attachment behavioral system.* According to Bowlby, the dynamics of the attachment system are similar to those of a homeostatic control system in which a goal state is maintained by the constant monitoring of endogenous or exogenous signals and continuous behavioral adjustment. In the case of the attachment system, the goal state is a sense of security that derives from the perceived availability of the primary attachment object. Striving for physical closeness, or *proximity seeking*, is one key feature of an attachment relationship. When the child appraises the caregiver as being nearby and responsive, he or she feels secure and, as a result, is likely to be playful and sociable. In this situation, the child is able to use the caregiver as a *secure base* from which he or she can freely explore. When the child senses a threat to the relationship, he or she experiences *separation distress* and attempts to use the attachment object as a *safe haven* (i.e., a source of security and comfort). According to Bowlby (1969), these emotional and behavioral dynamics serve an important evolutionary function. Specifically, they encourage proximity between child and caregiver that, in turn, helps to ensure the child's safety and protection and, ultimately, his or her inclusive fitness.

Although Bowlby (1969, 1980) was primarily interested in understanding the nature of the infant–caregiver relationship, he believed that attachment played a vital role in other kinds of intimate relationships across the life course. Nonetheless, it was not until 1987 that researchers began to systematically explore the possibility that attachment plays a critical role in the dynamics of romantic relationships (Hazan & Shaver, 1987). Based on their observations, Hazan and Shaver (1987) argued that romantic love is an attachment process. They observed, for example, that romantic love involves many of the same behavioral patterns that characterize the bond between infants and their caregivers. They noted that adults, like infants, feel safe and secure when the other person is present and distressed or restless in the absence of the other.

Even though the attachment behavioral system appears to be partly responsible for the feelings people experience as romantic love (see Hazan & Zeifman, 1999), it is unclear *why* the attachment system should be active in adult relationships. The existence of attachment in human romantic relationships raises a number of theoretical questions because adult attachment is a relatively rare phenomenon in mammalian species. Many animals are able to get by adequately without forming deep, emotional connections to their mates. It is noteworthy that the relational behavior of bonobo chimpanzees, our closest evolutionary relatives, is similar to ours in many respects. Bonobos display obvious signs of affection, such as holding one another and kissing. Moreover, during intercourse, which is often *ventro-ventral* (i.e., the so-called missionary position), bonobos often gaze into one another's eyes. Despite the similarities between bonobos and humans, bonobos do not exhibit long-term pair-bonds. Their affection is relatively short-lived, and they readily participate in sexual contact with multiple partners of both sexes without exhibiting strong signs of mate guarding, jealously, or exclusivity.

HYPOTHESES ABOUT THE EVOLUTION OF LOVE

The striking differences in the romantic behavior of humans and that of our closest evolutionary relatives raises the question of why the attachment system continues to play a role in human relationships but not in those of species closely related to us. In this section we review three hypotheses that have been proposed to explain the evolution of attachment in romantic relationships. Although these hypotheses are often discussed independently of one another in the literature, they are not mutually exclusive, and each hypothesis has the potential to inform our understanding of the evolution of love.

The Paternal-Care Hypothesis

> Our early ancestors acquired tendencies to form an emotional bond between a male and one or more females because the end result was to provide nurture and protection for several years for their exceptionally helpless young. (Mellen, 1981, p. 139)

Most discussions of the function of attachment center on the possibility that attachment enabled fathers to play a greater role in caregiving—care that would have been essential given that humans are born without the capacity to feed, protect, or defend themselves. According to the *paternal-care hypothesis*, the bond that develops between mates may enhance inclusive fitness by supplying an additional source of protection and care for infants (Belsky, 1999; Fraley & Shaver, 2000; Gubernick, 1994; Hazan & Zeifman, 1999; Mellen, 1981). In support of this hypothesis, within-species evidence indicates that offspring have a higher likelihood of surviving to adulthood if they are reared in a family unit in which the mother and father are pair-bonded. The contributions of males to promoting the survival of their young are sometimes indirect and minimal (e.g., guarding territory against predators). This nominal kind of caregiving assistance may be a simple consequence of mating effort—an effect of males' attempts to win over females as a means of gaining further sexual access—rather than a purposeful act to help one's offspring (Seyfarth, 1978; Smuts & Gubernick, 1992). On the other hand, males can be quite direct and invested in caregiving efforts by actively playing with young, providing resources, or carrying young. In any case, in humans, support from a spouse has been found to have a positive association with birthweight and infant survival rates (Collins, Dunkel-Schetter, Lobel, & Scrimshaw, 1993). Thus any additional help the father can provide may contribute to his offspring's fitness by helping to distribute the burden of child care across two parents instead of one.

In addition to providing care, bonded males may also provide defense from unrelated males who pose a danger to their offspring (van Schaik & Janson, 2000). This is critical because examples of infanticide and child abuse committed by nonpaternal males are prevalent in many mammal species, including nonhuman primates (Hiraiwa-Hasegawa & Hasegawa, 1994), lions (Pusey & Packer, 1994), and humans (Daly & Wilson, 1994). In fact, some writers have postulated that monogamous mating systems evolved in some species as an infanticide prevention strategy (van Schaik & Kappeler, 1997). It is believed that killing another male's offspring can be a beneficial reproductive strategy for an intruding male because it hastens the females' sexual receptivity and heightens the chance that the intruder can then sire his own children with her (Sommer, 1994). Incidents of males killing their own offspring are very low. For instance, infant victims are only directly related to their killers 5% of the time or less (Sommer, 1994). This suggests that infanticide is a strategic or selective tactic used to increase reproductive success.

Heightened violence toward genetically unrelated children has been documented in humans as well. Even when controlling for other risk factors (e.g., low socioeconomic status, maternal age), children living in two-parent homes with a stepfather are 40 times more at risk for abuse than children in two-parent homes with both biological parents (Daly & Wilson, 1985). Furthermore, men appear to refrain from hurting their own children while simultaneously abusing stepchildren who live in the same household (Daly & Wilson, 1985). Mothers also treat their children differently depending on whether the father is present or absent. For instance, the absence of the father sometimes leads mothers to lose interest in their children at an earlier age and corresponds to increases in observed child mortality rates (Draper & Harpending, 1988).

Divorce patterns also support the idea that the pair-bond between parents exists to facilitate child rearing throughout a child's vulnerable years. Fisher (1992) found that, on average, divorce rates tend to peak 4 years into marriage. Based on these data, Fisher developed an evolutionary account of why divorce often occurs when it does. Because human infants are most vulnerable in infancy (i.e., before the age of 4), the need for both parents' presence and protection is reduced after this stage. In sum, if infants have a lower chance of survival without the care and defense of both parents, selection pressures may have facilitated pair-bonding between the mates, a process that would enable a greater degree of paternal investment.

The Neoteny Hypothesis

Another possible explanation for the existence of pair-bonds in humans is the *neoteny* or *developmental-immaturity hypothesis* (Fraley & Shaver, 2000). The neoteny hypothesis is rooted in the idea that changes in the timing of developmental processes (i.e., heterochrony) are one of the major mechanisms of evolution (deBeer, 1958). It is generally held that the timing of physical development has been delayed in humans due to our ever-evolving and complex brain, which eventually became too large to fit through the birth canal (Fisher, 1992). In fact, our brains are thought to have tripled in size within the last 3 million years (Coppens, 1994). To facilitate the growth of the human brain, it was necessary for human babies to enter the world in an immature state and spend a large portion of time developing outside the womb.

One consequence of this shift in developmental timing is that humans are much more developmentally neotenous (i.e., child-like) than other primates. Compared to other primates, we remain relatively hairless, our teeth erupt at a late age, and our sexual maturation is delayed—taking twice as long as that of chimpanzees (Montagu, 1989; Poirier & Smith, 1974). Moreover, our internal systems, including the liver, kidneys, and immune system, also take a substantially longer time to become fully functional than they do in other mammals (Fisher, 1992). According to the neoteny hypothesis (Fraley & Shaver, 2000), the existence of attachment in human adults is another example of our delayed maturation. Specifically, although the attachment system is normally "turned off" in other mammals as they mature, the fact that developmental timing is broadly delayed in humans suggests that the attachment system may continue to be sensitive—even in adulthood—to certain signals and readily activated in contexts that resemble the infant–parent relationship (e.g., caring, safe, or physically intimate interactions).

It is important to note that neoteny is thought to be relevant for explaining a variety of psychological and behavioral traits in humans—not just adult attachment. For example, Bjorklund (1997) has observed that although adult play is common to many mammalian species, it tends to be limited to courtship contexts in nonhumans. Only in humans, he argues, is adult play manifested in such a diverse range of contexts. According to Bjorklund (1997), the extended period of human development enables children to learn more about their world and improve their skills in coping with environmental changes and, more broadly, enables greater behavioral flexibility.

The Concealed-Ovulation Hypothesis

In many primate species, it is obvious when females are in estrus (i.e., when they are ovulating). For example, female baboons exhibit prominent sexual swellings that advertise their receptiveness to males (Jolly, 1972). According to the *concealed-ovulation hypothesis*, the shift from outward signs of estrus to concealed ovulation played a substantial role in the development of monogamy in humans (Alexander & Noonan, 1979; Strassman, 1981; Turke, 1984). According to this view, the outward signs of fertility that were present in our primate ancestors (e.g., odor changes, sexual swellings) were lost, while female buttocks, hips, and breasts increased in size to mimic sexual receptivity (Margulis & Sagan, 1991; Szalay & Costello, 1991). Because males were unable to determine whether or not females were ovulating, they were compelled to engage in constant mate guarding to ensure paternity certainty, and their constant presence consequently facilitated the development of a pair-bond. Theoretically, the shift to pair-bonding might have amounted to a win–win situation for both sexes. Females benefited by receiving more support, protection, and other resources from males. Meanwhile, males benefited by ensuring paternity certainty.

Although the role of concealed ovulation in the development of monogamy has been discussed by many writers (see Sillén-Tullberg & Møller, 1991), some scholars have cast doubt on the hypothesis (Hrdy, 1988). An important implication of the concealed-ovulation hypothesis is that hidden ovulation not only makes it more difficult for a male to know when a female is ovulating but also theoretically enables men and women to mate freely throughout the cycle. However, Hrdy (1988) has pointed out that many female primates can make adjustments to the times at which they are receptive regardless of whether they exhibit concealed ovulation. Under some circumstances, female primates may engage in sex during times of non-estrus as a means of gaining support or resources when those resources are scarce. For example, Parish (1994) observed that bonobos participated in sexual contacts to a greater degree when food was limited, suggesting that bonobos, who are generally sexually promiscuous, sometimes use sex to obtain access to limited resources.

Sillén-Tullberg and Møller (1991) conducted an important study on the relationship between monogamy and concealed ovulation in a broad sample of primate species. They found that concealed ovulation may have promoted monogamy. It should be noted that monogamy was explicitly defined in their study as a *sexually monogamous* (i.e., a sexually exclusive) mating system. Sexual monogamy is a good proxy for pair-bonding, but it is important theoretically to separate the social organization of mateships from the nature of the bond that might exist between mates. In some of the data, reported in a subsequent section, we reexamine the concealed-ovulation hypothesis by explicitly focusing on adult attachment rather than sexual monogamy.

A COMPARATIVE ANALYSIS OF ADULT ATTACHMENT

At face value, each of the hypotheses we have reviewed seems plausible. For example, it is difficult to imagine an evolutionary reality in which concealed ovulation did not play some role in the mating behavior of animals. Nonetheless, these hypotheses have been difficult to evaluate for two reasons. First, as can be inferred from our brief review of the literature, much of the research conducted on these issues has focused on a highly selective sampling of information about a single species (e.g., humans) or comparisons among only a handful of species. In fact, beyond questions regarding the evolution of love, most research in comparative psychology has focused only on comparisons between two species (see Garland & Adolph, 1994, for a discussion of the limitations of this approach). These comparisons are limited from an evolutionary perspective because, at the species level, the effective *n* is only 2.

Beyond this limitation, most scholarly discussions of these hypotheses have adopted a format more common to the humanities than the natural sciences. The classic approach to scholarship in the humanities is to begin with a thesis (e.g., the neotenous characteristics of humans are one reason why people exhibit attachment in their adult romantic relationships) and marshal evidence that supports the thesis. Unfortunately, this approach is bound to "work" even if the thesis is incorrect. To see how this might be the case, consider Figure 4.1. Let us assume that there is no relationship between pair bonding and paternal care. If there is no association between these variables, the proportion of species exhibiting pair-bonding that also have paternal care will be equal to the proportion of species that exhibit pair-bonding but that do not have paternal care. Notice that, even if no association exists between these variables, there will still be plenty of examples of species that are pair-bonders and that show paternal care ($n = 10$), as well as species that exhibit neither pair-bonding nor paternal care ($n = 40$). The fact that it is possible to identify species (such as humans) that show both pair-bonding and paternal care does not imply that these two traits are functionally related.

A more systematic way to examine hypotheses concerning the functions of adult attachment would be to quantify the variables in question (i.e., pair-bonding, paternal care, developmental immaturity, concealed ovulation) and study their covariation across *multiple* species (i.e., species that, a priori, may or may not exhibit patterns consistent with these hypotheses). Doing so would overcome the limitations of small sample sizes in compara-

Paternal care	Pair bonded: No	Pair bonded: Yes
No	Consistent 40	Inconsistent 10
Yes	Inconsistent 40	Consistent 10

FIGURE 4.1. An illustration of the availability of data that seemingly confirm a hypothesis (shaded cells) despite the fact that the overall pattern is inconsistent with that hypothesis.

tive research while also helping to ensure that the species under investigation are not selected in a manner biased toward one or another conclusion. In the next section we report findings from a series of comparative studies undertaken to explore the evolution of attachment in romantic relationships.

The Functions of Love

In previous research, we addressed the paternal care and neoteny hypotheses in a broad sample of mammals and primates (see Fraley, Brumbaugh, & Marks, 2005). Specifically, we drew two large samples of species, one of mammals and the other of primates, and, using comparative methods, quantified several morphological, social, and developmental variables relevant to these species. Our objective was to determine how these various factors were related to one another across species and, more important, to determine which characteristics were associated with pair-bonding. If pair-bonding facilitates the care and protection of offspring, there should be a positive correlation across species between pair-bonding and paternal involvement in child rearing. We classified species as exhibiting paternal care if the father was involved in any aspect of rearing the offspring after birth, such as providing food for offspring, building a nest or den, protecting the young, and providing food for the mate while she tends to the young. In addition, if neoteny is one of the factors that leads to attachment in adult relationships, there should be a positive correlation between pair-bonding and developmental immaturity as quantified, for example, by the proportion of the lifespan spent in the family of origin or gestation time. In this chapter we summarize some of our findings from the primate sample we reported in Study 2 of Fraley et al. (2005). However, we supplement those data with additional, more recent data relevant to the concealed-ovulation hypothesis.

In Study 2 of Fraley et al. (2005), we collected data on 66 anthropoid primate species that had been studied previously by Sillén-Tullberg and Møller (1991). For each species, we recorded whether it exhibited *social monogamy*—an indicator of adult attachment. Animals are typically classified as being socially monogamous if mates spend a great deal of time together (i.e., engage in proximity seeking), if there are signs of mate guarding, if mates engage in extensive physical contact, and if there are signs of separation distress (see Carter, DeVries, & Getz, 1995, for example). As previously discussed, these features are central to the definition of adult attachment in the social psychological literature on close relationships (see Fraley & Davis, 1997; Hazan & Zeifman, 1999). We also recorded developmental information about the species, such as average gestation time, age of puberty, the number of offspring or litter size, and the average lifespan. Consistent with the paternal-care hypothesis, we found that paternal care was most prevalent among pair-bonded primates (*r* = .22). We also found that primate species that were more neotenous were more likely to exhibit pair-bonding. For example, primate species exhibiting pair-bonding were more likely to have longer lifespans (*r* = .16), longer gestation times (*r* = .21), take longer to leave the home or nest (*r* = .51), and reach puberty at a later age (*r* = .11). The correlation between pair-bonding and a composite of these neoteny variables was .20.

To examine the concealed-ovulation hypothesis, we used data on the expression of sexual swellings published by Sillén-Tullberg and Møller (1991) and compared them with our classifications of whether primates were pair-bonded or not. The correlation between pair-bonding and the expression of sexual swellings was negative (*r* = –.39). Primate species that were pair-bonded were less likely to exhibit sexual swellings than species that did not exhibit pair-bonding.

In summary, these data are compatible with each of the three hypotheses regarding the evolution of love. We should note, however, that the correlation across species between neoteny and paternal care was .19. This is compatible with the position that the immaturity of offspring may be a factor that leads to the development of paternal care. Moreover, the correlation between concealed ovulation and paternal care was .10, raising the possibility that the development of concealed ovulation in species may have led to a heightened degree of paternal investment in offspring.

The Evolution of Love

The comparative data reviewed thus far help to clarify the potential evolutionary functions of adult attachment. Nonetheless, they do not address evolution per se. One way to address the function of attachment is to use phylogenetic analyses to reconstruct the evolutionary development of these distinct traits. The objective of a phylogenetic analysis is to reconstruct the evolution of a trait through historical time. To do so, evolutionary biologists often rely on the principle of parsimony (see Felsenstein, 2003). Specifically, an attempt is made to identify a pattern of trait evolution that minimizes the number of times a trait independently evolved (i.e., evolved in a manner that leads to divergence from a most recent ancestor). For example, if one were trying to explain the distribution of the trait illustrated in Figure 4.2, the reconstruction shown in the left-hand panel would be considered the most likely because it involves fewer instances of evolutionary change (one change, between ancestral nodes I and H) than the reconstruction shown in the right-hand panel (four changes). In the present research, we reconstructed the evolution of adult attachment using the MacClade software package (Version 4.06; Maddison & Maddison, 2001), a tool for phylogenetic analysis that allows one to explore evolutionary hypotheses and reconstruct phylogenies based on different characters of interest. The

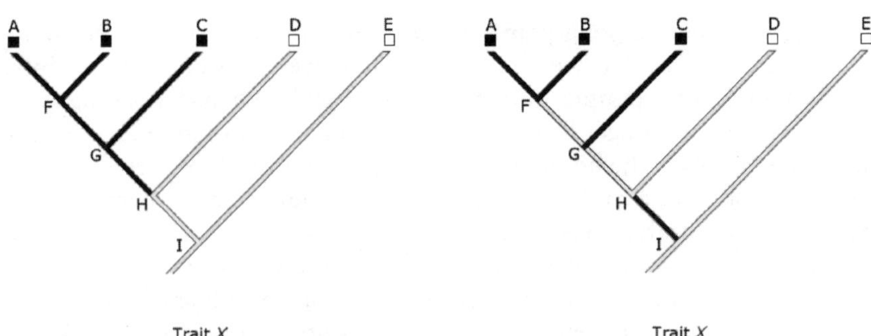

FIGURE 4.2. Examples of different evolutionary reconstructions of a trait. The reconstruction on the left is considered more parsimonious because it requires only one evolutionary change to explain the distribution of the trait among living species. The reconstruction on the right is considered less parsimonious because it requires four changes to explain the same distribution of trait values.

results are illustrated in Figure 4.3. (For more detail concerning phylogenetic methods, see Fraley et al., 2005.)

As can be seen, pair-bonding is relatively rare in primates, being present in only 19% of species studied. Thus adult attachment is exceptional, even among humans' closest relatives. It is also noteworthy that pair-bonding

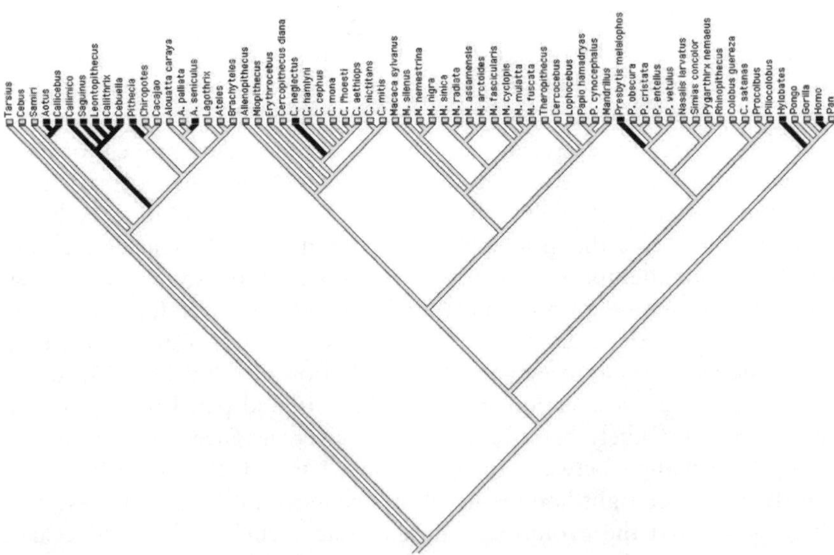

FIGURE 4.3. Reconstructions of the evolution of adult attachment across a sample of anthropoid primates. Dark branches represent the presence of adult attachment.

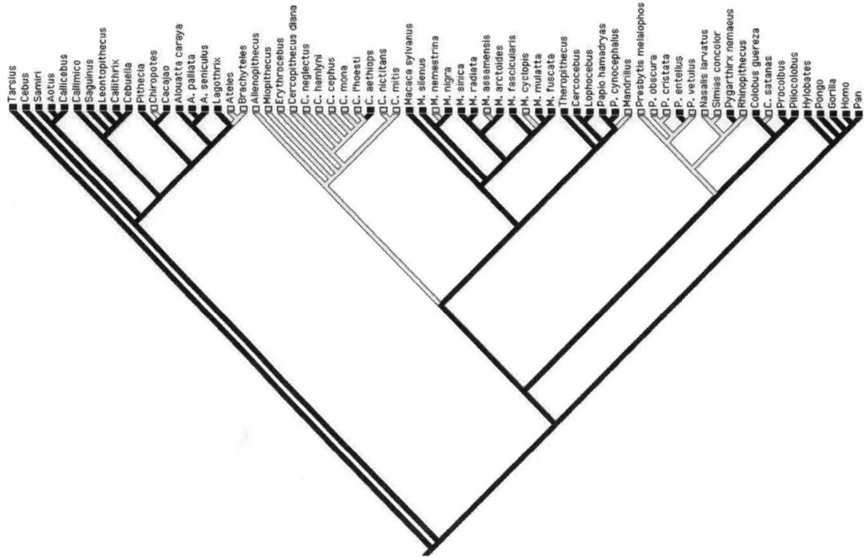

FIGURE 4.4. Reconstructions of the evolution of paternal care across a sample of anthropoid primates. Dark branches represent the presence of paternal care.

is a relatively recent "invention" in the evolutionary landscape of primates. In other words, there are few places along the evolutionary tree where pair-bonding reaches deeply into the past. This pattern suggests that pair-bonding may have evolved largely independently in different primate lineages. In other words, it does not appear to function as a *homologous* trait—one that is common to species because it was present in the ancestor shared by those species. Instead, pair-bonding may have arisen on independent occasions due to similar selection pressures acting on different primate species.

Figures 4.4, 4.5, and 4.6 illustrate the evolutionary reconstructions for paternal care, neoteny, and ovulatory signals, respectively. It is noteworthy that paternal care appears to have earlier evolutionary origins than pair-bonding, which suggests that, if there is a causal relationship between pair-bonding and paternal care, it is more likely that pair-bonding emerged following the evolution of paternal care rather than the other way around. A similar pattern exists for neoteny and the display of ovulatory signals. It is also of interest that, although there is considerable variation in the neotenous qualities across primates, the branch containing humans and our closest relatives appears to be the most neotenous. In other words, although humans are the most neotenous species in the sample, our neotenous qualities are shared with other closely related species.

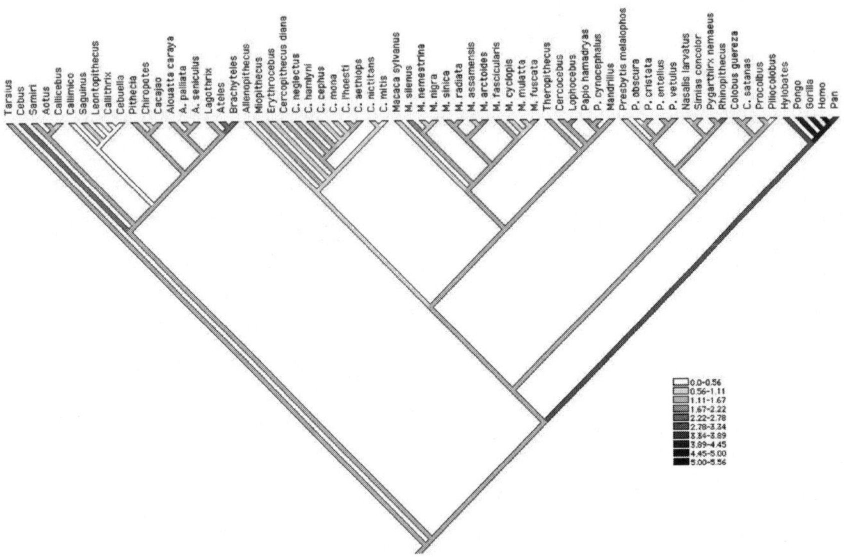

FIGURE 4.5. Reconstructions of the evolution of neoteny across a sample of anthropoid primates. Darker branches represent greater neoteny, according to an aggregated measure of lifespan, gestation time, time at which children leave the family of origin, and age of menarche.

One of the valuable aspects of reconstructing the evolution of traits is that those reconstructions allow one to determine whether the traits evolved together in a functional way. If two traits are functionally related, then not only should those traits covary across species but the evolutionary changes in one trait should also be mirrored in the other. It is necessary to evaluate this assumption carefully, because it is possible for two traits to covary across species even if they have no functional relationship. For example, covariation between traits may exist simply because species that possessed both traits descended from a common ancestor that also possessed those traits (i.e., correlation due to homology). To provide a more rigorous evaluation of the paternal care and neoteny hypotheses, we computed phylogenetically independent contrasts—contrasts that essentially "control" for the phylogenetic relationships among species, allowing hypotheses about homologous versus functional associations to be examined (see Felsenstein, 2003). After controlling for genetic relatedness, we found that pair-bonding may have coevolved with paternal care. On the other hand, the association between pair-bonding and neoteny does not seem to be a functional one, but instead likely stems from common ancestry (see Fraley et al., 2005, for more information).

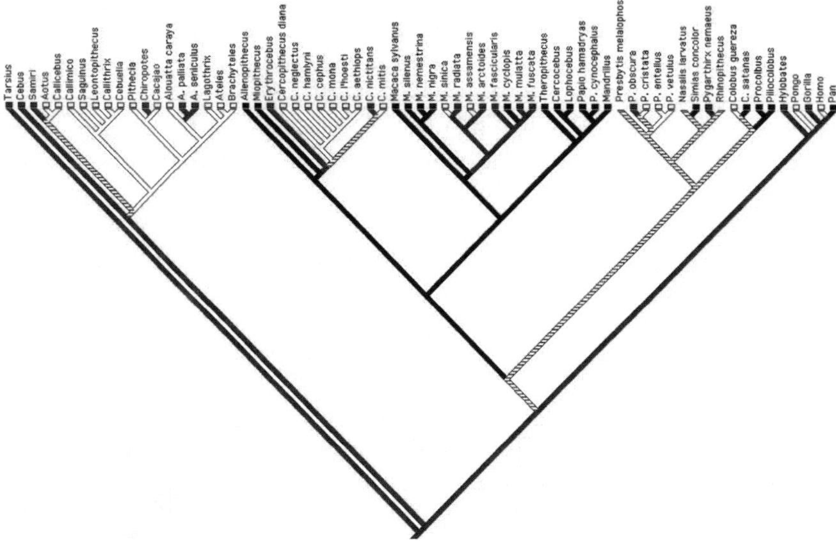

FIGURE 4.6. Reconstructions of the evolution of the visibility of ovulatory signals across a sample of anthropoid primates. Darker branches represent more visible sexual swellings. Hatched branches represent equivocal reconstructions (i.e., branches that could assume two or more values on the basis of the parsimony criterion). Data based on those reported by Sillén-Tullberg & Møller (1991).

WITHIN-SPECIES VARIATION IN HUMAN MATING SYSTEMS

The comparative data presented thus far are based on between-species comparisons. We believe these data are important for understanding the broader context in which love may have evolved. Nonetheless, there is much to be learned by considering evolutionary issues within the human branch of the evolutionary tree. In the sections that follow, we discuss cultural variation in human mating patterns and some of the factors that shape this diversity. We first describe the numerous forms that human mating strategies assume, then we consider some possible contextual influences on human mating, and finally we review implications of the three hypotheses regarding within-human variability in mating.

We begin by noting that discussing variability in attachment raises a thorny theoretical issue. According to Bowlby's attachment theory (Bowlby, 1969) and subsequent extensions of the theory into the realm of adult romantic relationships (e.g., Hazan & Shaver, 1987), the attachment system is a normative one—a system that is present and active in all humans. Nonetheless, just as not all primates exhibit attachments to their mates, neither do all humans. From an attachment-theoretical perspective, this observation does not necessarily imply that the attachment system is inactive in such individuals. It is possible, for example, that the attachment bond has yet to form in such cases. Hazan and her colleagues suggest that romantic relationships of less than 2 years' duration rarely function as attachment relationships (Hazan, Gur-Yaish, & Campa, 2004). Moreover, some individuals, despite being in a romantic relationship for an extended period of time, may engage in a variety of defensive maneuvers that prevent them from establishing a deep emotional connection with their partner. For example, Fraley and Davis (1997) and Fraley and Shaver (1997) found that highly dismissing adults were less likely to rely on their romantic partners as attachment figures.

The important point here is that, even though there is variation in the extent to which humans "attach" to their mates, this variation does not imply that the presence of the attachment system itself is variable in humans. It does suggest, however, that the extent to which attachment is manifested in a relationship can vary across people or cultures. The fact that such variation exists suggests that much can be learned about the function of attachment by studying variation in the manifestation of attachment within humans.

Variability in Human Mating Systems

Because it is unusual for cultural anthropologists to discuss "attachment" per se, in the following sections we focus on variation in human *mating systems*—the social organization of marriages or mateships—as an indicator of variation in attachment. Specifically, we consider *monogamous* mating systems—marriages in which two people are legally bound together—as a proxy for adult attachment. This should not be taken to imply that all marriages in a monogamous mating system constitute attachments, but we suspect that they are more likely to be attachments than the marriages that characterize other kinds of mating systems.[1]

Although monogamous relationships are accepted in the majority of human societies, there are a variety of other *polygamous* mating systems (i.e., marriages involving more than two people) that exist as well. One kind of polygamous system is that of *polygyny*—a marriage of more than one woman to one man. Another kind is *polyandry*, in which more than one man is married to one woman. Some mating systems are *polygynandrous*—a group marriage of mixed sexes. Murdock's *Ethnographic Atlas* (1967) indicates that only 16% of the world's societies recognize monogamy exclusively. Moreover, although the majority (over 83%; see Murdock, 1967) of cultures *allow* polygamous relationships, these relationships are not necessarily practiced. Polygyny was practiced openly in the United States between 1852 and 1890, though it occurred primarily within the Mormon population in Utah (Smith & Kunz, 1976). The least common form of polygamy, polyandry, is permitted in only 0.5% of cultures worldwide (Murdock, 1967).

What Kinds of Factors Influence the Type of Mating System a Society Adopts?

The diversity of human mating systems raises the question of why a society would be more likely to adopt one kind of strategy rather than another. In this section, we review evidence suggesting that a number of factors play a role in shaping the organization of human mating systems, including values and religion, economics, and the distribution of food and other resources.

Values and Religion

The cultural values held during specific periods in history can have a sizable influence on romantic relationships. For instance, in the late 19th century, the Victorian era's sexually repressive principles vehemently enforced sexual morality and moderation in sexual activity (Pivar, 1973). Many cultural values are sanctioned by the dominant religious institutions in a society. The influence of religion on the social organization of mating is well illustrated by the finding that, in a sample of Ghanaian women, 43% of Muslims practiced polygyny, whereas only 25% of Catholics and 24% of Protestants were involved in a polygynous marriage (Klomegah, 1997). Moreover, religious systems influence whether or not people marry, divorce, and have extramarital affairs. For example, in a recent meta-analysis, Mahoney, Pargament, Tarakeshwar, and Swank (2001) found that 62% of nonreligious individuals were divorced at least once compared with 49% of those who were religiously affiliated. Furthermore, Cochran, Chamlin, Beeghley, and Fenwick (2004) report that membership in a Protestant denomination is strongly and inversely related to engaging in extramarital affairs. In summary, belief systems and societal norms play a substantial role in determining the forms that relationships between sexual partners assume.

For Love or Money?

In addition to ideology, resource distribution is another driving force in the variation in human mating systems. Polygamy is strongly driven by conditions in which men control a large share of resources relative to women, thus allowing them to support numerous dependent brides. Ohadike (1968), for example, found that women who married polygynously had less formal education, a lower quality of residence, and less prestigious occupations than women who did not. Klomegah (1997) also noted a negative relationship between education and polygyny, implying that financially dependent women are more likely to enter polygynous mating structures.

In a study of human economics and marriage trends in East African families, Borgerhoff Mulder, George-Cramer, Eshleman, and Ortolani (2001) pointed out the importance of *bridewealth* (i.e., payments of cash or livestock made by the groom or groom's father to the bride's relatives on engagement). Borgerhoff Mulder and her colleagues (2001) found that higher levels of bridewealth were negatively related to divorce rates and that variation in bridewealth payments was a function of the supply-and-demand ratio of marriageable women. Furthermore, differences in women's "value," whether defined with respect to fertility or labor investment, drove the size of bridewealth payments and, consequently, the later likelihood of divorce.

Nourishment before Nurturance

In addition to values and economics, natural ecological conditions, such as the ratio of the sexes, geography, and food availability can also affect romantic relationships. Farming practices and the distribution of food are thought to have especially important influences on mating practices. For instance, subsistence farming requires dedication to the land that one harvests and entails a lack of mobility that limits access to the number of mates one can obtain. Under these conditions, there appears to be a higher incidence of monogamy than polygamy (Fisher, 1992; Miller, 1998).

The role of "home range" and food availability has also been demonstrated in nonhuman primates. For example, monogamy has been found to occur most frequently in primate species in which females are solitary and roam in a small geographic area, thus allowing them to be easily monopolized and guarded by just one male (Komers & Brotherton, 1997). Furthermore, in some primates, the availability of food often determines the distribution of females, which in turn affects the distribution of males. When females search for food independently, monogamy is likely to result; however, when females look for food in groups, polygyny is more likely (Miller, 1998). Food shortages can also result in shifts in sexual behavior. Evidence of this process comes from research on the sexually coercive practices of our close relative, the bonobo chimpanzee. Parish (1994) found that bonobos increased sexual contacts when food was limited, suggesting, as mentioned earlier, that bonobos use sex to obtain access to valued resources.

When Polygamy Turns into Monogamy and Vice Versa

The fact that mating systems are influenced by such a diverse array of factors implies that they are fairly fluid and dynamic entities, which can be ambiguous at times and easily changed at others. Because feelings of love or favoritism toward one individual can destroy the defined structure of polygamous marriages, there may be an inborn tendency for people to form attachments to specific others. For example, jealousy is often an issue within polygynous marriages, particularly when older wives envy newer, younger wives who receive more attention and whose children may receive more care from the father (Elbedour, Onwuegbuzie, Caridine, & Abu-Saad, 2002). Feelings of jealousy may arise if wives perceive that their husband is spending more leisure time with another wife (Hassouneh-Phillips, 2001). Al-Krenawi and Graham (1999) found that, in a case study of one particular polygynous marriage, arguments frequently occurred due to jealousy and favoritism. Al-Krenawi and Graham (1999) also reported that each wife in this marriage believed that, deep down, the husband loved her and not the others. Sleeping arrangements also caused strife in this marriage: Women felt disgraced when their husband was intimate with another wife. The extent of hostility between wives is well illustrated by the prevalence of physical aggression between women in polygynous marriages. Obukwe (2002) found that disagreements among women in polygynous marriages in Nigeria were the most frequently cited cause for human bites to the face.

Even when there is not just one partner to be shared among many mates, feelings of love and jealousy tend to arise. For example, in the polygynandrous Kerista commune, which existed from 1971 to 1991 in San Francisco, California, there were occasional incidents in which attachment-like feelings emerged, despite the fact that members practiced what they called "polyfidelity"—fidelity to numerous partners at once. According to a website maintained by ex-Keristans, sleeping arrangements were rotated on a nightly basis, and preferences for specific individuals were frowned on (Winegar, 2002). The Keristas discouraged preferential treatment or sexual exclusivity, implying that members ran the risk of forming pair bonds within the group unless they systematically rotated their sleeping arrangements. A similar example comes from an atypical religious community in upstate New York founded by John Humphrey Noyes—the Oneida Commune. From 1848 to 1881, this polygynandrous group maintained a sexually communal group marriage, shared child-rearing responsibilities, and held property in common. When the group dissolved in the late 1800s, partially because of extreme antagonism from the surrounding community, many of the members immediately paired off and married monogamously, suggesting that the seeds of such attachments had already formed, despite the polygynandrous mating structure that had been enforced.

Favoritism within polygamous mating systems exemplifies how bonding processes between two individuals can supersede the confines of a specific mating system, raising the possibility that the tendency to fall in love and bond with a specific individual is an inevitable feature of human experience. However, an opposing argument could be made that monogamous mating systems are susceptible to polygamous influence as well. In fact, national survey estimates suggest that at least 20–25% of all Americans have extramarital sex while involved in monogamous marriages (Greeley, 1994; Wiederman, 1997). Some writers have argued that extra-pair copulations may have evolved because infidelity promotes reproductive success in both sexes, increasing men's total number of offspring and increasing women's likelihood of receiving good quality genes (Buss, 2000). The fact that love can emerge in polygamous contexts and that infidelity can emerge in monogamous ones underscores the potential value in treating the evolution of desire and love as separate questions for research (see also chapters by Berscheid, Chapter 16, and Diamond, Chapter 11, this volume).

Beyond Culture: Individual Differences in Relational Orientations

In the previous section we discussed some of the cultural, demographic, economic, and ecological factors that might determine whether a culture is monogamous or polygamous. Beyond questions regarding cultural systems, it is important to recognize that, even within a culture, there is variation in the orientations people adopt toward relationships. For example, some people, when asked, will readily explain that they are seeking a long-term mate—someone with whom they can have children and spend the rest of their lives. Other people indicate that they are not interested in settling down and are concerned only with the sexual aspect of relationships rather than the long-term bonds they might offer.

Psychologists have drawn attention to this kind of variation, sometimes referring to sociosexual orientation (e.g., Simpson & Gangestad, 1991), long-term versus short-term mating strategies (e.g., Buss & Schmidt, 1993), or secure attachment (i.e., the extent to which one is willing to engage in a close, committed, and trusting relationship with another individual; Hazan & Shaver, 1987; Kirkpatrick, 1998). In this section we return to the three hypotheses with which we opened the chapter and attempt to evaluate them—granted in a rather speculative manner—with respect to what is known (and what could be known, given future research) about individual differences in people's relationship orientations.

Within-Human Variation in Paternal Care

Our comparative analyses of paternal care and monogamy showed that long-term mating strategies, such as social monogamy, are associated with greater levels of paternal care. The existence of paternal care in mammals suggests that there were selection pressures for males to invest in their offspring. If no negative consequences stemming from a lack of paternal care existed, there would be no pressure for fathers to invest in their children. As mentioned in our discussion of paternal care, father presence versus absence can influence the survival of human infants. For example, paternal support promotes survival and positive health outcomes for children. Offspring with unavailable fathers have lower birthweights (Padilla & Reichman, 2001) and a higher incidence of health disadvantages compared with children with available fathers (Reading, 2003). When their biological father is not present, infants also have a greater chance of being abused or murdered (Daly & Wilson, 1985, 1994).

In addition to affecting physical health, father absence also affects behavioral and psychological health in offspring. For instance, Zvizdic and Butollo (2001) found that children who had lost their fathers to war were more likely to be depressed. Numerous researchers have studied the link between behavioral problems and father absence. In general, the trend for both sexes is toward more rule breaking (Bereczkei & Csanaky, 1996) and temper tantrums (Livson & Peskin, 1980). Importantly, as it pertains to our interests, father presence can affect social behaviors as well. For example, Balharova and Sporcrova (2002) found that boys with no father in the household showed poorer social functioning in the classroom. Because of these numerous behavioral and psychological effects, some authors have proposed that father absence has a direct influence on children's neurohormonal development (Bereczkei & Csanaky, 1996). This proposal is compatible with findings that females who do not have an available dad during childhood go through puberty at a younger age (Maestripieri, Roney, DeBias, Durante, & Spaepen, 2004), as well as enter menarche earlier than those with present fathers (Quinlan, 2003). This kind of evidence regarding pubertal timing in girls and behavior in boys has led some researchers to look for an evolutionary explanation of why these patterns may exist.

Evolutionary theories of socialization and life histories have been proposed to explain the effects of paternal care on developmental outcomes in humans (e.g., Belsky, 1999; Draper & Harpending, 1988; Kirkpatrick, 1998). According to these theories, children are sensitive to the nuances of their early caregiving environments and adopt reproductive strategies later in life based on their childhood experiences. Supporting evidence for this idea exists in the behaviors and life outcomes of both sexes. As mentioned previously, girls who have absent fathers tend to mature earlier (Maestripieri et al., 2004; Quinlan, 2003), engage in intercourse at a younger age (Aro & Taipale, 1987), and tend to have their first pregnancy earlier (Quinlan, 2003). Shorter first marriages and a heightened probability of divorce also characterize females whose fathers were absent in childhood (Glenn & Kramer, 1987; Quinlan, 2003). For boys who experience a lack of paternal care in childhood, the life outlook and trajectory is also somewhat troubled. For example, such boys have more temper problems (Livson & Peskin, 1980) and are more likely to be aggressive and take risks (Bereczkei & Csanaky, 1996; Rainwater, 1966).

When children have little paternal care, the outcomes are likely to include behavioral problems, earlier sexual activity, more negativity toward the opposite sex, and shorter relationships. Conversely, children raised in homes with both parents are characterized by a more favorable relationship pattern, including a delay in sexual activity and a greater desire to form long-term bonds in adulthood (Hetherington, 1972). These associations point to the possibility that early childhood experiences guide one's reproductive strategy later in life (Belsky, 1999; Draper & Harpending, 1982). Specifically, if children perceive that their social environment is unreliable or unstable, they may adjust their strategy toward forming short-term, unstable adult sexual relationships. Kirkpatrick (1998, 2005) has proposed that individual differences in attachment security are due to a similar process. In other words, attachment security reflects a childhood in which one has learned that the environment is reliable. This secure perspective then leads the person to adopt long-term mating strategies and invest highly in his or her own offspring. On the other hand, avoidant attachment may lead to the development of opportunistic, short-term mating tactics in which the number of mating partners is emphasized over the quality of those relationships (Belsky, 1999).

Within-Human Variation in Concealed Ovulation

The concealed-ovulation hypothesis predicts that human pair-bonds may have arisen when females lost their signs of estrus and essentially forced males to stay by their side most of the time to ensure paternity certainty. Unfortunately for our purposes, there is not much evidence of variability in the degree of ovulatory signals in humans. However, although women do not have sexual swellings to advertise their ovulatory periods, there is some evidence that men can distinguish ovulating women by scent (Kuukasjarvi et al., 2004). Furthermore, it is possible that some women display their sexual receptivity in other ways. Evidence for this possibility, though indirect, comes from studies conducted on the correspondence between monthly ovulation and women's fleeting sexual preferences. In an innovative series of studies, Gangestad and his colleagues have discovered that women are especially attracted to the smell of symmetrical men over asymmetrical men (Gangestad & Thornhill, 1998) when they are ovulating. Women are also more attracted to social dominance and competitiveness in men during ovulation (Gangestad, Simpson, Cousins, Garver-Apgar, & Christensen, 2004). Taken together, these findings indicate that women may be motivated, perhaps without knowing it, to engage selectively in extra-pair copulations at the precise time when those copulations are most likely to result in conception.

In addition to possessing these strategic preferences, women have also been found to act on them. For example, women are more likely to engage in extra-pair copulations during ovulation (Baker & Bellis, 1995; Meuwissen & Over, 1992). Researchers who study this phenomenon often theorize that women's increased desire for masculine men and tendency to cheat during ovulation is due to the genetic payoff of reproducing with dominant, healthy men (Gangestad et al., 2004). These findings may have implications for the concealed-ovulation hypothesis.

If women are more likely to desire and have sex during ovulation, their behavioral sexual displays, like their preferences, may vary as a function of their ovulatory cycle. For example, women may flirt more, make sexual advances, or dress in a more provocative way during ovulation as a way to entice men. Buss (1994) has emphasized the role of appearance-altering techniques used by women to attract the opposite sex, such as cosmetics, high-heeled shoes, and padded or constrictive clothing. Moreover, these tactics often mimic youthfulness and fertility. For instance, cosmetics give a healthy glow, padded bras enhance breast size, and girdles create a slim waistline while emphasizing the fullness of the hips. All of these physical alterations correspond to signs of fertility in women. If the concealed-ovulation hypothesis is correct, women might use these enhancement techniques to a greater degree when they are ovulating.

In sum, variability in ovulatory signals does not occur to a conspicuous degree in humans; all women lack the prominent sexual swellings and most of the other signals of ovulation that our primate relatives exhibit. However, data on changes in female sexuality during the fertility cycle indicate that ovulation may not be *fully* concealed. Although naturally occurring physical signs of ovulation have been lost in humans, women may use behavioral signs of ovulation to advertise their receptivity. These behavioral signals, to the extent that they exist, may covary negatively with pair-bonding tendencies in humans. As far as we know, this hypothesis has not yet been tested.

Within-Human Variation in Neoteny

The neoteny hypothesis proposes that the delayed maturation of humans results in the attachment system remaining active during adulthood. This hypothesis is difficult to evaluate from a within-species perspective because most humans tend to mature at similar rates. Nonetheless, in this section we examine the variability that does exist in human developmental timing and consider how immature features in human adults may correlate with attachment processes.

As discussed in the section on paternal care in humans, father absence leads to earlier physical maturation in humans, especially in females (Maestripieri et al., 2004; Quinlan, 2003). Thus there is some variability in girls' pubertal timing and menarche onset. We also discussed how the early onset of physical development leads to a higher likelihood of short-term mating strategies and divorce. Therefore, it appears that developing earlier (i.e., being less neotenous) is related to establishing briefer or more transient pair-bonds in adulthood. On the other hand, if development is not hastened (e.g., in females who were reared with their fathers present), long-term pair-bonds are more likely to be established in adulthood. This series of events lends credence to the possibility that, within humans, developmental neoteny is a factor in the formation of pair-bonds. Specifically, when a person matures slowly, he or she may be more likely to establish long-term pair-bonds in adulthood. For later-maturing people, the attachment system, which originally evolved as an adaptation related to childhood survival, may remain active and carry over into romantic relationships. Conversely, rapid development may lead to the suppression or deactivation of the attachment system at a younger age, thus discouraging the formation of enduring pair-bonds in adulthood.

Further evidence regarding neoteny's possible role in pair-bonding can be found in the research on father absence and paternal investment. Johnston, Hagel, Franklin, Fink, and Grammer (2001) discovered that men who have more masculine facial features invest less in their children. If men who are more masculine in appearance, and presumably more developed (i.e., less neotenous), are poorer caregivers, this implies that they may also be less likely to form pair-bonds with the mothers of their offspring. Another finding regarding neotenous facial features is that, overall, people of both sexes find adult faces with baby-like characteristics (i.e., large eyes) to be most attractive (Cunningham, Roberts, Barbee, Druen, & Wu, 1995). Faces that look childish may be more appealing because they elicit nurturant feelings, but they might also be attractive because neotenous features signal that a person is a good candidate for a long-term relationship.

Because a lack of body hair is a sign of developmental immaturity, a person's degree of neoteny can also be measured by the amount of body hair he or she possesses. In a study of women's preferences for facial hair, Freedman (1979) found that women preferred men without beards when judging them in terms of their potential to be good fathers. Furthermore, in the same study, bald men were also expected to make better fathers and were seen as more trustworthy. These findings highlight the way in which people with different levels of body hair are evaluated or perceived by others. The neoteny hypothesis, however, would predict that people with different levels of body hair would vary in their *own* orientations toward relationships. We are currently investigating this hypothesis in some of our empirical research.

In addition to being measured in terms of external physical features, neoteny can also be assessed by examining how playful people are (see Bjorklund, 1997). In accordance with the neoteny hypothesis, playfulness in relationships has been found to be positively associated with relationship functioning. For instance, Metz and Lutz (1990) observed that couples who were undergoing marital therapy were the most deficient in play behavior within the relationship. Aron, Norman, Aron, McKenna, and Heyman

(2000) found that couples' relationship quality was higher if they jointly participated in novel and exciting activities. Betcher (1981) also claims that play promotes bonding and stabilizes marriages.

Findings from attachment research also bear on the issue of behavioral immaturity and its relation to pair-bonding. Of the attachment styles studied in adults, the anxious pattern seems the least mature. For example, people who are high in anxiety tend to cope poorly with pressure (Feeney, 1998), to express more anger during stress (Rholes, Simpson, & Orina, 1999) and separations (Fraley & Shaver, 1998), and to desire extreme closeness with partners (Hazan & Shaver, 1987). This kind of behavior can be viewed as "childish" in the sense that infants tend to have underdeveloped coping and emotion-regulation skills, to throw temper tantrums, and to be highly dependent on caregivers. Importantly, this kind of behavior is associated with a strong desire to be close to others and to "merge" with them completely (Hazan & Shaver, 1987), suggesting that anxious adults are also oriented toward long-term, exclusive relationships. Although there is evidence that anxious adults may not be particularly successful at making those relationships function well (see Simpson, Ickes, & Grich, 1999), there is little doubt that they long for them.

CONCLUSIONS

Although the evolutionary functions of attachment are relatively clear in infant–caregiver relationships, it has been unclear what functions, if any, attachment serves in the context of adult mating relationships. In this chapter we have used cross-species comparative methods to investigate the functional correlates of adult romantic attachment. Our comparative analyses suggest that there are a number of social, developmental, and morphological traits that distinguish pair-bonded species from those that do not exhibit pair-bonding. We sought to complement our between-species data with information on within-species variation in human mating strategies. Ultimately, the study of evolution and behavior will be enriched by investigating both between- and within-species differences. We hope this chapter helps to fill the gaps in our knowledge of the evolution and adaptive functions of attachment in adult romantic relationships.

NOTE

1. Even monogamous relationships are susceptible to infidelity, thus undermining the view that humans are truly sexually exclusive (Barash & Lipton, 2001). We do not wish in this chapter to enter into the debate over whether humans are "designed" to be sexually faithful. We believe it is possible for people to be attached

to one another even if they are not sexually faithful. In this respect, whenever possible, we think it best to focus on *social monogamy* as an indicator of adult attachment as opposed to *sexual monogamy.* The form of the relationship between two individuals might have little to say ultimately about the sexual behavior of those individuals.

REFERENCES

Al-Krenawi, A., & Graham, J. R. (1999). The story of Bedouin-Arab women in a polygamous marriage. *Women's Studies International Forum, 22,* 497–509.

Alexander, R. D., & Noonan, K. M. (1979). Concealment of ovulation, parental care, and human social evolution. In N. A. Chagnon & W. Irons (Eds.), *Evolutionary biology and human social behavior: An anthropological perspective* (pp. 402–435). North Scituate, MA: Duxbury Press.

Aro, H., & Taipale, V. (1987). The impact of timing of puberty on psychosomatic symptoms among fourteen- to sixteen-year-old Finnish girls. *Child Development, 58,* 261–268.

Aron, A., Norman, C. C., Aron, E. N., McKenna, C., & Heyman, R. E. (2000). Couples' shared participation in novel and arousing activities and experienced relationship quality. *Journal of Personality and Social Psychology, 78,* 273–284.

Baker, R. R., & Bellis, M. A. (1995). *Human sperm competition: Copulation, masturbation, and infidelity.* London: Chapman & Hall.

Balharova, J., & Sporcrova, I. (2002). The father's role in formation of child's social attributes. *Psychologia a Patopsychologia Dietata, 37,* 36–50.

Barash, D. P., & Lipton, J. E. (2001). *The myth of monogamy: Fidelity and infidelity in animals and people.* New York: Freeman.

Belsky, J. (1999). Modern evolutionary theory and patterns of attachment. In J. Cassidy & P. R. Shaver (Eds.), *Handbook of attachment: Theory, research, and clinical applications* (pp. 151–173). New York: Guilford Press.

Bereczkei, T., & Csanaky, A. (1996). Mate choice, marital success, and reproduction in a modern society. *Ethology and Sociobiology, 17,* 17–35.

Betcher, R. W. (1981). Intimate play and marital adaptation. *Psychiatry: Journal for the Study of Interpersonal Processes, 44,* 13–33.

Bjorklund, D. F. (1997). The role of immaturity in human development. *Psychological Bulletin, 122,* 153–169.

Borgerhoff Mulder, M., George-Cramer, M., Eshleman, J., & Ortolani, A. (2001). A study of East African kinship and marriage using a phylogenetically-based comparative method. *American Anthropologist, 103,* 1059–1082.

Bowlby, J. (1969). *Attachment and loss: Vol. 1. Attachment.* New York: Basic Books.

Bowlby, J. (1980). *Attachment and loss: Vol. 3. Loss: Sadness and depression.* New York: Basic Books.

Bowlby, J., Robertson, J., & Rosenbluth, D. (1952) A two-year old goes to hospital. *Psychoanalytic Study of the Child, 7,* 82–94.

Buss, D. M. (1994). *The evolution of desire: Strategies of human mating.* New York: Basic Books.

Buss, D. M. (2000). *The dangerous passion: Why jealousy is as necessary as love and sex.* New York: Free Press.

Buss, D. M., & Schmitt, D. P. (1993). Sexual strategies theory: An evolutionary perspective on human mating. *Psychological Review, 100*, 204–232.

Carter, C. S., DeVries, A. C., & Getz, L. L. (1995). Physiological substrates of mammalian monogamy: The prairie vole model. *Neuroscience and Biobehavioral Reviews, 19*, 303–314.

Cochran, J.K., Chamlin, M. B., Beeghley, L., & Fenwick, M. (2004). Religion, religiosity, and nonmarital sexual conduct: An application of reference group theory. *Sociological Inquiry, 74*, 102–127.

Collins, N. L., Dunkel-Schetter, C., Lobel, M., & Scrimshaw, S. C. (1993). Social support in pregnancy: Psychosocial correlates of birth outcomes and postpartum depression. *Journal of Personality and Social Psychology, 65*, 1243–1258.

Coppens, Y. (1994). East side story: The origin of humankind. *Scientific American, 270*, 88–95.

Cunningham, M. R., Roberts, A. R., Barbee, A. P., Druen, P. B., & Wu, C. (1995). "Their ideas of beauty are, on the whole, the same as ours": Consistency and variability in the cross-cultural perception of female physical attractiveness. *Journal of Personality and Social Psychology, 68*, 261–279.

Daly, M., & Wilson, M. (1985). Child abuse and other risks of not living with both parents. *Ethology and Sociobiology, 6*, 197–210.

Daly, M., & Wilson, M. (1994). Stepparenthood and the evolved psychology of discriminative parental solicitude. In S. Parmigiani & F. S. vom Saal (Eds.), *Infanticide and parental care* (pp. 121–134). Chur, Switzerland: Harwood Academic.

deBeer, G.(1958). *Embryos and ancestors* (3rd ed.). Oxford, UK: Clarendon Press.

de Waal, F., & Lanting, F. (1997). *Bonobo: The forgotten ape*. Berkeley: University of California Press.

Diamond, L. M. (2003). What does sexual orientation orient? A biobehavioral model distinguishing romantic love and sexual desire. *Psychological Review, 110*, 173–192.

Draper, P., & Harpending, H. (1982). Father absence and reproductive strategy. *Journal of Anthropological Research, 38*, 255–273.

Draper, P., & Harpending, H. (1988). Sociobiological perspectives on the development of human reproductive strategies. In K. M. MacDonald (Ed.), *Sociobiological perspectives on human development* (pp. 340–372). New York: Springer.

Elbedour, S., Onwuegbuzie, A. J., Caridine, C., & Abu-Saad, H. (2002) The effect of polygamous marital structure on behavioral, emotional, and academic adjustment in children: A comprehensive review of the literature. *Clinical Child and Family Psychology Review, 5*, 255–271.

Feeney, J. A. (1998). Adult attachment and relationship-centered anxiety: Responses to physical and emotional distancing. In J. A. Simpson & W. S. Rholes (Eds.), *Attachment theory and close relationships* (pp. 189–218). New York: Guilford Press.

Feeney, J. A. (1999). Adult romantic attachment and couple relationships. In J. Cassidy & P. R. Shaver (Eds.), *Handbook of attachment: Theory, research, and clinical applications* (pp. 355–377). New York: Guilford Press.

Felsenstein, J. (2003). *Inferring phylogenies*. Sunderland, MA: Sinauer.

Fisher, H. E. (1992). *The anatomy of love*. New York: Norton.

Fraley, R. C., Brumbaugh, C. C., & Marks, M. J. (2005). The evolution and function of adult attachment: A comparative and phylogenetic analysis. *Journal of Personality and Social Psychology, 89*, 731–746.

Fraley, R. C., & Davis, K. E. (1997). Attachment formation and transfer in young adults' close friendships and romantic relationships. *Personal Relationships, 4*, 131–144.

Fraley, R. C., & Shaver, P. R. (1997). Adult attachment and the suppression of unwanted thoughts. *Journal of Personality and Social Psychology, 73*, 1080–1091.

Fraley, R. C., & Shaver, P. R. (1998). Airport separations: A naturalistic study of adult attachment dynamics in separating couples. *Journal of Personality and Social Psychology, 75*, 1198–1212.

Fraley, R. C., & Shaver, P. R. (2000). Adult romantic attachment: Theoretical developments, emerging controversies, and unanswered questions. *Review of General Psychology, 4*, 132–154.

Freedman, D. G. (1979). *Human sociobiology.* New York: Free Press.

Gangestad, S. W., Simpson, J. A., Cousins, A. J., Garver-Apgar, C. E., & Christensen, P. (2004). Women's preferences for male behavioral displays change across the menstrual cycle. *Psychological Science, 15*, 203–206.

Gangestad, S. W., & Thornhill, R. (1998). Menstrual cycle variation in women's preference for the scent of symmetrical men. *Proceedings of the Royal Society of London B, 262*, 727–733.

Garland, T., Jr., & Adolph, S. C. (1994). Why not to do two-species comparative studies: Limitations on inferring adaptation. *Physiological Zoology, 67*, 797–828.

Glenn, N., & Kramer, K. (1987). The marriages and divorces of the children of divorce. *Journal of Marriage and the Family, 49*, 811–825.

Greeley, A. (1994). Marital infidelity. *Society, 31*, 9–13.

Gubernick, D. J. (1994). Biparental care and male–female relations in mammals. In S. Parmigiani & F. S. vom Saal (Eds.), *Infanticide and parental care* (pp. 427–464). Chur, Switzerland: Harwood Academic.

Hassouneh-Phillips, D. (2001). Polygamy and wife abuse: A qualitative study of Muslim women in America. *Health Care for Women International, 22*, 735–748.

Hazan, C., Gur-Yaish, N., & Campa, M. (2004). What does it mean to be attached? In W. S. Rholes & J. A. Simpson (Eds.), *Adult attachment: Theory, research, and clinical applications* (pp. 55–85). New York: Guilford Press.

Hazan, C., & Shaver, P. (1987). Romantic love conceptualized as an attachment process. *Journal of Personality and Social Psychology, 52*, 511–524.

Hazan, C., & Zeifman, D. (1999). Pair-bonds as attachments: Evaluating the evidence. In J. Cassidy & P. R. Shaver (Eds.), *Handbook of attachment: Theory, research, and clinical applications* (pp. 336–354). New York: Guilford Press.

Heinicke, C. M., & Westheimer, I. (1966). *Brief separations.* New York: International Universities Press.

Hetherington, E. (1972). Effects of paternal absence on personality development in adolescent daughters. *Developmental Psychology, 7*, 313–326.

Hiraiwa-Hasegawa, M., & Hasegawa, T. (1994). Infanticide in non-human primates: Sexual selection and local resource competition. In S. Parmigiani & F. S. vom Saal (Eds.), *Infanticide and parental care* (pp. 137–154). Chur, Switzerland: Harwood Academic.

Hrdy, S. B. (1988). The primate origins of human sexuality. In G. Stevens & R. Bellig (Eds.), *The evolution of sex* (pp. 101–132). San Francisco: Harper & Row.

Johnston, V. S., Hagel, R., Franklin, M., Fink, B., & Grammer, K. (2001). Male facial attractiveness: Evidence for hormone mediated adaptive design. *Evolution and Human Behavior, 21*, 251–267.

Jolly, A. (1972). *The evolution of primate behavior.* New York: Macmillan.

Kirkpatrick, L. A. (1998). Evolution, pair-bonding, and reproductive strategies: A reconceptualization of adult attachment. In J. A. Simpson & W. S. Rholes (Eds.), *Attachment theory and close relationships* (pp. 353–393). New York: Guilford Press.

Kirkpatrick, L. A. (2005). *Attachment, evolution and the psychology of religion.* New York: Guilford Press.

Klomegah, R. (1997). Socio-economic characteristics of Ghanaian women in polygynous marriages. *Journal of Comparative Family Studies, 28*, 73–88.

Komers, P. E., & Brotherton, P. N. M. (1997). Female space use is the best predictor of monogamy in mammals. *Proceedings of the Royal Society of London B, 264*, 1261–1270.

Kuukasjarvi, S., Eriksson, C. J., Koskela, W., Mappes, T., Nissinen, K., & Rantala, M. J. (2004). Attractiveness of women's body odors over the menstrual cycle: The role of oral contraceptives and receiver sex. *Behavioral Ecology, 15*, 579–584.

Livson, N., & Peskin, H. (1980). Perspectives on adolescence from longitudinal research. In J. Adelson (Ed.), *Handbook of adolescent psychology* (pp. 47–98). New York: Wiley.

Maddison, W. P., & Maddison, D. R. (2001). *MacClade 4: Analysis of phylogeny and character evolution* [Version 4.06]. Sunderland, MA: Sinauer.

Maestripieri, D., Roney, J. R., DeBias, N., Durante, K., & Spaepen, G. M. (2004). Father absence, menarche and interest in infants among adolescent girls. *Developmental Science, 7*, 560–566.

Mahoney, A., Pargament, K. I., Tarakeshwar, N., & Swank, A. B. (2001). Religion in the home in the 1980's and 1990's: A meta-analytic review and conceptual analysis of links between religion, marriage, and parenting. *Journal of Family Psychology, 15*, 559–596.

Margulis, L., & Sagan, D. (1991). *Mystery dance: On the evolution of human sexuality.* New York: Summit Books.

Mellen, S. L. (1981). *The evolution of love.* San Francisco: Freeman.

Metz, M. E., & Lutz, G. (1990). Dyadic playfulness differences between sexual and marital therapy couples. *Journal of Psychology and Human Sexuality, 3*, 169–182.

Meuwissen, I., & Over, R. (1992). Sexual arousal across phases of the human menstrual cycle. *Archives of Sexual Behavior, 21*, 101–119.

Miller, G. F. (1998). A review of sexual selection and human evolution: How mate choice shaped human nature. In C. Crawford & D. Krebs (Eds.), *Handbook of evolutionary psychology: Ideas, issues, and applications* (pp. 87–130). Mahwah, NJ: Erlbaum.

Montagu, A. (1989). *Growing young* (2nd ed.). Grandy, MA: Bergin & Garvey.

Murdock, G. P. (1967). *Ethnographic atlas.* Pittsburgh, PA: University of Pittsburgh Press.

Obukwe, O. N. (2002). A study of human bite injuries to the face. *Central African Journal of Medicine, 48*, 68–71.

Ohadike, P. O. (1968). A demographic note on marriage, family, and family growth in

Lagos, Nigeria. In J. C. Caldwell & C. Okonjo (Eds.), *The population of tropical Africa* (pp. 379–392). London: Longmans Green.

Padilla, Y. C., & Reichman, N. E. (2001). Low birthweight: Do unwed fathers help? *Children and Youth Services Review, 23*, 427–452.

Parish, A. R. (1994). Sex and food control in the "uncommon chimpanzee": How bonobo females overcome a phylogenetic legacy of male dominance. *Ethology and Sociobiology, 15*, 157–179.

Pivar, D. J. (1973). *Purity crusade and sexual morality and social control, 1868–1900.* Westport, CN: Greenwood Press.

Poirier, F. E., & Smith, E. O. (1974). Socializing functions of primate play. *American Zoologist, 14*, 275–287.

Pusey, A. E., & Packer, C. P. (1994). Infanticide in lions: Consequences and counter-strategies. In S. Parmigiani & F. S. vom Saal (Eds.), *Infanticide and parental care* (pp. 277–300). Chur, Switzerland: Harwood Academic.

Quinlan, R. J. (2003). Father absence, parental care, and female reproductive development. *Evolution and Human Behavior, 24*, 376–390.

Rainwater, L. (1966). Crucible of identity: The Negro lower-class family. *Daedalus: Journal of the American Academy of Arts and Sciences, 95*, 172–216.

Reading, R. (2003). Mortality, severe morbidity and injury in children living with single parents in Sweden: A population-based study. *Child: Care, Health and Development, 29*, 316–317.

Rholes, W. S., Simpson, J. A., & Orina, M. N. (1999). Attachment and anger in an anxiety-provoking situation. *Journal of Personality and Social Psychology, 76*, 940–957.

Seyfarth, R. M. (1978). Social relationships among adult male and female baboons: I. Behaviour during sexual consortship. *Behaviour, 64*, 204–226.

Shaver, P. R., Hazan, C., & Bradshaw, D. (1988). Love as attachment: The integration of three behavioral systems. In R. J. Sternberg & M. L. Barnes (Eds.), *The psychology of love* (pp. 68–99). New Haven, CT: Yale University Press.

Sibley, C. G., & Ahlquist, J. E. (1984). The phylogeny of the hominoid primates, as indicated by DNA–DNA hybridization. *Journal of Molecular Evolution, 20*, 2–15.

Sillén-Tullberg, B., & Møller, A. P. (1991). The relationship between concealed ovulation and mating systems in anthropoid primates: A phylogenetic analysis. *American Naturalist, 141*, 1–25.

Simpson, J. A., & Gangestad, S. (1991). Individual differences in sociosexuality: Evidence for convergent and discriminant validity. *Journal of Personality and Social Psychology, 60*, 870–883.

Simpson, J. A., Ickes, W., & Grich, J. (1999). When accuracy hurts: Reactions of anxious-ambivalent dating partners to a relationship-threatening situation. *Journal of Personality and Social Psychology, 76*, 754–769.

Smith, J. E., & Kunz, P. R. (1976). Polygyny and fertility in nineteenth century America. *Population Studies, 30*, 465–480.

Smuts, B. B., & Gubernick, D. J. (1992). Male–infant relationships in nonhuman primates: Paternity certainty or mating effort? In B. Hewlett (Ed.), *Father–child relations* (pp. 1–30). Hawthorne, NY: Aldine.

Sommer, V. (1994). Infanticide among the langurs of Jodhpur: Testing the sexual selection hypothesis with a long-term record. In S. Parmigiani & F. S. vom Saal (Eds.),

Infanticide and parental care (pp. 155–198). Chur, Switzerland: Harwood Academic.

Strassman, I. (1981). Sexual selection, paternal care and concealed ovulation in humans. *Ethology and Sociobiology, 2*, 31–40.

Szalay, F. S., & Costello, R. K. (1991). Evolution of permanent estrus displays in hominids. *Journal of Human Evolution, 20*, 439–464.

Turke, P. W. (1984). Effects of ovulatory concealment and synchrony on protohominid mating systems and parental roles. *Ethology and Sociobiology, 5*, 33–44.

van Schaik, C. P., & Janson, C. H. (2000). Infanticide by males: Prospectus. In C. P. van Schaik & C. H. Janson (Eds.), *Infanticide by males and its implications* (pp. 1–6). Cambridge, UK: Cambridge University Press.

van Schaik, C. P., & Kappeler, P. M. (1997). *Infanticide risk and the evolution of male–female association in primates. Proceedings of the Royal Society of London B, 264*, 1687–1694.

Wiederman, M. W. (1997). Extramarital sex: Prevalence and correlates in a national survey. *Journal of Sex Research, 34*, 167–174.

Winegar, (2002). *Kerista.comune: Historical home of the Kerista commune*. Retrieved February 7, 2004, from http://www.kerista.com/index.html.

Zvizdic, S., & Butollo, W. (2001). War-related loss of one's father and persistent depressive reactions in early adolescents. *European Psychologist, 6*, 204–214.

5

An Attachment Perspective on Abusive Dynamics in Intimate Relationships

KIM BARTHOLOMEW
and COLLEEN J. ALLISON

In this chapter we review dominant approaches to understanding relationship abuse. Feminist perspectives propose that partner abuse stems from patriarchal norms that dictate that men should dominate and control women. In contrast, various psychological perspectives consider why some individuals (and not others) act abusively in their intimate relationships as a function of such individual factors as childhood experiences, social skills, personality, and psychopathology. Attachment theory is one such psychological perspective. In particular, researchers have explored how particular forms of attachment insecurity may put individuals at risk for acting abusively toward intimate partners. Although considerable theory and research have shown the limitations of feminist models of abuse, little attention has been given to the limitations of individually focused psychological perspectives on abuse. We hope to demonstrate the inadequacy of such individual perspectives, with a particular focus on previous work guided by attachment theory.

We argue instead that partner abuse should be considered from a relational or dyadic perspective. Thus we ask why some relationships become abusive whereas others do not. Research on the interactional processes of violent couples shows the promise of such a systemic approach. We review some initial work suggesting the value of attachment theory in conceptualizing the dyadic foundations of abuse. Attachment theory may also contribute to a unifying framework for psychological and interactional approaches to partner violence. Finally, we consider the clinical implications of an attachment-informed dyadic analysis of partner violence.

A FEMINIST PERSPECTIVE ON PARTNER ABUSE

A feminist perspective on domestic violence addresses a primary question: Why do men beat their wives? (Bograd, 1988, p. 13). The feminist answer to this question is that men internalize patriarchal norms that lead them to believe they have the right to dominate and control women. "Men who assault their wives are actually living up to cultural prescriptions that are cherished in Western society—aggressiveness, male dominance and female subordination" (Dobash & Dobash, 1979, p. 24). From this perspective, violence against women is primarily a societal problem and not a problem of individual behavior or pathology. To quote Bograd (1988, p. 17), wife assault is assumed to result from "the normal psychological and behavioral patterns of most men." Psychological explanations of violent behavior are avoided because they may be used to excuse the behavior of male perpetrators.

From a strict feminist perspective, female victims play no role in the development of violent relationships. Because all men have the potential to be violent, it is not seen as useful to consider why some women become victims of male violence and others do not. In fact, psychological analyses of women victims are condemned because of the potential for such explanations to "blame the victim." However, consideration is given to the difficulties women face in leaving violent relationships, with particular focus on factors such as economic constraints and fear of further violence. Research from this perspective has also documented physical and mental health costs of women's victimization.

There are many problems with patriarchal accounts of partner violence, especially as applied to Western countries, in which the vast majority of research has been conducted. First, if violence against women is a norm, why are only a minority of men violent? Moreover, there is no evidence that men's right to dominate women is a current societal norm; rather, only a small minority of men condone violence against women (Simon et al., 2001). The assumption that male violence serves to enforce and maintain male domination of women is inconsistent with a growing body of literature that male violence toward women is associated with a *lack* of power in intimate relationships. For example, husbands' perceptions of low relationship power and income discrepancies in favor of wives are associated with violence of husbands toward wives (e.g., Anderson, 1997; Sagrestano, Heavey, & Christensen, 1999). Moreover, men who are violent toward their partners (relative to those who are not) are less likely to uphold masculine ideals of self-confidence and independence (e.g., Murphy, Meyer, & O'Leary, 1994) and less likely to endorse masculine gender schemas (e.g., Sugarman & Frankel, 1996).

Feminist perspectives also have great difficulty accounting for much of the established evidence on partner violence: high rates of women's violence (e.g., Archer, 2000), high rates of violence in same-sex relationships (e.g., Bartholomew, Landolt, & Oram, 1999; Lie, Schilit, Bush, Montague, & Reyes, 1991), and high mutuality of violence in many relationships (e.g., Magdol et al., 1997). The common claims that women's violence is a form of self-defense and that only men's violence is injurious do not hold up to empirical scrutiny (e.g., Archer, 2000; DeKeseredy & Schwartz, 1998). For more detailed critiques of this perspective on partner violence, at least as applied to violence in Western societies, please see Dutton (1994; Dutton & Nicholls, 2005) and George (2003).

PSYCHOLOGICAL PERSPECTIVES ON PARTNER ABUSE

Psychological perspectives on partner violence have typically addressed the question, Why are some men violent toward their partners? Although patriarchy may be seen as the social context in which other factors operate, sociocultural explanations are viewed as insufficient because they fail to explain why only a minority of men are violent toward female partners.

Many psychosocial variables have been hypothesized to influence partner violence, including a history of violence in the family of origin (e.g., Kwong, Bartholomew, Henderson, & Trinke, 2003); substance abuse (Leonard, 1993); individual-difference variables, such as dependency, self-esteem (e.g., Murphy et al., 1994), and negative emotionality (Moffitt, Robins, & Caspi, 2001); personality disorders (e.g., Dutton, 1995); poor communication and problem-solving skills (e.g., Anglin & Holtzworth-Munroe, 1997), and negative attributions for partner behaviors (e.g., Holtzworth-Munroe & Hutchinson, 1993). The majority of research has been aimed at understanding why some men are violent toward their partners. However, similar approaches can be, and have been, applied to women's violence toward men and to violence by both men and women in same-sex relationships. Moreover, many researchers have constructed and tested models of how various psychosocial factors may combine to predict partner violence. For example, Leonard and Senchak (1996) tested a social-interactional model predicting husband aggression over the first year of marriage, a model that included family history, personality, communication, and substance use as variables.

Less attention has been given to psychosocial predictors of victim behavior in violent relationships. Moreover, the work that has been done has tended to focus on the psychological impact of victimization on women (Giles-Sims, 1998). However, some work has addressed the family backgrounds associated with victimization by an intimate partner (e.g., Kwong et al., 2003) and the psychological predictors of women's ability to leave abusive relationships (e.g., Rusbult & Martz, 1995).

Psychosocial perspectives on partner abuse have many advantages. These perspectives help to explain why only some individuals are violent within their intimate relationships and, to a lesser extent, why only some individuals stay in relationships in which they are abused. Many of the constructs studied can be applied to both genders and to both heterosexual and same-sex relationships. Thus these perspectives allow for an empirical examination of whether the predictors of violence vary depending on the gender of the perpetrator and the nature of the relationship. They also lend themselves to exploring whether there might be subtypes of aggressors who show different profiles of background characteristics, personality dimensions, psychopathology, and violence-related attitudes (e.g., Holtzworth-Munroe & Stuart, 1994). Moreover, whereas feminist approaches to partner violence have tended to focus on marital relationships, the key arena in which patriarchal norms are expected to be manifested, psychological approaches have also explored partner violence in dating and cohabiting relationships, in which violence is most common. However, psychological approaches tend to be limited by a failure to consider the dyadic or relational context in which partner abuse develops and takes place. In particular, they have typically focused on either perpetrators or victims of violence in isolation, without acknowledging that abuse takes place within a relationship between two people. We demonstrate these limitations by briefly reviewing the literature on partner violence guided by an attachment perspective. We pay particular attention to work conducted by our collaborators and ourselves.

AN ATTACHMENT PERSPECTIVE ON PARTNER ABUSE

Drawing on theorizing by Bowlby (1984), researchers have conceptualized relationship abuse as an exaggerated and dysfunctional form of protest behavior (Bartholomew, Henderson, & Dutton, 2001). In intimate relationships, the attachment figure is the partner against whom the protest is directed. Thus anger toward a partner is expected to be precipitated by attachment-related threats, such as interpersonal conflict and fears of rejection, separation, and abandonment. Individuals high in attachment anxiety are expected to be hypersensitive to such threats because they are more likely than those low in anxiety to perceive ambiguous partner behaviors in threatening terms. Anxious individuals who have failed to effectively communicate their need for reassurance to a relationship partner in more functional ways may then strike out in abusive anger or even violence to gain or regain proximity to an attachment figure. Moreover, anxious individuals who also have a strong approach orientation (or low avoidance), or those with ambivalent or preoccupied attachment orientations, may be especially likely to strike out in anger when they perceive a relationship threat. This perspective on partner violence is consistent with the finding that relationship violence typically takes place in the context of couple conflict (e.g., Cascardi & Vivian, 1995), and that perpetrators of partner violence are characterized by high dependency and psychological vulnerability (e.g., Murphy et al., 1994).

Attachment avoidance has been linked with hostility, with a hostile attribution bias, and with a lack of forgiveness toward partners (e.g., Kobak & Sceery, 1988; Mikulincer, 1998; Shaver & Mikulincer, 2003). Therefore, it might be expected that avoidance would also be predictive of partner abuse. However, the defining feature of attachment avoidance is a tendency to withdraw when anxious or threatened, with the goal of deactivating the attachment system and maintaining personal control (Mikulincer, Florian, Cowan, & Cowan, 2002). Correspondingly, avoidance is associated with controlling the expression of anger (Mikulincer, 1998). As a result, we would not generally expect avoidance to engender extreme and dysfunctional protest behavior. Rather, the tendency to withdraw when threatened would seem contrary to the active protest behavior shown in aggressive acts.

An attachment-based conceptualization of partner violence is not gender specific; however, typically this framework has been applied to understanding male violence against women. Consistent with expectations, studies have demonstrated links between anxious attachment (assessed in various ways) and male-to-female partner violence (e.g., Dutton, Saunders, Starzomski, & Bartholomew, 1994; Holtzworth-Munroe, Stuart, & Hutchinson, 1997). Moreover, studies that have considered other forms of partner violence have yielded similar patterns of findings. For example, attachment anxiety (and especially a preoccupied orientation) is associated with women's violence toward male partners (Henderson, Bartholomew, Trinke, & Kwong, 2005) and with men's violence toward male partners (Bartholomew, Oram, & Landolt, 2000).

Although most attachment-guided work in the field of partner violence has focused on the perpetration of violence, attachment theory has also been used to guide research on victims of relationship abuse (e.g., Dutton & Painter, 1993; Henderson, Bartholomew, & Dutton, 1997). The attachment bonds that form between partners in intimate relationships make it difficult to leave such relationships, even highly dysfunctional and distressing ones. Moreover, victims of partner abuse are likely to be anxiously attached as a consequence of abuse and perhaps also as a prior risk factor for involvement in an abusive relationship. This anxiety is then expected to exacerbate the normative fear of separation and loss involved in ending a long-term attachment relationship. It has also been suggested that threatening situations might strengthen attachment bonds, even when the attachment figure is the source of threat (Bowlby, 1969; Dutton & Painter, 1993). Such traumatic bonding may, paradoxically, make leaving abusive relationships especially difficult.

Most research investigating the potential role of attachment in partner violence has focused on one gender and only one direction of violence (from male to female). For example, in our earliest work in this field, we looked at links between attachment patterns and perpetrated violence in a sample of men only (Dutton et al., 1994), and we looked at links between attachment patterns and success in separating from abusive male partners in a sample of women only (Henderson et al., 1997). However, recent work based on a more inclusive approach suggests that gender and direction of abuse may not necessarily moderate associations between attachment and violence variables. Thus, in a diverse community sample, preoccupied attachment was correlated with both the receipt and perpetration of relationship aggression, for both men and women (Henderson et al., 2005). Similarly, in a sample of male and female undergraduates, Bookwala and Zdaniuk (1998) found that preoccupied and fearful attachment were significantly associated with reciprocal dating violence for both men and women.

EVALUATION OF PSYCHOLOGICAL APPROACHES

Psychological research on partner violence, including research guided by an attachment perspective, has contributed substantially to our understanding of why, given the same normative environment, only some individuals become violent in their intimate relationships. Also, this research has deepened our understanding of why some individuals stay in abusive relationships and what is involved in the process of leaving such relationships.

Unfortunately, most psychological approaches to understanding partner violence have not taken the relational context of partner violence into account. Thus studies of perpetrators of violence (most often male perpetrators) and recipients of violence (most often female recipients) tend to be conducted in isolation. This failure to consider both partners in violent relationships has resulted in some questionable interpretations of data. In cross-sectional studies, for example, high attachment anxiety (or a preoccupied attachment orientation) has quite consistently been found to be associated with male violence and with female victimization. The typical interpretation of such findings is that anxious males are more prone to violence and that male violence tends to undermine the security of women. Thus only the male perpetrator is seen as having any role in the development of a violent relationship. Moreover, identical cross-sectional results for women and men are interpreted as indicating opposite causal relations: Male insecurity causes violence perpetration, and receipt of violence causes female insecurity. For a similar observation about the interpretation of findings that link social-skills deficits in men and women to marital violence, see Anglin and Holtzworth-Munroe (1997). Such gender-biased interpretations of data are the legacy of the patriarchal model, which defines partner violence in terms of male violence against women and explicitly rejects the possibility that a female victim of abuse has any role in the development of an abusive relationship.

DYADIC BASIS OF RELATIONSHIP FUNCTIONING AND PARTNER ABUSE

In the research literature on intimate relationships, there is considerable evidence that both partners contribute to the quality of their relationship. Evidence of assortative mating suggests that partners select one another based on preexisting qualities and traits. For example, men and women with histories of antisocial behavior tend to become partnered with one another (Krueger, Moffitt, Caspi, Bleske, & Silva, 1998). Moreover, individual qualities of *both* partners contribute to relationship dynamics and relationship outcomes. For example, both partners' negative emotionality independently predicts relationship quality (e.g., Robins, Caspi, & Moffitt, 2000). Studies also indicate that partner similarity on values and expectations predict relationship outcomes (e.g., Fowers & Olson, 1986). However, the strongest predictors of marital outcomes are interactional processes, processes that arise out of the joint behavior of partners in a relationship (for reviews, see Bradbury, Fincham, & Beach, 2000; Karney & Bradbury, 1995). Similarly, there is some evidence in the attachment literature that both partners' attachment orientations contribute to relationship outcomes (for a review, see Feeney, 2003). For example, in a large sample of married couples, wives' and husbands' attachment orientations independently predicted each partner's marital satisfaction (Banse, 2004). Moreover, there was some evidence of interactive effects, such that particular combinations of wife and husband attachment were predictive of satisfaction.

Given the general acceptance of the dyadic basis of relationship behaviors and experiences in the study of dating and marital relationships, it is striking that such relational models have not gained a higher profile in research on partner violence. However, considerable data in the violence field point to the role of both partners in the development of violent relationships. Notably, studies have documented that power imbalances in heterosexual relationships (in favor of the male or female partner) are associated with partner violence by both male and female partners (e.g., Coleman & Straus, 1990). Other studies have indicated that characteristics of both partners are associated with marital violence, for example, problem-solving skills (Anglin & Holtzworth-Munroe, 1997). With such cross-sectional data, however, it is possible that just one partner has determined the course of the violent relationships, with the other partner simply responding to the violent partner. However, studies examining partners' family backgrounds suggest that violence in the family of origin is predictive of both women's and men's violence and of victimization, as well as perpetration (e.g., Ehrensaft et al., 2003; Kwong et al., 2003). Moreover, having experienced violence in a prior dating relationship appears to increase the risk of violence in a subsequent dating relationship (e.g., Gwartney-Gibbs, Stockard, & Bohmer, 1987), and there is modest continuity in the experience of abuse across relationships (Robins, Caspi, & Moffitt, 2002). Finally, negative emotionality at age 18 has been found to predict subsequent partner violence, again for both genders (Moffitt, Krueger, Caspi, & Fagan, 2000). If only men influenced the development of abusive heterosexual relationships, we would not expect background or personality characteristics of women to be associated with their likelihood of becoming involved in and staying in abusive relationships.

The well-established finding that violence in intimate relationships is often bi-directional also suggests the need to consider the dyadic context of partner violence. In about half of relationships with any violence, both members of the couple report violence (e.g., Morse, 1995; Stets & Straus, 1990a). Moreover, there are strong associations between partner reports of severity of violence. For example, in a large community sample of young adult couples, there was a correlation of .67 between male and female partners' abuse perpetration (Moffitt et al., 2001). We have found that similar levels of abuse reciprocity characterize male same-sex relationships (Regan, Bartholomew, Oram, & Landolt, 2002). If both members of a couple are violent (especially if this violence is not self-defensive), then it is necessary to consider the backgrounds and dispositions of both partners and how they interact to fully understand the development of relationship violence. To focus only on one identified perpetrator (usually the male partner in heterosexual relationships) in relationships with bidirectional violence is inherently limiting. Moreover, severe violence (especially male severe violence) is considerably more likely to occur in mutually abusive relationships than in relationships with unidirectional abuse (e.g., Ehrensaft, Moffitt, & Caspi, 2004). For example, in a national U.S. survey, the likelihood of severe male violence was much higher when the female partner was also severely violent than when the female partner was not violent: The relative odds were 10:1

for dating relationships, 3:1 for cohabiting relationships, and almost 2:1 in marital relationships (Stets & Straus, 1990b).

The documented reciprocity of violence in many relationships is at odds with the stereotype that such relationships invariably involve distinct abuser and victim roles. This stereotype is made explicit in the feminist perspective on partner violence, which assumes that men are always perpetrators and women are always victims. If this were the case, we would not expect to find reciprocity of violence in heterosexual relationships, nor would we expect the most severe violence to occur in mutually violent relationships. Nonetheless, from aggregate data on violence reciprocity, we cannot rule out the possibility that individual partners act as abuser and victim at different points in time. A few in-depth, qualitative studies have explored the dynamics of abusive relationships (e.g., Allison, Bartholomew, Mayseless, & Dutton, 2005; Cruz & Firestone, 1998; Stanley, Bartholomew, Taylor, Landolt, & Oram, in press). Consistent with interpersonal models in which negativity is expected to be reciprocal and mutually reinforcing in relationships (e.g., Kiesler, 1983), these studies document that mutual violence often takes place within violent incidents and that it is often difficult to distinguish between the abuser and victim roles. To provide just one graphic example, a female participant identified as a victim of violence in one of our early studies (Henderson et al., 1997) described conflicts in which both partners were fully engaged and in which the abusive behavior of both partners tended to escalate. In the most extreme violent incident described, she admitted to instigating the incident by stabbing her partner in the back because he refused to keep arguing with her after they had been up almost all night fighting (he was trying to relax with the paper before leaving for work). Although her male partner predictably reciprocated by beating her badly, this woman's description of her relationship suggested that she was a fully equal partner in the abusive dynamics.

Perhaps the strongest support to date for the hypothesis that both partners contribute to the development of abusive relationships comes from a longitudinal study of a birth cohort born in Dunedin, New Zealand, in 1972–1973 (Ehrensaft et al., 2004). A range of developmental risk factors were used to predict involvement in three types of relationships—no violence, nonclinical levels of violence, or clinical levels of violence—at the 26-year follow-up. Men in the clinical group were distinctive in terms of their histories of hyperactivity, attention deficit, conduct disorder, and personality pathology. In contrast, women in both the nonclinical and clinical abuse groups were characterized by a history of childhood conduct disorders. Thus relationship abuse was likely to escalate to clinical levels only when the male partner had a history of psychopathology *and* the female partner was prone to aggression. The clinical group also showed the highest levels of both male and female violence, suggesting reciprocity of abuse. Further, the findings for the nonclinical abuse group (characterized by higher levels of female than male violence) suggested that when the female partner was prone to aggression but the male partner was not, violence was unlikely to escalate. Another study that focused on the 21-year follow-up of the Dunedin cohort indicated that both male and female negative emotionality independently predicted abuse perpetration and receipt (Moffitt et al., 2001). Notably, there were significant perpetrator and victim effects, even after controlling for reciprocity of abuse. Thus, for instance, women's negative emotionality predicted their abuse perpetration independently of their male partners' abuse.

In summary, findings indicate that similar variables are associated with male and female violence, that the predictors of perpetration and receipt of violence are generally identical (necessarily so, given high rates of reciprocity), and that characteristics of both partners are predictive of relationship violence. Such findings highlight the need to move beyond a narrow focus on male perpetrators and female victims of partner abuse (e.g., Moffitt et al., 2000).

INTERACTIONAL APPROACHES TO PARTNER VIOLENCE

The dyadic context of partner violence has been directly investigated in studies of the interaction and communication processes in violent relationships. These studies are designed to reveal the interpersonal context in which aggression takes place. As a group, interaction studies of violent couples suggest that violence may arise out of a general pattern of relational dysfunction, with the most distinctive feature being reciprocity of negative affect. For example, in one of the earliest interaction studies of physically abusive couples, Burman, Margolin, and John (1993) found that violent couples were distinguished by high levels of reciprocity of hostile affect, involving both husbands and wives. Similarly, Cordova, Jacobson, Gottman, Rushe, and Cox (1993) found that both women and men in violent relationships (defined in terms of men's violence only) were inclined toward strong negative reciprocity as assessed on an interaction task. Moreover, based on sequential analyses of verbal descriptions of violent incidents, Jacobson et al. (1994) found that both husbands and wives in violent couples (also defined in terms of male violence) were likely to be violent in response to partner violence and emotional abuse. These findings are directly contrary to the patriarchal model of male violence in which men are believed to dominate and control their wives through violence. That model would presume that husbands' aggression is reinforced by wives' compliance, leading to the prediction that wives in violent relationships would be less likely to reciprocate negativity than their spouses or than wives in nonviolent relationships.

Consistent with the negative reciprocity findings, some studies have indicated that violent couples are distinguished from distressed but nonviolent couples by high levels of negativity and verbal aggressiveness on the part of both partners (e.g., Burman et al., 1993; Jacobson et al., 1994). Notably, even in studies of couples chosen for severe male-to-female violence, female partners also demonstrate high levels of anger and negativity in conflict interactions. For example, Jacobson et al. (1994) compared distressed-violent and distressed-nonviolent couples interacting in a laboratory setting. Based on observational measures, wives showed higher levels of provocative anger than husbands in the distressed-nonviolent couples, whereas husbands' provocative anger rose almost to the level of wives' in the violent couples. Thus violent marriages seem to be characterized by two partners who are angry, belligerent, and contemptuous of each other.

Until recently, researchers who conduct interactional studies of partner violence have not questioned the assumption that partner violence is fundamentally a matter of men abusing women. We are not aware of any interaction studies that have looked at couples identified for same-sex violence or for female-to-male violence. Rather, the goal of this work has been to understand the relationship context, including wife behaviors, in which male battering occurs (Jacobson, 1994). However, given the high reciprocity of partner abuse, even in couples identified for high levels of male-to-female violence, many of the couples studied are also characterized by moderate to severe female violence. For example, although Jacobson et al. (1994) selected violent-distressed couples based on severe male-to-female violence, almost half of couples would have qualified for the violent couple group based on wife violence.

In summary, both prospective studies of partner violence (Ehrensaft et al., 2004) and interaction studies of violent couples (e.g., Jacobson et al., 1994) converge on the conclusion that severe violence is most likely to occur when both partners are prone to abusive behavior. More specifically, distressed couples (in some cases, with female violence) are characterized by high levels of negative expressivity on the part of women, coupled with avoidant, defensive, or withdrawing behavior on the part of male partners. When, in contrast, both members of a couple are high on negative expressivity, reciprocity of negative affect may escalate into male violence and generally more serious partner violence. This pattern is quite evident in work on the demand-withdrawal pattern of interaction: Whereas distressed but nonviolent couples are characterized by high levels of female demand and male withdrawal, domestically violent couples are characterized by high levels of both female demand/male withdrawal and male demand/female withdrawal (Babcock, Waltz, Jacobson, & Gottman, 1993; see also Stanley et al., in press, for a discussion of this pattern in male same-sex relationships). This pattern of findings has often been interpreted as indicating that male partners are the driving force behind marital violence, because only their behavior distinguishes between distressed couples who are and are not severely violent. For example, Jacobson et al. (1994) conclude that "Indeed, everything we found in our analyses of violent arguments is consistent with the notion that it is the men who are driving the system" (p. 987). Such interpretations are biased toward holding men solely responsible for the dynamics of abusive relationships, despite clear evidence to the contrary. Our interpretation of these findings is more balanced: Relationships are likely to escalate to severe violence only when *both* members of a couple reciprocate negativity on the part of their partners and act in an attacking and belligerent manner.

With few exceptions (e.g., Babcock, Jacobson, Gottman, & Yerington, 2000), interactional approaches to partner violence have been aimed at exploring the interpersonal context of violence without paying attention to psychosocial variables that might affect partners' likelihood of adopting particular interaction strategies. As would be expected from general interpersonal principles (e.g., Kiesler, 1983), it appears that negative reciprocity is generally required for couples to escalate to clinical levels of abuse. However, interaction studies do not address why only some women and men reciprocate hostility in their intimate relationships. Based on the longitudinal findings of Ehrensaft et al. (2004) and Moffitt et al. (2001), we can extrapolate that such mutually reinforcing negative dynamics are predictable from developmental and personality characteristics of both partners. Attachment theory may be helpful in creating a conceptual link between these psychological and interactional approaches to partner violence.

A DYADIC ATTACHMENT PERSPECTIVE ON PARTNER ABUSE

Although attachment theory is an intrinsically interpersonal theory, much of attachment research has focused on how individual differences in attachment affect individuals' psychological and social functioning. Considerably less attention has been paid to how both partners' attachment orientations interact in the development of a given relationship and how, in turn, relationship experiences influence each partner's attachment orientation. As argued by Mikulincer and colleagues (2002), the attachment-related emotions, cognitions, and behaviors of each individual in a relationship will be dependent on the corresponding emotions, cognitions, and behaviors of their partner (see also Feeney, 2003). Individuals bring particular attachment-related tendencies to a relationship (expectations, interaction goals, strategies for affect regulation, etc.), but the combination of both partners' tendencies results in a self-regulating couple system that is more than the sum of its parts. From a systemic perspective, a given relational behavior can be fully understood only within the context of the couple system. By applying this thinking to the study of partner violence, attachment theory has the potential to integrate psychological perspectives that focus on individual contributors to partner violence with interactional perspectives that focus on the interpersonal context in which violence occurs.

As far as we know, just five studies have included both partners in exploring the associations between individual differences in attachment and partner violence (Allison et al., 2005; Babcock et al., 2000; Kesner & McKenry, 1998; Landolt & Dutton, 1997; Roberts & Noller, 1998). However, in two of these studies, female partners' data were used solely to understand male perpetration of partner violence. Kesner and McKenry (1998) found associations between men's and women's attachment insecurity and male perpetration of partner abuse in a community sample of heterosexual couples. They did not consider how the attachment orientations of both partners might be associated with female perpetration of abuse or with different patterns of couple violence (e.g., reciprocal or one-sided violence). Based on women's descriptions of couple conflict, Babcock et al. (2000) reported that only preoccupied men responded to their female partner's withdrawal with violence. Based on observation and coding of men's facial, vocal, and body expressions in a couple interaction task, preoccupied and dismissing men displayed more dominance than secure men, and dismissing men were uniquely high on stonewalling (distancing behaviors). However, the wives' attachment orientations were not considered in these analyses, and it is not even clear whether Babcock et al. (2000) collected attachment data from their female participants. Moreover, the women's behaviors in the interaction task were not reported, which is unusual for a study of marital interaction. These omissions are especially noteworthy given that we know from a previous publication (Jacobson et al., 1994) that the majority of women in this sample had perpetrated violence against their partners. Thus it is unfortunate that Babcock and colleagues (2000) did not take advantage of the opportunity to look at the interactive processes associated with couple violence.

In contrast, Landolt and Dutton (1997), Roberts and Noller (1998), and Allison et al. (2005) adopted more systemic approaches to exploring partner violence. Landolt and Dutton (1997) looked at psychological and relational predictors of partner abuse in a sample of male same-sex couples. Results indicated that anxious attachment (both fearful and preoccupied) on the part of both partners was associated with a given partner's abusiveness. In fact, the attachment pattern of a recipient of abuse was just as predictive of victimization as was the attachment pattern of the perpetrator. Moreover, the same profile of attachment and other psychological variables (including borderline personality organization and anger proneness) characterized both members of gay couples with high levels of abuse. However, this study was limited by the arbitrary identification of one partner as the abuser and the other as the victim, in spite of high reciprocity of abuse across partners, and by a failure to consider how partners' attachment patterns might interact in predicting abusive behavior.

Roberts and Noller (1998) avoided these limitations in their study of attachment, communication, and partner violence in heterosexual couples. As expected, high attachment anxiety was predictive of partner violence for men and women. Moreover, the association between anxiety over abandonment and use of violence was significant only if a partner high in attachment anxiety was partnered with someone high in attachment avoidance. These findings suggest that individuals high in attachment anxiety may actively seek greater closeness in their relationships, while their avoidant partners may withdraw from the anxious partner's needy, demanding, or clingy behavior. When their attempts to engage their avoidant partners fail, anxious individuals may sometimes strike out violently in an attempt to force their partners to pay attention and move closer to them. However, rather than drawing closer, avoidant partners are likely to respond to such demands with further distance, setting in motion a self-perpetuating positive feedback loop.

Allison et al. (2005) took a qualitative approach to exploring the attachment dynamics of a sample of 23 couples identified for male partner violence. The attachment orientations of both partners were coded using the four-prototype model of attachment (Bartholomew, 1990; Bartholomew & Horowitz, 1991), and interviews in which partners individually described their intimate relationship were qualitatively analyzed in order to uncover dynamics associated with partner violence. We observed that partner violence was often part of a coherent strategy to regulate closeness. In particular, we observed two strategies that were consistently used to regulate closeness: *pursuing* and *distancing*. Pursuing involved attempts to gain and/or maintain closeness to a partner, whereas distancing involved attempts to decrease closeness to a partner. Violence was generally enacted only when previous strategies failed to bring a partner closer or to push a partner away. Moreover, the same relational behaviors could reflect different strategies, depending on the motivations of the individual and the relational context. For example, engagement in an extramarital affair was sometimes a pursuing strategy—attempting to regain attention from a partner or to elicit jealousy—and at other times a distancing strategy, attempting to disengage from a partner who made excessive emotional demands.

There was a tendency for the distance-regulation strategies, including violence, to be associated with certain attachment orientations: pursuing with preoccupied attachment and distancing with fearful and dismissing attachment. However, the dynamics of these relationships could not be understood simply in light of one individual's attachment profile. Rather, they required an examination of the interplay of both partners' attachment profiles. We observed two common interpersonal patterns in these couples: pursuing/distancing and pursuing/pursuing. The pursuing/distancing pattern tended to occur in couples with incompatible attachment needs (i.e., closeness vs. distance), similar to the demand/withdrawal pattern noted by Christensen and colleagues (Christensen & Heavey, 1990; Sagrestano, Heavey, & Christensen, 1998). Consistent with Roberts and Noller's (1998) and Babcock et al.'s (2000) findings, we generally observed this pattern when individuals with preoccupied tendencies were partnered with more avoidant (fearful or dismissing) individuals. Preoccupied partners sometimes struck out violently when their attachment anxiety was activated by relational events and nonviolent pursuit strategies failed (e.g., requests for attention, attempts to communicate, verbal abuse, expressions of jealousy). In turn, avoidant partners felt engulfed and overwhelmed by their partner's pursuit and attempted to distance themselves through emotional, verbal, and physical disengagement. When their nonviolent distancing strategies failed, avoidant partners sometimes reacted with violence to push their partners away. Thus at times both preoccupied and avoidant partners resorted to violence when their partners failed to respond to their other attempts to regulate the degree of emotional and physical closeness. In contrast, the pursuing/pursuing pattern tended to occur in couples in which both partners showed moderate to high levels of preoccupation. Feeney (2003) has described this pattern as "mutual attack-and-retreat" (p. 151). This type of interaction is also consistent with previous evidence that violent couples are characterized by high reciprocity of negativity and hostility. When both partners showed preoccupied tendencies, they tended to compete for support and attention from each other. Moreover, neither partner was able to recognize or meet his or her partner's needs, leading to mutual frustration and, at times, aggression.

In summary, the few studies to investigate the role of attachment in violent couples suggest that the intra- and interpersonal needs and goals associated with particular attachment patterns may give rise to violence when partners are not able to satisfy one another's needs through other means. Partner violence as a pursuit behavior is consistent with prior attachment-based conceptualizations of violence as a dysfunctional form of protest behavior. However, the observation that partner violence can also occur as a means of creating distance from a partner, an idea first proposed by Roberts and Noller (1998), suggests that this conceptualization may be incomplete. Rather, partner violence may reflect attempts to increase or decrease distance, depending on individual interaction goals and the dyadic context.

We expect that the links between attachment and violence are considerably more complex than our previous analysis would suggest. In particular, it will be essential for future work to explicate the specific mediators between attachment goals and violent incidents, including relational triggers of violence and the attributional processes and communication patterns of both partners. More generally, our focus on abuse as a form of attachment behavior is clearly too narrow. Not only may attachment needs directly drive abusive behaviors but attachment may also play an indirect role in the development and maintenance of abusive relationships. For example, the relationship expectations and attribution biases associated with forms of attachment insecurity may be helpful in explaining the willingness of some individuals to establish relationships that exhibit clear signs of problems from the outset, as well as their willingness to stay in relationships that have become highly dysfunctional. For example, preoccupied individuals may be at heightened risk for establishing and staying in problematic relationships because of their high emotional dependency (e.g., Alonso-Arbiol, Shaver, & Yarnoz, 2002) and their tendency to idealize romantic partners (Bartholomew & Horowitz, 1991). Within romantic relationships, preoccupied individuals may be especially prone to experience conflict and abuse because of their negative appraisals of partner behaviors (e.g., Collins, 1996) and even because of their apparent interpretation of high relationship conflict as indicating intimacy and engagement (Pietromonaco & Feldman Barrett, 1997). These processes are also expected to hinder the ability of romantic partners to negotiate the inevitable challenges of close relationships. Moreover, attachment concepts may be helpful in understanding instances in which abuse is not directly serving attachment needs. For example, hostile attributional styles and lack of empathy associated with insecure attachment may be predictive of retaliatory or vengeful violence (Mikulincer, 1988; Mikulincer & Shaver, 2005).

Attachment theory can provide a theoretical framework for understanding links between childhood family experiences and subsequent experiences with partner violence. However, no attachment-guided studies to date have fully incorporated a consideration of family and relational history into the study of violent couples. We predict that individuals whose attachment histories have fostered some degree of attachment security and a relatively positive orientation toward close relationships are highly unlikely to become involved in violent relationships. We would not expect such individuals to become entrenched in the interpersonal dynamics associated with violent relationships, and we would expect such individuals to leave relationships in which a romantic partner begins to show abusive behavior. Although we have not systematically addressed this issue in our work, in all of our studies that have included histories of attachment relationships, we have yet to come across an individual in a severely abusive relationship (male or female, perpetrator and/or victim) who did not report a dysfunctional family background.

Another promising direction for future work is the role of caregiving in the development of abusive relationships (see Collins, Guichard, Ford, & Feeney, Chapter 7, this volume, for another discussion of caregiving). We expect that a consideration of caregiving needs, as related to but conceptually distinct from attachment needs, will broaden and clarify our understanding of abusive dynamics. We predict that both partners in violent relationships tend to be characterized by global deficits in support seeking and caregiving: deficits in the ability to effectively ask for care, in the ability to perceive and appropriately respond to a partner's need for care, and even in the ability to accept and benefit from partner care. In addition, we speculate that compulsive caregiving by one partner toward the other may play an important role in some abusive relationships. In relationships in which a partner's attachment needs are chronically frustrated, caregiving may indirectly fulfill attachment needs and may even serve to inhibit the activation of the attachment system. Again, it will be essential to consider how caregiving and attachment motivations and behaviors of both partners interact.

CLINICAL IMPLICATIONS

Feminist perspectives on partner violence have largely shaped treatment programs for partner abuse. Thus therapists, clinical researchers, and lawmakers focus almost exclusively on the violent behavior of male partners in heterosexual relationships. Although treatments have been informed, to some degree, by findings regarding the psychological correlates of male violence, they have rarely taken into consideration findings regarding the dyadic context of partner violence. They have disregarded the empirical evidence that heterosexual partner abuse is often reciprocal and that both partners are involved in the development and maintenance of abusive dynamics. It is notable that in dealing with couples experiencing distress, marital therapists routinely locate the problem within the dyad rather than within one individual in the dyad. Yet in the case of partner abuse, the dominant treatment approach involves only the male partner and focuses only on his abuse perpetration.

We believe it is problematic, and potentially unethical, to treat only the male partners in violent relationships. Focusing exclusively on men as batterers blames men for partner violence that is likely to be the result of reciprocal interactions, and it fails to address the issue of female-to-male partner violence. Treated men are likely to remain in relationships with women who may be just as or more violent than themselves. Furthermore, treating only the male partner encourages the women to externalize their abusive behaviors and to make stable, global, and internal attributions about men's violent behavior. This seems likely to put men at increased risk for female-to-male violence, which may in turn put women at continued risk for male-to-female violence. Ironically, one of the major reasons for not treating both partners in a violent couple is concern for the safety of women victims. Ensuring client safety is an ethical imperative for therapists. However, given the compelling evidence that men, as well as women, are at risk for receipt of violence from a partner, safety concerns should also be extended to men in these relationships. Moreover, even were we to accept (and we do not) that conjoint treatment puts only women at increased risk for violence, there are procedures for minimizing safety risks (see Stith, Rosen, & McCollum, 2003; Stith, Rosen, McCollum, & Thomsen, 2004).

Given the shaky theoretical foundations of treatment that targets men as batterers, it is not surprising that there is little empirical support for the effectiveness of this mode of treatment (e.g., Babcock, Green, & Robie, 2004). Yet the assumptions underlying this approach have become entrenched in government policy, in the criminal justice system, and, correspondingly, in treatment protocols. In a review of U.S. standards for batterer intervention programs, Austin and Dankwort (1999) reported that couple counseling was judged to be an inappropriate initial intervention in 25 of the 31 states that had developed standards for batterer treatment. This is particularly troubling in light of Babcock et al.'s (2004) meta-analysis of the effectiveness of batterer treatment programs. Effect sizes were at best .34 for quasi-experimental research designs, and at worst .09 for experimental research designs (generally using a Duluth or cognitive-behavioral therapy model). In contrast, Smith, Glass, and Miller (1980, as cited in Babcock et al., 2004) reported an average effect size across psychotherapy studies of .85. Clearly there is room for incorporating a more relational perspective in treatment for partner violence.

There is a small but growing trend toward incorporating couple treatment into more traditional approaches to treating partner violence. For instance, Heyman and Schlee (2003) presented evidence that their physical aggression couples treatment (PACT), a 14-session program including both intrapersonal and interpersonal aspects, was as effective as gender-specific treatment. In this treatment, therapists take a "no blame" (p. 138) stance to gain the trust of both partners, thereby enhancing the therapeutic alliance. Attachment theory would seem to be uniquely suited to such an approach because it includes both intrapersonal and interpersonal aspects of emotion, cognition, and behavior. Sonkin and Dutton (2003) proposed that gender-specific male batterer programs could profitably be grounded in an attachment perspective; but they did not suggest attachment-based conjoint treatment. Interestingly, Johnson (1996) has suggested that emotionally focused marital therapy (EFT), based on attachment theory, should be considered only after abusive partners have completed more traditional treatment programs for violence. However, we see no reason why the safety procedures developed in the context of other treatment approaches could not also be used in the context of EFT for partner abuse.

Therapists who treat couples from an attachment perspective aim to provide a secure base and safe haven in therapy to foster the creation of a secure bond in distressed couples. Such an approach acknowledges the importance of having attachment figures who are dependable and predictable, even in adulthood (e.g., Johnson, 2003). Moreover, viewing the occurrence of partner violence within an attachment framework can assist therapists to lead their clients to a stance that is not blaming (Heyman & Schlee, 2003), while still emphasizing the importance of taking personal responsibility for abusive behavior. In fact, Hamel (2005) suggests specific interventions for treating partner violence that draw on an attachment perspective: (1) highlighting the role of attachment orientations in conflict and violence, (2) establishing a secure base in therapy, (3) defining clear but reasonable relationship boundaries that will allow partners to pursue both their closeness and independence needs, and (4) identifying irrational beliefs that have arisen out of current and previous relationships.

Stith et al. (2004) have recently developed and investigated multicouple treatment for partner violence. Such an approach may be useful because it gives couples the opportunity to view the impact of negative and positive interactions in other couples who are similar to themselves. Thus partners may come to view their own interactions more objectively. In fact, qualitative feedback obtained from clients indicated that they valued hearing about other couples' experiences with partner abuse, appreciated the support they gave and received in the group, and felt that they benefited from both active and passive learning from other couples. Moreover, clients commented on the importance of the "vicarious communication" (Stith et al., 2004, p. 316) that occurred when other group members raised issues they themselves were afraid to raise with their own partners. These advantages appear to parallel those claimed by clinicians who practice multiple family therapy. Preliminary evidence suggests that multicouple treatment groups for couple violence may offer benefits over and above those of individual couple treatment. For instance, Stith et al. (2004) found that marital aggression decreased and marital satisfaction increased for couples who participated in a multicouple treatment condition, but not for those who participated in individual couple treatment or a comparison condition. This pattern held for both men and women. Moreover, the 6-month recidivism rate for men in the multicouple condition was significantly lower than for men in the other conditions. The inclusion of an attachment perspective in multicouple treatment for partner abuse may further enhance this treatment approach. For instance, we believe that it would be feasible and potentially beneficial to conduct EFT for couples in a multicouple format.

QUALIFICATIONS AND FINAL THOUGHTS

Our work on partner violence has taken place in a decidedly Western context. As far as we know, all of the published research on partner violence guided by an attachment perspective and all of the published research looking at both members of violent couples has been done in Western cultures. More specifically, the overwhelming majority of this work has been conducted in the United States, Canada, United Kingdom, Australia, or New Zealand. These countries share some important features: strong norms against male violence toward women, equitable roles of men and women within marital relationships (e.g., Coleman & Straus, 1990), the freedom to choose romantic partners, and relatively easy access to divorce. In these conditions, feminist models may be less helpful in explaining partner abuse, and psychosocial models such as attachment theory may be applicable. However, in cultural contexts in which male violence toward women is condoned, in which men hold more power than women, and in which individuals (and especially women) have less control over their marital relationships, an attachment perspective may have less to offer, and feminist models may become more useful.

Concerns have repeatedly been raised in the field of domestic violence that psychological and interactional perspectives on partner abuse may undermine responsibility for inappropriate behavior and shift responsibility to the victim. Although such concerns are understandable, we feel they are misguided. Our goal is to understand how and why abusive dynamics develop in some intimate relationships, with the hope that this understanding will inform prevention and treatment efforts. We see no contradiction between holding individuals responsible for their behavior (especially in a legal sense) and attempting to understand that behavior, whether in terms of individuals' backgrounds and characteristics or in terms of the relational context in which aggression occurs. A psychological understanding of a behavior does not condone the behavior. We believe that all partners should be held fully responsible for any abuse they perpetrate in their relationships and that violent women should be held to the same standard of responsibility as violent men. Anything less perpetuates the very gender-based biases that feminists have worked so hard to overcome.

We are confident that developing a more accurate and complete understanding of partner violence will ultimately serve all victims of partner violence, regardless of gender. In contrast, willfully ignoring the potential role of both partners in the development of violent relationships, in spite of overwhelming evidence, will only serve to slow progress toward the collective goal of reducing the incidence of partner violence. We therefore encourage researchers and clinicians alike to draw on empirical findings about partner violence in the development and study of new and more effective approaches to prevention and treatment. In particular, we are hopeful that a systemic model of partner violence guided by attachment theory will integrate previous research findings, point to fruitful new directions of study, and help guide the design of more effective interventions for couples experiencing violence.

REFERENCES

Allison, C. J., Bartholomew, K., Mayseless, O., & Dutton, D. G. (2005). *Love as a battlefield: Attachment and relationship dynamics in couples identified for male partner violence.* Unpublished manuscript, Simon Fraser University, Vancouver, British Columbia, Canada.

Alonso-Arbiol, I., Shaver, P. R., & Yarnoz, S. (2002). Insecure attachment, gender roles, and interpersonal dependency in the Basque Country. *Personal Relationships, 9,* 479–490.

Anderson, K. L. (1997). Gender, status, and domestic violence: An integration of feminist and family violence approaches. *Journal of Marriage and the Family, 59,* 655–669.

Anglin, K., & Holtzworth-Munroe, A. (1997). Comparing the responses of maritally violent and nonviolent spouses to problematic marital and nonmarital situations: Are the skill deficits of physically aggressive husbands and wives global? *Journal of Family Psychology, 11,* 301–313.

Archer, J. (2000). Sex differences in aggression between heterosexual partners: A meta-analytic review. *Psychological Bulletin, 126,* 651–680.

Austin, J. B., & Dankwort, J. (1999). Standards for batterer programs: A review and analysis. *Journal of Interpersonal Violence, 14,* 152–168.

Babcock, J. C., Green, C. E., & Robie, C. (2004). Does batterers' treatment work? A meta-analytic review of domestic violence treatment. *Clinical Psychology Review, 23,* 1023–1053.

Babcock, J. C., Jacobson, N. S., Gottman, J. M., & Yerington, T. P. (2000). Attachment, emotional regulation, and the function of marital violence: Differences between secure, preoccupied, and dismissing violent and nonviolent husbands. *Journal of Family Violence, 15,* 391–409.

Babcock, J. C., Waltz, J., Jacobson, N. S., & Gottman, J. M. (1993). Power and violence: The relation between communication patterns, power discrepancies, and domestic violence. *Journal of Consulting and Clinical Psychology, 61,* 40–50.

Banse, R. (2004). Adult attachment and marital satisfaction: Evidence for dyadic configuration effects. *Journal of Social and Personal Relationships, 21,* 273–282.

Bartholomew, K. (1990). Avoidance of intimacy: An attachment perspective. *Journal of Social and Personal Relationships, 7,* 147–178.

Bartholomew, K., Henderson, A. J. Z., & Dutton, D. G. (2001). Insecure attachment and abusive intimate relationships. In C. Clulow (Ed.), *Adult attachment and couple work: Applying the "secure base" concept in research and practice* (pp. 43–61). London: Routledge.

Bartholomew, K., & Horowitz, L. M. (1991). Attachment styles among young adults: A test of a four-category model. *Journal of Personality and Social Psychology, 61,* 226–244.

Bartholomew, K., Landolt, M. A., & Oram, D. (1999, August). *Abuse in male same-sex relationships: Prevalence, incidence, and injury.* Paper presented at the annual convention of the American Psychological Association, Boston.

Bartholomew, K., Oram, D., & Landolt, M. (2000, August). *Attachment and abuse in male same-sex relationships.* Paper presented at the annual convention of the American Psychological Association, Washington, DC.

Bograd, M. (1988). Feminist perspectives on wife abuse: An introduction. In M.

Bograd & K. Yllo (Eds.), *Feminist perspectives on wife abuse* (pp. 11–26). Beverly Hills, CA: Sage.

Bookwala, J., & Zdaniuk, B. (1998). Adult attachment styles and aggressive behavior within dating relationships. *Journal of Social and Personal Relationships, 15,* 175–190.

Bowlby, J. (1969). *Attachment and loss: Vol. 1. Attachment.* New York: Basic Books.

Bowlby, J. (1984). Violence in the family as a disorder of the attachment and caregiving systems. *American Journal of Psychoanalysis, 44,* 9–27.

Bradbury, T. N., Fincham, F. D., & Beach, S. R. H. (2000). Research on the nature and determinants of marital satisfaction: A decade in review. *Journal of Marriage and the Family,* 6, 964–981.

Burman, B., Margolin, G., & John, R. S. (1993). America's angriest home videos: Behavioral contingencies observed in home reenactments of marital conflict. *Journal of Consulting and Clinical Psychology,* 6, 28–39.

Cascardi, M., & Vivian, D. (1995). Context for specific episodes of marital violence: Gender and severity of violence differences. *Journal of Family Violence, 10,* 265–293.

Christensen, A., & Heavey, C. (1990). Gender and social structure in the demand/withdraw pattern of marital conflict. *Journal of Personality and Social Psychology, 59,* 73–81.

Coleman, D. H., & Straus, M. A. (1990). Marital power, conflict, and violence in a nationally representative sample of American couples. In M. A. Straus & R. J. Gelles (Eds.), *Physical violence in American families: Risk factors and adaptations to violence in 8,145 families* (pp. 287–304). New Brunswick, NJ: Transaction.

Collins, N. (1996). Working models of attachment: Implications for explanation, emotion, and behavior. *Journal of Personality and Social Psychology, 71,* 810–832.

Cordova, J. V., Jacobson, N. S., Gottman, J. M., Rushe, R., & Cox, G. (1993). Negative reciprocity and communication in couples with a violent husband. *Journal of Abnormal Psychology, 102,* 559–564.

Cruz, J. M., & Firestone, J. M. (1998). Exploring violence and abuse in gay male relationships. *Violence and Victims, 13,* 159–173.

DeKeseredy, W. S., & Schwartz, M. D. (1998). *Woman abuse on campus: Results from the Canadian national survey.* Thousand Oaks, CA: Sage.

Dobash, R. E., & Dobash, R. P. (1979). *Violence against wives: A case against the patriarchy.* New York: Free Press.

Dutton, D. G. (1994). Patriarchy and wife assault: The ecological fallacy. *Violence and Victims, 9,* 125–140.

Dutton, D. G. (1995). *The batterer: A psychological profile.* New York: Basic Books.

Dutton, D. G., & Nicholls, T. L. (2005). The gender paradigm in domestic violence research and theory: The conflict of theory and data. *Aggression and Violent Behavior, 10,* 680–714.

Dutton, D. G., & Painter, S. L. (1993). Emotional attachment in abusive relationships: A test of traumatic bonding theory. *Violence and Victims, 8,* 105–120.

Dutton, D. G., Saunders, K., Starzomski, A. J., & Bartholomew, K. (1994). Intimacy-anger and insecure attachment as precursors of abuse in intimate relationships. *Journal of Applied Social Psychology, 24,* 1367–1386.

Ehrensaft, M. K., Cohen, P., Brown, J., Smailes, E., Chen, H., & Johnson, J. G. (2003). Intergenerational transmission of partner violence: A 20-year prospective study. *Journal of Consulting and Clinical Psychology, 71*, 741–753.

Ehrensaft, M. K., Moffitt, T. E., & Caspi, A. (2004). Clinically abusive relationships in an unselected birth cohort: Men's and women's participation and developmental antecedents. *Journal of Abnormal Psychology, 113*, 258–271.

Feeney, J. A. (2003). The systemic nature of couple relationships: An attachment perspective. In P. Erdman & T. Caffrey (Eds.), *Attachment and family systems* (pp. 139–163). New York: Brunner-Routledge.

Fowers, B. J., & Olson, D. H. (1986). Predicting marital success with PREPARE: A predictive validity study. *Journal of Marital and Family Therapy, 12*, 403–413.

George, M. J. (2003). Invisible touch. *Aggression and Violent Behavior, 8*, 23–60.

Giles-Sims, J. (1998). The aftermath of partner violence. In J. L. Jasinski & L. M. Williams (Eds.), *Partner violence: A comprehensive review of 20 years of research* (pp. 44–72). London: Sage.

Gwartney-Gibbs, P. A., Stockard, J., & Bohmer, S. (1987). Learning courtship aggression: The influence of parents, peers, and personal experiences. *Family Relations, 36*, 276–282.

Hamel, J. (2005). *Gender inclusive treatment of intimate partner abuse: A comprehensive approach*. New York: Springer.

Henderson, A. J. Z., Bartholomew, K., & Dutton, D. G. (1997). He loves me; he loves me not: Attachment and separation resolution of abused women. *Journal of Family Violence, 12*, 169–191.

Henderson, A. J. Z., Bartholomew, K., Trinke, S., & Kwong, M. J. (2005). When loving means hurting: An exploration of attachment and intimate abuse in a community sample. *Journal of Family Violence, 20*, 219–230.

Heyman, R. E., & Schlee, K. (2003). Stopping wife abuse via physical aggression couples treatment. *Journal of Aggression, 7*, 135–157.

Holtzworth-Munroe, A., & Hutchinson, G. (1993). Attributing negative intent to wife behavior: The attributions of maritally violent versus nonviolent men. *Journal of Abnormal Psychology, 102*, 206–211.

Holtzworth-Munroe, A., & Stuart, G. (1994). Typologies of male batterers: Three subtypes and the differences among them. *Psychological Bulletin, 116*, 476–497.

Holtzworth-Munroe, A., Stuart, G., & Hutchinson, G. (1997). Violent versus nonviolent husbands: Differences in attachment patterns, dependency, and jealousy. *Journal of Family Psychology, 11*, 314–331.

Jacobson, N. S. (1994). Rewards and dangers in researching domestic violence. *Family Process, 33*, 81–95.

Jacobson, N. S., Gottman, J. M., Waltz, J., Rushe, R., Babcock, J., & Holtzworth-Munroe, A. (1994). Affect, verbal content, and psychophysiology in the arguments of couples with a violent husband. *Journal of Consulting and Clinical Psychology, 62*, 982–988.

Johnson, S. M. (1996). *The practice of emotionally focused marital therapy: Creating connection*. New York: Brunner/Mazel.

Johnson, S. M. (2003). Introduction to attachment: A therapist's guide to primary relationships and their renewal. In S. M. Johnson & V. E. Whiffen (Eds.), *Attachment processes in couple and family therapy* (pp. 3–17). New York: Guilford Press.

Karney, B. R., & Bradbury, T. N. (1995). The longitudinal course of marital quality and stability: A review of theory, method, and research. *Psychology Bulletin, 188*, 3–34.

Kesner, J. E., & McKenry, P. C. (1998). The role of childhood attachment factors in predicting male violence toward female intimates. *Journal of Family Violence, 13*, 417–432.

Kiesler, D. J. (1983). The 1982 interpersonal circle: A taxonomy for complementarity in human transactions. *Psychological Review, 90*, 185–214.

Kobak, R. R., & Sceery, A. (1988). Attachment in late adolescence: Working models, affect regulation, and representations of self and others. *Child Development, 59*, 135–146.

Krueger, R. F., Moffitt, T. E., Caspi, A., Bleske, A., & Silva, P. A. (1998). Assortative mating for antisocial behavior: Developmental and methodological implications. *Behavior Genetics, 28*, 173–185.

Kwong, M. J., Bartholomew, K., Henderson, A. J. Z., & Trinke, S. (2003). The intergenerational transmission of relationship violence. *Journal of Family Psychology, 17*, 288–301.

Landolt, M. A., & Dutton, D. G. (1997). Power and personality: An analysis of gay male intimate abuse. *Sex Roles, 37*, 335–359.

Leonard, K. E. (1993). Drinking patterns and intoxication in marital violence: Review, critique, and future directions for research. In S. E. Martin (Ed.), *Alcohol and interpersonal violence: Fostering interdisciplinary research* (NIAAA Research Monograph No. 24, NIH Publication No. 93-3496). Rockville, MD: National Institutes of Health.

Leonard, K. E., & Senchak, M. (1996). Prospective prediction of husband marital aggression within newlywed couples. *Journal of Abnormal Psychology, 105*, 369–380.

Lie, G., Schilit, R., Bush, J., Montague, M., & Reyes, L. (1991). Lesbians in currently aggressive relationships: How frequently do they report aggressive past relationships? *Violence and Victims, 6*, 121–135.

Magdol, L., Moffitt, T. E., Caspi, A., Newman, D. L., Fagan, J., & Silva, P. A. (1997). Gender differences in partner violence in a birth cohort of 21-year-olds: Bridging the gap between clinical and epidemiological approaches. *Journal of Consulting and Clinical Psychology, 65*, 68–78.

Mikulincer, M. (1998). Adult attachment style and individual differences in functional versus dysfunctional experiences of anger. *Journal of Personality and Social Psychology, 74*, 513–524.

Mikulincer, M., Florian, V., Cowan, P., & Cowan, C. (2002). Attachment security in couple relationships: A systemic model and its implications for family dynamics. *Family Process, 41*, 405–434.

Mikulincer, M., & Shaver, P. R. (2005). Attachment theory and emotions in close relationships: Exploring the attachment-related dynamics of emotional reactions to relational events. *Personal Relationships, 12*, 149–168.

Moffitt, T. E., Krueger, R. F., Caspi, A., & Fagan, J. (2000). Partner abuse and general crime: How are they the same? *Criminology, 38*, 199–232.

Moffitt, T. E., Robins, R. W., & Caspi, A. (2001). A couples analysis of partner abuse with implications for abuse-prevention policy. *Criminology and Public Policy, 1*, 5–36.

Morse, B. J. (1995). Beyond the Conflict Tactics Scale: Assessing gender differences in partner violence. *Violence and Victims, 10*, 251–272.

Murphy, C. M., Meyer, S., & O'Leary, K. D. (1994). Dependency characteristics of partner assaultive men. *Journal of Abnormal Psychology, 103*, 729–735.

Pietromonaco, P. R., & Feldman Barrett, L. (1997). Working models of attachment and daily social interactions. *Journal of Personality and Social Psychology, 73*, 1409–1423.

Regan, K., Bartholomew, K., Oram, D., & Landolt, M. (2002, July). *Reciprocity of physical violence in male same-sex relationships.* Paper presented at the International Conference on Personal Relationships, Halifax, Nova Scotia, Canada.

Roberts, N., & Noller, P. (1998). The associations between adult attachment and couple violence: The role of communication patterns and relationship satisfaction. In J. A. Simpson & W. S. Rholes (Eds.), *Attachment theory and close relationships* (pp. 317–350). New York: Guilford Press.

Robins, R. W., Caspi, A., & Moffitt, T. E. (2000). Two personalities, one relationship: Both partners' personality traits shape the quality of their relationship. *Journal of Personality and Social Psychology, 79*, 251–259.

Robins, R. W., Caspi, A., & Moffitt, T. E. (2002). It's not just who you're with, it's who you are: Personality and relationship experiences across multiple relationships. *Journal of Personality, 70*, 925–964.

Rusbult, C. E., & Martz, J. M. (1995). Remaining in an abusive relationship: An investment model analysis of nonvoluntary dependence. *Personality and Social Psychology Bulletin, 21*, 558–571.

Sagrestano, L., Heavey, C., & Christensen, A. (1998). Theoretical approaches to understanding sex differences and similarities in conflict behavior. In D. Canary & K. Dindia (Eds.), *Sex differences and similarities in communications: Critical essays and empirical investigations of sex and gender in interaction* (pp. 287–302). Mahwah, NJ: Erlbaum.

Sagrestano, L. M., Heavey, C. L., & Christensen, A. (1999). Perceived power and physical violence in marital conflict. *Journal of Social Issues, 55*, 65–79.

Shaver, P. R., & Mikulincer, M. (2003, May). *Attachment, compassion, and altruism.* Paper presented at the Conference on Compassionate Love, Normal, IL.

Simon, T. R., Anderson, M., Thomson, M. P., Crosby, A. E., Shelley, G., & Sacks, J. J. (2001). Attitudinal acceptance of intimate partner violence among U. S. adults. *Violence and Victims, 16*, 115–126.

Sonkin, D. J., & Dutton, D. (2003). Treating assaultive men from an attachment perspective. *Journal of Aggression, Maltreatment, and Trauma, 7*, 105–133.

Stanley, J., Bartholomew, K., Taylor, T., Landolt, M., & Oram, D. (in press). An exploration of partner violence in male same-sex relationships. *Journal of Family Violence.*

Stets, J. E., & Straus, M. A. (1990a). Gender differences in reporting marital violence and its medical and psychological consequences. In M. A. Straus & R. J. Gelles (Eds.), *Physical violence in American families: Risk factors and adaptations to violence in 8,145 families* (pp. 151–165). New Brunswick, NJ: Transaction.

Stets, J. E., & Straus, M. A. (1990b). The marriage license as a hitting license: A comparison of assaults in dating, cohabiting, and married couples. In M. A. Straus & R. J. Gelles (Eds.), *Physical violence in American families: Risk factors and adaptations to violence in 8,145 families* (pp. 227–244). New Brunswick, NJ: Transaction.

Stith, S. M., Rosen, K. H., & McCollum, E. E. (2003). Effectiveness of couples treatment for spouse abuse. *Journal of Marital and Family Therapy, 29*, 407–426.

Stith, S. M., Rosen, K. H., McCollum, E. E., & Thomsen, C. J. (2004). Treating intimate partner violence within intact couple relationships: Outcomes of multi-couple versus individual couple therapy. *Journal of Marital and Family Therapy, 30*, 305–318.

Sugarman, D. B., & Frankel, S. L. (1996). Patriarchal ideology and wife assault: A meta-analytic review. *Journal of Family Violence, 11*, 13–40.

6

Sex Differences in Jealousy

A Matter of Evolution or Attachment History?

KENNETH N. LEVY, KRISTEN M. KELLY, and EJAY L. JACK

Jealousy is a powerful and painful emotion with pernicious effects on romantic relationships (White & Mullen, 1989). It has been implicated as the leading cause of spouse battering and homicide across many cultures (Daly & Wilson, 1988; Gibbens, 1958; Wolfgang, 1958). Historically, jealousy has been conceptualized as a consequence of low self-esteem or even neurosis (Mathes, Phillips, Skowron, & Dick, 1982; Pines & Aronson, 1983). Nearly two-thirds of romantic couples reported that jealousy posed a significant problem in their relationship, sometimes leading to assaults or battery (Gayford, 1975, 1979). Research has linked spousal abuse, rapes, and stalking behavior to feelings of jealousy (Davis, Ace, & Andra, 2000; Dutton, van Ginkel, & Landolt, 1996; Tjaden & Thoennes, 1998). If jealousy can be understood through developmental analysis rather than attributed to biological evolution, it might be easier to manage through education and clinical treatment. Although evolutionary psychologists (e.g., Thornhill & Palmer, 2000) have argued that evolutionary analyses of sex differences in socially undesirable behaviors do not imply that the behaviors cannot be socially controlled, viewing these behaviors as strongly attributable to evolved genetic mechanisms clearly makes them seem virtually inevitable and hence difficult to change.

Evolutionary psychologists have distinguished between two kinds of jealousy: sexual and emotional (e.g., Buss, Larsen, Westen, & Semmelroth, 1992). Sexual jealousy is evoked by a perceived threat concerning a partner's sexual infidelity, whereas emotional jealousy arises from a perceived threat of a partner's emotional infidelity. Sexual jealousy is reportedly more common in men than in women. Across a wide variety of cultures, men are more likely than women to divorce partners who are sexually unfaithful (Betzig, 1989) and even to batter and kill such partners (Daly & Wilson, 1988). Given the seriousness and pervasiveness of these effects of male sexual jealousy, it is important to understand its causes and dynamics. In this chapter we argue that attachment theory provides a framework for understanding jealousy and for changing attitudes and beliefs in ways that may reduce the tragic consequences of jealousy that occurs in the context of romantic relationships.

THE EVOLUTIONARY EXPLANATION OF SEX DIFFERENCES IN JEALOUSY

David Buss and his colleagues have offered an evolutionary explanation of sex differences in jealousy. They and other proponents of the evolutionary perspective assert that men and women evolved different sexual strategies (Buss, 1995; Daly & Wilson, 1988; Daly, Wilson, & Weghorst, 1982; Symons, 1979). For male mammals, gamete production is relatively inexpensive, because sperm are continuously and copiously produced. For female mammals, however, gamete production is more limited, there being only a few hundred gametes that become mature over a female's relatively short reproductive life cycle. Thus, even at the time of fertilization, women have contributed a greater proportion of net resources to future offspring than men have; women typically go on to invest more bodily resources in nursing and caring for offspring than men do. From these facts, evolutionary psychologists conclude that there is likely to be conflict between men and women due to differences in their mating strategies (Buss, 1995). Men can maximize their evolutionary fitness by impregnating as many women as possible while investing as little as possible in rearing any individual offspring. In contrast, women can maximize their fitness by carefully choosing a mating partner who will maximize their offspring's survival by providing support, protection, and "good genes" that get passed on to offspring. For women, it matters a great deal that some men more than others may be willing to provide the extended support and biparental care that increase the likelihood of offspring survival and health.

These differences in reproductive strategies are thought by evolutionary psychologists to produce inherent sex differences in types of jealousy. Whereas women bear the greater reproductive costs, the fact that fertilization occurs inside a woman's body means that men have always faced a profound adaptive problem not faced by women: uncertainty of paternity. Women are virtually certain which offspring are their own, but DNA studies indicate that between 9 and 13% of children have a putative father who is not the man who impregnated their mother (Baker & Bellis, 1995). Being uncertain of paternity presents substantial reproductive costs to men in the form of time, energy, nuptial gifts, and opportunity costs. The adaptive problem of uncertain paternity is exacerbated in species such as ours in which males often engage in postfertilization parental investment (Trivers, 1972). A man risks investing resources in a putative child who is not (genetically speaking) his own, thereby investing in another male's offspring while reducing his own evolutionary fitness. Evolutionary psychologists believe that male sexual jealousy evolved as a solution to this problem (Wilson & Daly, 1992).

In contrast, although women do not experience much uncertainty with regard to maternity, they do risk losing time, resources, and commitment from a man if he deserts her or channels investments to alternative mates (Trivers, 1972). Therefore, the evolutionary story says, women exercise more vigilance to prevent other women from absconding with their mates, rather than responding to specific acts of sexual infidelity, because a man's continued presence aids in successfully rearing offspring. Consistent with this notion that men are more bothered by sexual infidelity and women by emotional infidelity or loss of interest and commitment, research has found that men across a wide variety of cultures are more likely than women to divorce partners who are sexually unfaithful (Betzig, 1989) and possibly to batter or even kill partners who are unfaithful (Daly & Wilson, 1988). Conversely, women manifest greater distress while imagining their male partner's emotional infidelity (Buss et al., 1992), viewed as an important warning sign that their mate may withdraw his resources from the relationship and child.

In two large-sample tests of this line of reasoning, Buss et al. (1992) found that men tend to view sexual infidelity as more distressful than women do, and women tend to view emotional infidelity as more distressful. They also found that men displayed greater physiological distress than did women while imagining a mate's sexual infidelity, as reflected by increased electromyographic activity (i.e., muscle tension), increased electrodermal response (indicating autonomic arousal), and elevated heart rate.

These findings have been replicated by other researchers in the United States, Germany, the Netherlands, and China (Buunk, Angleiter, Oubaid, & Buss, 1996; Geary, Rumsey, Bow-Thomas, & Hoard, 1995; Wiederman & Allgeier, 1993). Buss and his colleagues (Buss, Kirkpatrick, Shackelford, &

Bennett, 1996) interpret the cross-cultural replicability of the sex differences as good evidence for their basis in genes and evolution.

ALTERNATIVES TO THE EVOLUTIONARY PERSPECTIVE

A number of researchers have challenged the evolutionary interpretation of sex differences in jealousy (DeSteno & Salovey, 1996a; Harris, 2003; Harris & Christenfeld, 1996; Rabinowitz & Valian, 2000). First, although cross-cultural data are crucial for testing the evolutionary hypothesis, they alone are not sufficient to support it. Second, it is especially important to rule out plausible alternative explanations in quasi-experimental studies such as these, in which biological sex serves as the independent variable, because men and women obviously cannot be randomly assigned to male and female conditions. In such studies, unmeasured variables are major threats to the validity of results and can lead to accepting spurious findings (Abelson, 1995). Third-variable correlations often cannot be accounted for, so it is quite possible that the replicable sex differences in types of jealousy are a result of other, nongenetic variables. Third, although a higher percentage of men than women report being more distressed by sexual infidelity, in many studies the majority of both genders are more distressed by emotional infidelity (Buss et al., 1992; Buunk et al., 1996; Geary et al., 1995; Wiederman & Allgeier, 1993). For instance, American men are equally divided on which form of infidelity is more distressing; the majority of Chinese, Dutch, and German men find emotional infidelity more distressing (see Buller, 2005, for a review). Thus Buss's theory does not fully or conclusively explain the data, and there are a number of reasonable alternative hypotheses. An evolutionary perspective on sex differences in jealousy cannot, without invoking additional constructs, explain these international differences within the sexes. Finally, evolutionary psychologists make "predictions" about events that have already occurred, based on assumptions and inferences about environments that generally cannot be tested. For instance, Eagly and Wood (1999) found a great deal of cross-cultural variability in the relative contributions of men and women to subsistence, with women sometimes contributing more. This variability makes it difficult to infer from evidence at hand what conditions prevailed for our ancestors.

TESTS OF ALTERNATIVE THEORIES

DeSteno and Salovey (1996a, 1996b) and Harris and Christenfeld (1996) considered most of the alternative explanations of sex differences in jealousy. Harris and Christenfeld's (1996) "rational belief hypothesis" suggests that sex differences may be based on a difference between the sexes in how they interpret evidence of infidelity, that is, a difference in reasoning or in operative rationality. They argue that, for cultural reasons, men are more likely to believe that women engage in sexual behavior when in love; and conversely, women are more likely to believe that men engage in sexual behavior independently of love. Thus men are more bothered by sexual infidelity because it signals that their mate has fallen in love with another man. Women, in contrast, may be bothered by sexual infidelity less than by emotional infidelity because sexual infidelity alone does not necessarily mean that her mate has fallen in love with someone else. These authors found support for their hypothesis in a survey of 137 people (Harris & Christenfeld, 1996). DeSteno and Salovey (1996a) proposed a "double-shot hypothesis." They contended that beliefs about types of infidelity are not as separable as might be expected. Instead, they argued, sex differences are due to different beliefs about the conditional probabilities that either sexual or emotional infidelity implies the occurrence of the other kind of infidelity. They found that both men and women selected the infidelity event that they believed was more likely to signal the concurrence of the other type of infidelity as well. Additionally, women more than men believed that emotional infidelity implied sexual infidelity. Thus the forced-choice dichotomy used by Buss and colleagues to study jealousy may not actually separate two interrelated kinds of jealousy.

It is important to realize, however, that the rational-belief and double-shot hypotheses do not explain cultural variation in sex differences in types of jealousy (Buss, Larsen, & Westen, 1996). Buss and colleagues noted that both hypotheses wrongly imply that socialization rather than genetics is the causal agent responsible for observed sex differences. They pointed out that biologically evolved sex differences might, in fact, explain the processes responsible for the rational-belief and double-shot phenomena. In support of their arguments, a recent series of empirical studies controlling for the correlated nature of infidelity types failed to replicate the findings reported by Harris and Christenfeld (1996) and DeSteno and Salovey (1996; Buss et al., 1999). The continued failure to resolve the debate between groups of theorists who favor an evolutionary explanation of sex differences in jealousy and groups who favor a nonbiological explanation suggests a need for a theory that explains both between- and within-sex differences, that distinguishes between socially and genetically mediated conditional probabilities of various implications of acts of infidelity, and that reveals why men often find sexual infidelity more distressing than emotional infidelity, whereas women often find emotional infidelity more distressing.

Rabinowitz and Valian (2000) and Eagly and Wood (1999) offered additional alternative explanations for sex differences in jealousy. They suggested that the differences are rooted in social and economic structures and the associated internalization of and adherence to gender roles. Although

Eagly and Wood (1999) provided evidence for certain parts of their critique of evolutionary psychological theories (showing, for example, that there is a great deal of cross-cultural variability in the relative contributions of men and women to subsistence, with women sometimes contributing more), there have been no direct tests of their account of sex differences in jealousy.

ATTACHMENT PROCESSES AS THE ALTERNATIVE EXPLANATION

Bowlby's (1969, 1973, 1980) attachment theory offers a parsimonious alternative explanation for the existence of sex differences in jealousy. According to the theory, the affective bond that develops between the child and caretaker affects the child's emerging self-concept and view of the social world. Bowlby (1969) conceptualized human motivation in terms of "behavioral systems," a concept borrowed from ethology, and proposed that attachment-related behavior in infancy (e.g., clinging, crying, smiling, monitoring caregivers, and developing a preference for a few reliable caregivers or "attachment figures") is part of a functional biological system that increases the likelihood of protection from predation, provides comfort during times of stress, and offers a foundation for social learning. Central to attachment theory is the concept of internal working models—mental representations formed through repeated transactions with attachment figures. These working models subsequently act as heuristic guides through the world of relationships and organize personality development.

Based on Bowlby's theory, Ainsworth and her coworkers (Ainsworth, Blehar, Waters, & Wall, 1978) identified three major styles of attachment in infancy—secure, avoidant, and anxious-ambivalent—and traced these styles to caregivers' behavior. Subsequently, Hazan and Shaver (1987) extended Ainsworth's framework to the study of romantic love, which they conceptualized as an attachment process. They created a pencil-and-paper measure of adult attachment styles, which asked respondents to say which of three descriptions of relationship styles fit them best: secure, avoidant, or anxious-ambivalent. In a host of studies conducted since 1987, this brief measure and various extensions of it have significantly predicted relationship outcomes (e.g., satisfaction, breakups, commitment), patterns of coping with stress, couple communication, and even phenomena such as religious experiences and patterns of career development (see reviews by Shaver & Hazan, 1993, and Mikulincer & Shaver, 2003).

Bartholomew (Bartholomew & Horowitz, 1991) revised Hazan and Shaver's (1987) three-category classification scheme, proposing a four-category model that differentiated between two types of avoidant adults: fearful and dismissive. Consistent with Bowlby's (1969) analysis of working models of self and relationship partners, the four categories could be arrayed in a two-dimensional space, with one dimension being "model of self" (positive vs. negative) and the other being "model of others" (positive vs. negative). For secure individuals, the models of self and other are both positive. For anxious-ambivalent (or preoccupied, to use Bartholomew and Horowitz's term) individuals, the model of others is positive (i.e., relationships are attractive), but the model of self is not. For dismissing individuals, the reverse is true: The somewhat defensively maintained model of self is positive, whereas the model of others is not (i.e., intimacy in relationships is regarded with caution or avoided). Fearful individuals have relatively negative models of both self and others.

Attachment research indicates that attachment styles are mainly attributable to experiences in close relationships, not to genes. Numerous studies have linked children's developing attachment patterns to patterns of parenting behavior (see Main, 1995, for a review), but researchers have failed to find genetic influences on children's attachment styles (e.g., Bokhorst et al., 2003). The stability or instability of attachment patterns across the childhood and adolescent years is largely attributable to stability or instability of relationships with attachment figures during that same period (see Fraley, 2002, for a review). Moreover, adult romantic attachment styles are related to people's descriptions of childhood relationships with parents (e.g., Levy, Blatt, & Shaver, 1998) and can change systematically over time as a function of relationship experiences (e.g., Kirkpatrick & Hazan, 1994). In addition, behavior genetic studies of relationship styles in adult twins show that these styles are attributable more to environmental factors than to genetic factors (e.g., Waller & Shaver, 1992).

Although there are no replicable sex differences in attachment security measured in infancy or in adulthood, there are sex differences among the insecure styles that may help explain sex differences in jealousy. More men than women have an insecure dismissive-avoidant attachment style (e.g., Bartholomew & Horowitz, 1991; Levy et al., 1998; Shaver et al., 1996). Dismissive-avoidant individuals tend to be unemotional, to deny their needs for intimacy, to be strongly invested in autonomy, and to exhibit greater sexual promiscuity (e.g., Bartholomew & Horowitz, 1991; Brennan & Shaver, 1995; Schachner & Shaver, 2002, 2004; Simpson, 1990). However, this counterdependent and compulsively self-reliant style is not as strong as its possessors let on. Instead, it appears to be a defense against unconscious feelings of vulnerability (e.g., Bowlby, 1988; Mikulincer, Dolev, & Shaver, 2004).

ATTACHMENT STYLE AND SEX DIFFERENCES IN JEALOUSY

Recognizing the limitations discussed earlier concerning simple evolutionary models of sex differences in jealousy, we (Levy & Kelly, 2006) proposed an attachment theory perspective on sex differences in jealousy. We hypothesized that observed sex differences in types of jealousy were actually due to sex differences in adult romantic attachment style. First of all, we hypothesized, in line with most of the previous research, that there would be a significant sex difference in the type of jealousy that was experienced as most distressing. Second, we predicted a significant difference between men and women in the degree of dismissive attachment, with men being more dismissive than women. Although sex differences in attachment security in infancy and early childhood are not theoretically predicted in attachment theory, by late adolescence and early adulthood, sex differences in attachment are typically found when using the self-report romantic attachment measures typically employed by personality and social psychologists. More men are found to be dismissing, and more women are found to be preoccupied. Gender-specific parental socialization practices may contribute to these gender differences in attachment style. For example, research has shown that parents use more positive emotion words in conversation and joint play with their girl children than with their boy children (Dunn, Bretherton, & Munn, 1987; Fivush, Brotman, Buckner, & Goodman, 2000; Goodnow, 1988). Over time, the cumulative absences of such experiences may result in a greater likelihood of dismissive attachment for men. Additionally, with progressive development, gender roles may be increasingly internalized. However, the data are mixed with regard to the influence of gender roles. For example, Shaver et al. (1996) found that feminine gender roles were negatively correlated with avoidance; however, Servello and Bartholomew (1996) were unable to confirm a relationship between gender roles and dismissive attachment in men (although gender role was related to preoccupied attachment in women). These findings suggest a link between gender roles and attachment patterns but indicate that other factors are also likely to be influential in explaining sex differences in adult attachment.

Third, we expected a significant difference in reactions to different jealousy-provoking situations between people with different attachment styles. Specifically, we expected dismissive individuals to find sexual infidelity more distressing and securely attached individuals to find emotional infidelity more distressing. There are two main reasons for hypothesizing that dismissive individuals would find sexual infidelity more distressing. First, previous research has found that dismissive individuals, compared with people with the other attachment styles, tend to be more concerned with the sexual aspects of relationships than with emotional intimacy (Schachner & Shaver, 2004).[1] For example, dismissive men report more sexual interests in extradyadic relationships, more promiscuous behavior, and poaching the mates of others, and they are more likely to describe relationship partners in terms of physical and sexual attributes rather than internal and emotional ones (Allen & Baucom, 2004; Schachner & Shaver, 2002; Simpson & Gangestad, 1991). Additionally, dismissive men report a short-term, low investment, exploitive sexual strategy that includes engaging in sexual behavior to regulate negative affect and to control and coerce others (Davis, Shaver, & Vernon, 2004; Levy, 1990, 1999). Second, consistent with psychodynamic theories of projection, research has shown that dismissive individuals are more likely to engage in defensive projection of negative information about the self, which seems also to serve the secondary purpose of maintaining interpersonal distance (Mikulincer & Horesh, 1999). Taking these points together, we hypothesized that dismissive individuals would be more concerned about their partner's sexual investments than their partner's emotional investments. In addition, they were expected to be more likely to project their own motives and interests in extradyadic relationships onto their partners. Thus differences in jealousy that appear to be rooted in sex differences might actually reflect differences in attachment style. That is, dismissing individuals, who are more likely to be men, might be more likely to report jealousy regarding sexual infidelity. In contrast, secure individuals, regardless of sex, were hypothesized to be more likely to experience jealousy in response to a partner's emotional infidelity.

Using the Buss Infidelity Questionnaire (Buss et al., 1992) and Bartholomew's Relationship Questionnaire (Bartholomew & Horowitz, 1991), we assessed 416 undergraduate students enrolled in introductory psychology classes at two large northeastern urban universities. As predicted, we replicated Buss et al.'s (1992) finding of sex differences in jealousy reactions to sexual and emotional infidelity. Men were more likely to find sexual rather than emotional infidelity distressing, and women were more likely to find emotional infidelity rather than sexual infidelity distressing. In our study, this difference, shown in Table 6.1, was highly significant, $\chi^2(1) = 29.93$, $p < .001$.

Also, as predicted, we found a significant sex difference in the distribution of attachment types, $\chi^2(3) = 10.67$, $p < .01$. Men were more likely than

TABLE 6.1. Relation between Sex and Type of Jealousy Experienced as Most Distressing

	Sex			
Jealousy type	Male	Female	Row total	
Emotional	44 (18.1) (46.5%)	240 (81.9) (75.7%)	284	100%
Sexual	55 (44.4) (53.5%)	77 (53.3) (24.3%)	132	100%
Column total	99 (27.0%) 100.0%	317 (73.0%) 100.0%	416 100.0%	100%

Note: Cell entries are *n*'s, row percentages, and column percentages. $\chi^2(1) = 29.93$, $p < .001$. Data from Levy and Kelly (2006).

women to exhibit dismissive attachment, and women were slightly more likely than men to exhibit fearful attachment (Figure 6.1).

These results are consistent with previous research, in which men were more likely than women to be dismissingly avoidant in attachment style (Brennan, Shaver, & Tobey, 1991; Brennan & Morris, 1997; Levy et al., 1998; Shaver et al., 1996). Consistent with our (Levy & Kelly, 2006) main hypothesis that sex differences in jealousy would be explicable in terms of differences in attachment style, we found that dismissive individuals, who were more likely to be men, were also more likely to report distress regarding sexual infidelity (Figure 6.2).

In contrast, secure individuals, including secure men, reported more jealousy than did dismissive individuals in response to emotional infidelity (Figure 6.3). In line with our reasoning, we (Levy & Kelly, 2006) also found that the association between dismissive attachment and sexual jealousy was significant for both men and women, $\chi^2(3) = 27.84$, $p < .001$, and $\chi^2(3) = 16.29$, $p < .001$, respectively.

We computed odds ratios separately for each variable to evaluate the specific effects of sex and attachment style on jealousy. Overall, men were between three and four times more likely than women to endorse sexual jealousy. However, when odds ratios were computed separately by attachment style, the sex differences in jealousy for secure and preoccupied individuals were weak and not significant according to simple chi-square tests. The sex differences in jealousy were dramatically heightened, however, in the fearful and dismissive groups, with men being roughly 5 and 26 times, respectively, more likely to endorse sexual jealousy. A Mantel–Haenszel test showed that the odds ratios, taken together, were significantly greater than 1,

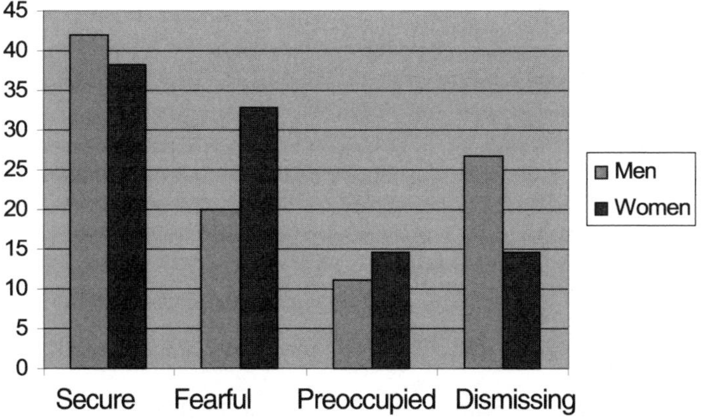

FIGURE 6.1. Percentage of each of four attachment styles in samples of men and women. Data from Levy and Kelly (2006).

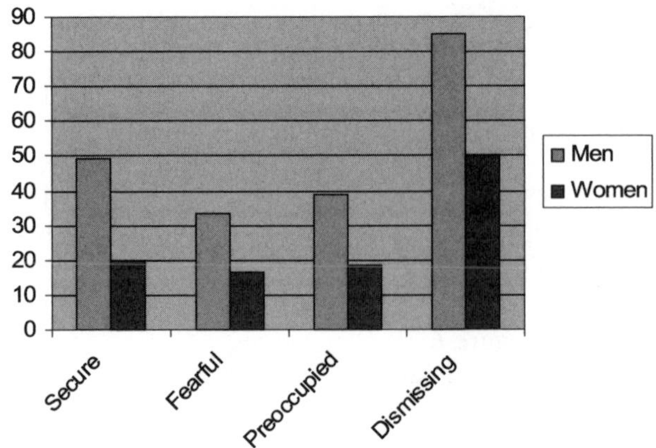

FIGURE 6.2. Percentage of respondents in each attachment-style category who were more distressed by sexual than by emotional infidelity. Data from Levy and Kelly (2006).

consistent with a main effect of sex on jealousy type, $\chi^2(1) = 24.07, p < .001$. However, the Breslow–Day test suggested significant heterogeneity between the stratified odds ratios, $\chi^2(3) = 8.03, p < .05$, consistent with a moderating effect of attachment style on the relationship between sex and jealousy type.

Odds ratio analyses also revealed the importance of attachment style overall, and within each sex, especially with regard to secure versus dismissing styles. Dismissive women, for example, were roughly 4 times more likely to endorse sexual jealousy than were their secure counterparts, whereas dismissive men were nearly 50 times more likely than secure men

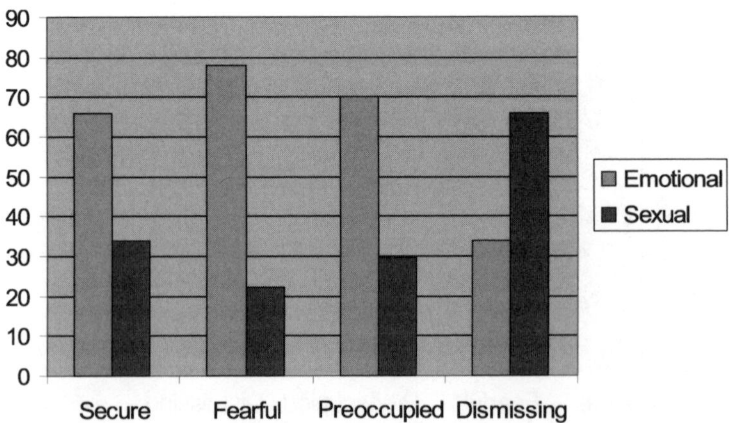

FIGURE 6.3. Percentage of respondents in each attachment-style category who were more distressed by sexual or by emotional infidelity. Data from Levy and Kelly (2006).

to endorse sexual jealousy. Simple chi-square analyses were significant for the relationship between overall attachment style and jealousy for both sexes.

To determine the relative strength of effect of each variable, as well as the significance of the moderating effect, we (Levy & Kelly, 2006) performed a series of sequential logistic regression analyses, which revealed that sex and attachment style were both significant predictors of jealousy individually and, after accounting for the effects of the other variable, consistent with independent main effects for each. The interaction term led to significant improvement in the model over and above sex and attachment style variables, suggesting significant moderation of the sex-jealousy relationship by attachment style. The full model, containing both variables and the interaction term, was statistically reliable when compared with a constant-only model, $\chi^2(7, n = 411) = 75.70, p < .001$, and performed well, correctly classifying 75% of cases according to jealousy type.

IMPLICATIONS AND CONCLUSIONS

Levy and Kelly's (2006) findings suggest that observed sex differences in jealousy are more complex than simple evolutionary models imply. Although Buss and colleagues (Buss et al., 1992; Buss, Larsen, & Westen, 1996) found that men are more likely than women to find sexual infidelity more distressing than emotional infidelity, there is no evidence that this replicable sex difference is due solely to biological sex. Levy and Kelly's findings indicate that adult romantic attachment style plays an important part in determining which kind of infidelity elicits more jealousy. Secure individuals, including secure men, are more likely to find emotional infidelity than sexual infidelity distressful, whereas dismissing individuals, especially dismissing men, are more likely to find sexual infidelity to be the bigger problem. The psychological and cultural/environmental mechanisms underlying sex differences in jealousy may be more important than evolutionary psychologists have supposed. Nevertheless, our findings do not completely rule out Buss's hypothesis, because a significant sex difference in jealousy type remained even after controlling for the contribution of attachment style. Both sex and attachment style differences made significant unique and interactive contributions to the distress caused by sexual and emotional infidelity. However, it is also important to keep in mind that sex differences may not operate as Buss and colleagues suggest but could be the function of a variable that covaries with sex, such as gender role identification (Rabinowitz & Valian, 2000).

We are not opposed to evolutionary perspectives in general: Attachment theory is, in fact, an evolutionary, ethological theory. However, we are concerned with the way evolutionary theory has been applied to explain a broad array of complex human behaviors in close relationships, such as romantic attraction, parenting, gender differences, and emotions such as jealousy. We believe that current discussions of evolved sex differences in jealousy could easily lead to a misunderstanding of evolutionary theory.

First, evolutionary theory holds that an organism's survival potential is enhanced by being supple and responsive to the environment rather than being as rigid as evolutionary psychologists typically portray it. Organisms need to be sensitive to cues from the environment, as well as flexible and adaptable in response to a wide range of environmental phenomena (Buller, 2005). For example, if maternal rejection is induced by a competitive social situation, offspring who develop aggressive, nonaltruistic, or "dismissing" personality styles may do better than those who are altruistic and cooperative (Belsky, 1999; Chisholm, 1999). On the other hand, infants brought up in a supportive social environment may benefit from developing a more altruistic, cooperative, and "secure" personality style. Therefore, it would not make evolutionary sense for either men or women to be locked into a particular mode of behavior (i.e., sexual jealousy vs. emotional jealousy).

Second, every human activity invariably involves inherited biological components, but evolution is possible only where there is variation among individuals. Any explanation that implies that an intraspecies or intragender behavior is invariant runs counter to basic principles of evolutionary theory.

Third, the existence of a behavior does not necessarily indicate that it evolved through natural selection. Cultural evolution does not depend on genetic change; it depends primarily on the development of new ideas and occurs much more quickly than biological evolution. Thus dramatic changes in how men and women behave have occurred during the past 25,000 years, although virtually no genetic changes have occurred during that time. Anthropological evidence, for example, suggests that patriarchy is a relatively recent phenomenon (Lerner, 1986) and thus cannot be accounted for by genetic explanations.

Fourth, evolutionary theory does not minimize the importance of environments to the extent implied in the explanations common in evolutionary psychology. Evolutionary psychological models tend to inflate the explanatory weight of biological processes. Instead of accepting such reductionistic notions, we need to look more closely at the environments in which genes and the processes they influence function. Both intrasex and interattachment-style variations for both kinds of jealousy we studied suggest that men have the same biological potential for emotional jealousy as do women and, conversely, that women have the same biological potential for sexual jealousy as do men. If evolutionary models are going to be of maximal value, they must specify the conditions and processes of organism–environment interactions through which genotypes are transformed into phenotypes. Genotypes are never expressed independently of environment.

In contrast, an attachment theory perspective provides a broad yet parsimonious explanation of sex differences in type of jealousy perceived as most distressing. Unlike simple evolutionary explanations, attachment theory can explain both between- and within-sex differences, as well as differentiate between environmentally and genetically based interpretations.

Another advantage of an attachment theoretical perspective on sex differences in jealousy is that it offers suggestions for prevention and intervention. An important goal of theoretical understanding is to enable change. That male sexual jealousy has been implicated as the leading cause of spouse battering and homicide across many cultures (Daly & Wilson, 1988) highlights the importance of understanding the dynamics of sexual jealousy. Unfortunately, the evolutionary perspective put forth by Buss and his colleagues offers little advice for reducing sexual jealousy in men. At its worst, it supplies a quietist justification for male violence by viewing it as rooted in nature. An attachment perspective, however, offers an understanding of jealousy that is rooted in internal working models of self and relationships based on past experiences. This perspective suggests a number of ways to reduce and prevent sexual jealousy in both men and women through establishing and enhancing secure attachment relationships throughout the lifespan. Good ideas about how to accomplish these goals can be found in writings by clinicians (e.g., Bowlby, 1988; Slade, 1999) and researchers (e.g., Gillath, Shaver, & Mikulincer, 2005; Mikulincer & Shaver, 2001).

In conclusion, jealousy is a complex and multidetermined emotional reaction (White & Mullen, 1989). Although evolutionary psychology can contribute to explaining between-sex differences in the elicitation of emotional versus sexual jealousy, it is limited in a number of respects. First, the evolutionary psychology perspective cannot systematically explain within-sex differences. Second, it cannot explain the full complexity of the emotional experience of jealousy. We believe that attachment theory offers a coherent and parsimonious explanation of kinds of jealous reactions with greater scope and better predictive power than explanations based in evolutionary psychology. Approaching the study and amelioration of jealousy from an attachment perspective helps us understand its sources, points to new research possibilities, offers suggestions for educational and clinical interventions, and promises to alleviate important social problems. Our own work leaves open a number of questions, such as why dismissing attachment is more common among men than women, which suggests that avoidant parenting interacts with either genetic factors or with societal sex-role stereotypes. If these remaining questions are tackled by researchers, we will be able to provide an even better set of guidelines for parents, educators, and clinicians.

NOTE

1. We do not want to suggest that secure individuals are not interested in the sexual aspects of relationships. In fact, research has shown that secure men and dismiss-

ive men report having comparable amounts of sex; however, secure men report having this sex in long-term committed relationships as a way of expressing intimacy and increasing closeness, whereas dismissive men report having sex in multiple, short-term uncommitted relationships as a way of conquering and coercing others (Brennan & Shaver, 1995; Davis, Shaver, & Vernon, 2004; Schachner & Shaver, 2004).

REFERENCES

Abelson, R. P. (1995). *Statistics as principled argument*. Hillsdale, NJ: Erlbaum.

Ainsworth, M. S., Blehar, M. C., Waters, E., & Wall, S. (1978). *Patterns of attachment: A psychological study of the Strange Situation*. Hillsdale, NJ: Erlbaum.

Allen, E. S., & Baucom, D. H. (2004). Adult attachment and patterns of extradyadic involvement. *Family Process, 43*, 467–488.

Baker, R. R., & Bellis, M. A. (1995). *Sperm competition: Copulation, masturbation, and infidelity*. London: Chapman & Hall.

Bartholomew, K., & Horowitz, L. (1991). Attachment styles among young adults: A four-category model of attachment. *Journal of Personality and Social Psychology, 61*, 226–241.

Belsky, J. (1999). Modern evolutionary theory and patterns of attachment. In J. Cassidy & P. R. Shaver (Eds.), *Handbook of attachment: Theory, research, and clinical applications* (pp. 141–161). New York: Guilford Press.

Betzig, L. (1989). Causes of conjugal dissolution: A cross-cultural study. *Current Anthropology, 30*, 654–676.

Bokhorst, C. L., Bakermans-Kranenburg, M. J., Fearon, R. M. P., van IJzendoorn, M. H., Fonagy, P., & Schuengel, C. (2003). The importance of shared environment in mother–infant attachment security: A behavioral genetic study. *Child Development, 74*, 1769–1782.

Bowlby, J. (1969). *Attachment and loss: Vol. 1. Attachment*. New York: Basic Books.

Bowlby, J. (1973). *Attachment and loss: Vol. 2. Separation*. New York: Basic Books.

Bowlby, J. (1980). *Attachment and loss: Vol. 3. Loss: Sadness and depression*. New York: Basic Books.

Bowlby, J. (1988). *A secure base*. New York: Basic Books.

Brennan, K. A., & Morris, K. A. (1997). Attachment styles, self-esteem, and patterns of seeking feedback from romantic partners. *Personality and Social Psychology Bulletin, 23*, 23–31.

Brennan, K. A., & Shaver, P. R. (1995). Dimensions of adult attachment, affect regulation, and romantic relationship functioning. *Personality and Social Psychology Bulletin, 21*, 267–283.

Brennan, K. A., Shaver, P. R., & Tobey, A. E. (1991). Attachment styles, gender, and parental problem drinking. *Journal of Social and Personal Relationships, 8*, 451–466.

Buller, D. J. (2005). *Adapting minds: Evolutionary psychology and the persistent quest for human nature*. Cambridge, MA: MIT Press.

Buss, D. M. (1995). Evolutionary psychology: A new paradigm for psychological science. *Psychological Inquiry, 6*, 1–30.

Buss, D. M., Kirkpatrick, L., Shackelford, T., & Bennett, K. (1999). *On the nature of sex differences in jealousy: Testing alternative hypotheses about origins*. Unpublished manuscript, University of Texas, Austin.

Buss, D. M., Larsen, R. J., & Westen, D. (1996). Sex differences in jealousy: Not gone, not forgotten, and not explained by alternative hypotheses. *Psychological Science*, *7*, 373–375.

Buss, D. M., Larsen, R. J., Westen, D., & Semmelroth, J. (1992). Sex differences in jealousy: Evolution, physiology, and psychology. *Psychological Science*, *3*, 251–255.

Buunk, B. P., Angleiter, A., Oubaid, V., & Buss, D. M. (1996). Sex differences in jealously in evolutionary and cultural perspective: Tests from the Netherlands, Germany, and the United States. *Psychological Science*, *7*, 359–363.

Chisholm, J. S. (1999). *Death, hope, and sex: Steps to an evolutionary ecology of mind and morality*. New York: Cambridge University Press.

Daly, M., & Wilson, M. (1988). *Homicide*. New York: Aldine de Gruyter.

Daly, M., Wilson, M., & Weghorst, S. J. (1982). Male sexual jealousy. *Ethology and Sociobiology*, *3*, 11–27.

Davis, D., Shaver, P. R., & Vernon, M. L. (2004). Attachment style and subjective motivations for sex. *Personality and Social Psychology Bulletin*, *30*, 1076–1090.

Davis, K. E., Ace, A., & Andra, M. (2000). Stalking perpetrators and psychological maltreatment of partners: Anger-jealousy, attachment insecurity, need for control, and break-up context. *Violence and Victims*, *15*, 407–425.

DeSteno, D. A., & Salovey, P. (1996a). Evolutionary origins of sex differences in jealousy: Questioning the "fitness" of the model. *Psychological Science*, *7*, 367–372.

DeSteno, D. A., & Salovey, P. (1996b). Genes, jealousy, and the replication of misspecified models. *Psychological Science*, *7*, 376–377.

Dunn, J., Bretherton, I., & Munn, P. (1987). Conversations about feeling states between mothers and their young children. *Developmental Psychology*, *23*, 132–139.

Dutton, D. G., van Ginkel, C., & Landolt, M. A. (1996). Jealousy, intimate abusiveness, and intrusiveness. *Journal of Family Violence*, *11*, 411–423.

Eagly, A. H., & Wood, W. (1999). The origins of sex differences in human behavior: Evolved dispositions versus social roles. *American Psychologist*, *54*, 408–423.

Fivush, R., Brotman, M. A., Buckner, P. J., & Goodman, S. H. (2000). Gender differences in parent–child emotion narratives. *Sex Roles*, *42*, 233– 253.

Fraley, C. R. (2002). Attachment stability from infancy to adulthood: Meta-analysis and dynamic modeling of developmental mechanisms. *Personality and Social Psychological Review*, *6*, 123–151.

Gayford, J. J. (1975). Wife battering: A preliminary survey of 100 cases. *British Medical Journal*, *1*, 194–197.

Gayford, J. J. (1979). Battered wives. *British Journal of Hospital Medicine*, *22*, 496–503.

Geary, D. C., Rumsey, M., Bow-Thomas, C. C., & Hoard, M. K. (1995). Sexual jealousy as a facultative trait: Evidence from the pattern of sex differences in adults from China and the United States. *Ethology and Sociobiology*, *16*, 355–383.

Gibbens, T. C. N. (1958). Sane and insane homicide. *Journal of Criminal Law, Criminology, and Police Science*, *49*, 110–115.

Gillath, O., Shaver, P. R., & Mikulincer, M. (2005). An attachment-theoretical approach to compassion and altruism. In P. Gilbert (Ed.), *Compassion: Conceptualizations, research, and use in psychotherapy* (pp. 121–147). London: Brunner-Routledge.

Goodnow, J. J. (1988). Children's household work: Its nature and functions. *Psychological Bulletin, 103*, 5–26.

Harris, C. R. (2003). A review of sex differences in sexual jealousy, including self-report data, psychophysiological responses, interpersonal violence, and morbid jealousy. *Personality and Social Psychology Review, 7*, 102–128.

Harris, C. R., & Christenfeld, N. (1996). Gender, jealousy, and reason. *Psychological Science, 7*, 364–366.

Hazan, C., & Shaver, P. R. (1987). Romantic love conceptualized as an attachment process. *Journal of Personality and Social Psychology, 52*, 511–524.

Kirkpatrick, L. A., & Hazan, C. (1994). Attachment styles and close relationships: A four-year prospective study. *Personal Relationships, 1*, 123–142.

Lerner, G. (1986). *The creation of patriarchy.* New York: Oxford University Press.

Levy, K. N. (1990). [Narrative descriptions of significant others]. Unpublished raw data.

Levy, K. N. (1999). Attachment style, representations of self and others, and affect regulation: Implications for the experience of depression (Doctoral dissertation, City University of New York, 1999). *Dissertation Abstracts International, 60*, 4895.

Levy, K. N., Blatt, S. J., & Shaver, P. R. (1998). Attachment style and parental representations. *Journal of Personality and Social Psychology, 74*, 407–419.

Levy, K. N., & Kelly, K. M. (2006). *Sex differences in jealousy: Evolutionary style or attachment style?* Manuscript submitted for review.

Main, M. (1995). Recent studies in attachment. In S. Goldberg, R. Muir, & J. Kerr (Eds.), *Attachment theory: Social, developmental, and clinical perspectives* (pp. 404–474). Hillsdale, NJ: Analytic Press.

Mathes, E. W., Phillips, J. T., Skowron, J., & Dick, W. E. (1982). Behavioral correlates of the interpersonal jealousy scale. *Educational and Psychological Measurement, 42*, 1227–1231.

Mikulincer, M., Dolev, T., & Shaver, P. R. (2004). Attachment-related strategies during thought-suppression: Ironic rebounds and vulnerable self-representations. *Journal of Personality and Social Psychology, 87*, 940–956.

Mikulincer, M., & Horesh, N. (1999). Adult attachment and the perception of others: The role of projective mechanisms. *Journal of Personality and Social Psychology, 76*, 1022–1034.

Mikulincer, M., & Shaver, P. R. (2003). The attachment behavioral system in adulthood: Activation, psychodynamics, and interpersonal processes. In M. P. Zanna (Ed.), *Advances in experimental social psychology* (Vol. 35, pp. 53–152). New York: Academic Press.

Pines, A., & Aronson, E. (1983). Antecedents, correlates, and consequences of sexual jealousy. *Journal of Personality, 51*, 108–136.

Rabinowitz, V. C., & Valian, V. (2000). Sex, sex differences, and social behavior. In P. Moller & D. LeCroy (Eds.), *Evolutionary perspectives on human reproductive behavior* (pp. 196–207). New York: New York Academy of Sciences.

Schachner, D. A., & Shaver, P. R. (2002). Attachment style and human mate poaching. *New Review of Social Psychology, 1*, 122–129.

Schachner, D. A., & Shaver, P. R. (2004). Attachment dimensions and sexual motives. *Personal Relationship*, *11*, 179–195.

Servello, S., & Bartholomew, K. (1996, August). *Sex, gender roles, and attachment patterns in young adults*. Paper presented at the International Conference on Personal Relationships, Banff, Alberta, Canada.

Shaver, P. R., & Hazan, C. (1993). Adult romantic attachment: Theory and evidence. In D. Perlman & W. Jones (Eds.), *Advances in personal relationships* (Vol. 4, pp. 29–70). London: Kingsley.

Shaver, P. R., Papalia, D., Clark, C. L., Koski, L. R., Tidwell, M. C., & Nalbone, D. (1996). Androgyny and attachment security: Two related models of optimal personality. *Personality and Social Psychology Bulletin*, *22*, 582–597.

Simpson, J. A. (1990). Influence of attachment styles on romantic relationships. *Journal of Personality and Social Psychology*, *59*, 971–980.

Simpson, J. A., & Gangestad, S. W. (1991). Influences of attachment styles on romantic relationships. *Journal of Personality and Social Psychology*, *59*, 971–980.

Slade, A. (1999). Attachment theory and research: Implications for the theory and practice of individual psychotherapy with adults. In J. Cassidy & J. R. Shaver (Eds.), *Handbook of attachment: Theory, research, and clinical applications* (pp. 575–594). New York: Guilford Press.

Symons, D. (1979). *The evolution of human sexuality*. New York: Oxford University Press.

Thornhill, R., & Palmer, C. T. (2000). *A natural history of rape: Biological bases of sexual coercion*. Cambridge, MA: MIT Press.

Tjaden, P., & Thoennes, N. (1998). *Stalking in America: Findings from the National Violence Against Women survey*. Denver, CO: Center for Policy Research.

Trivers, R. (1972). Parental investment and sexual selection. In B. Campbell (Ed.), *Sexual selection and the descent of man: 1871–1971* (pp. 136–179). Chicago: Aldine.

Waller, N. G., & Shaver, P. R. (1992). Importance of nongenetic influences on romantic love styles: A twin-family study. *Psychological Science*, *5*, 268–274.

White, G. L., & Mullen, P. E. (1989). *Jealousy: Theory, research, and clinical strategies*. New York: Guilford Press.

Wiederman, M. W., & Allgeier, E. R. (1993). Gender differences in sexual jealousy: Adaptationist or social learning explanation? *Ethology and Sociobiology*, *14*, 115–140.

Wilson, M. I., & Daly, M. (1992). The man who mistook his wife for a chattel. In J. Barkow, L. Cosmides, & J. Tooby (Eds.), *The adopted mind* (pp. 289–322). New York: Oxford University Press.

Wolfgang, M. E. (1958). *Patterns in criminal homicide*. Philadelphia: University of Pennsylvania Press.

Part III

Interplay between the Caregiving and Attachment Systems

7

Responding to Need in Intimate Relationships

Normative Processes and Individual Differences

NANCY L. COLLINS, ANAMARIE C. GUICHARD, MÁIRE B. FORD, and BROOKE C. FEENEY

There are many ways that romantic partners can express their love and commitment to each other, but providing responsive support and care to one another in times of need may play an especially important role in promoting relationship security and enhancing the health and emotional well-being of both members of a couple. Bowlby (1969/1982, 1988) recognized the profound importance of caregiving in adult close relationships, and he suggested that healthy and secure intimate relationships are possible only when relationship partners understand and respect each other's attachment needs and are aware of the crucial role they play as caregivers to one another. Nevertheless, romantic partners differ considerably in their willingness and ability to provide sensitive care to one another, and many intimate relationships fail to provide partners with the deep sense of emotional security that is necessary for optimal functioning. After all, responding to the needs of others is often a difficult task that involves a good deal of responsibility, as well as a substantial amount of cognitive, emotional, and sometimes tangible resources. Not everyone is equally skilled at providing responsive support, nor equally motivated to do so.

The complexity of caregiving in intimate relationships raises a number of important questions that have not been fully addressed in the adult attachment literature or in the broader social support literature. For example, what are the key features of effective caregiving in adult close relationships, and what types of skills, resources, and motivations are needed in order for a person to be truly responsive to the needs of others? Are there systematic individual differences in patterns of caregiving, and, if so, what are the personal and interpersonal mechanisms that explain these differences? To address these questions, we have used attachment theory as a framework for studying social support and caregiving processes in adult intimate relationships. In doing so, we have explored *normative processes* as well as *individual differences* in support-seeking and caregiving dynamics using a variety of research methods. Most of our work to date has centered on understanding the dynamics involved in responding to a relationship partner's expressions of distress. However, as we discuss later, a comprehensive view of caregiving must consider not only the way that relationship partners provide each other with comfort, reassurance, and support in times of adversity but also the ways in which they support each other's personal growth and autonomous exploration when not distressed. Throughout our work, we conceptualize social support as an *interpersonal process* that involves the mutual influence of care seekers and caregivers in dyadic interaction. In this chapter, however, we focus on the role of the caregiver because the nature of caregiving has received much less attention than the nature of care seeking in the adult attachment literature and in the broader social support literature.[1]

Our goal in this chapter is to elaborate on attachment theory's notion of caregiving behavior, to highlight aspects of our program of research in this area, and to integrate this work with the contributions of other researchers. We begin by describing the three major behavioral systems—attachment, exploration, and caregiving—that are relevant to understanding caregiving dynamics in couples. We then provide a detailed discussion of theory and research on the caregiving behavioral system. In doing so, we discuss the normative activation of the caregiving system, individual differences in the capacity for responsive care, and mechanisms that might explain these individual differences. Finally, we review current empirical work on caregiving in adult intimate relationships and point to directions for future research.

ATTACHMENT, EXPLORATION, AND CAREGIVING

Attachment theory provides an ideal framework for studying caregiving processes in intimate relationships because it provides a basis for understanding the complex dynamics involved in three interrelated aspects of human nature that are relevant to care-seeking and caregiving dynamics in couples: attachment, exploration, and caregiving (Bowlby, 1973, 1980, 1969/1982). The three systems are briefly described as a backdrop for our in-depth discussion of caregiving processes.

Attachment

Attachment theory regards the propensity to form strong emotional bonds with particular individuals as a basic component of human nature—present in infants and continuing through adulthood. According to the theory, individuals enter the world equipped with an innate attachment *behavioral system* that functions to promote the child's safety and survival through contact with nurturing caregivers. The attachment system becomes activated most strongly in adversity, so that when a child is frightened, anxious, tired, or ill, he or she will tend to seek protection, care, and assistance from a primary attachment figure, typically a parent (Bowlby, 1973, 1969/1982; Bretherton, 1985, 1987). Furthermore, the quality of the relationship that develops between a parent and child is expected to be largely determined by the parent's emotional availability and responsiveness to the child's needs (Ainsworth et al., 1978; Bowlby, 1973; Bretherton, 1985). The child's ability to rely on his or her attachment figure as a *safe haven* of comfort and support when distressed and a *secure base* for exploration when not distressed is considered to be a key component of secure attachment bonds and a key predictor of healthy emotional development.

Although attachment theory was originally developed to explain the nature of the relationship that develops between a child and a parent, Bowlby emphasized that the basic functions of the attachment system continue to operate across the lifespan and that attachment behavior is in no way limited to children (Bowlby, 1969/1982). Although the attachment system is likely to be less readily activated in adults than in children, attachment behavior can be seen whenever adults are faced with events that they perceive as stressful or threatening. For example, adults often seek proximity to the significant people in their lives (often romantic partners) in response to stress resulting from physical pain, fatigue, fear of new situations, feelings of attack or rejection by others, achievement problems or failures, and threat of loss. Attachment behavior and an associated increase in desire for care is considered to be the norm in these situations. Moreover, attachment theory emphasizes that the desire for comfort and support during times of adversity is neither childish nor immature. Indeed, Bowlby (1969/1982) argued that healthy self-reliance involves the "capacity to rely trustingly on others when occasion demands and to know on whom it is appropriate to rely" (p. 359).

Although the need for security is believed to be universal, adults as well as children will develop characteristic strategies for coping with distress and regulating feelings of security; and these strategies are thought to be contingent, at least in part, on an individual's history of regulating distress with attachment figures (Bartholomew, Cobb, & Poole, 1997; Kobak & Sceery, 1988; Mikulincer & Shaver, 2003). This idea has led researchers to identify systematic individual differences in *attachment style* in infants and adults (Ainsworth et al., 1978; Bartholomew & Horowitz, 1991; Hazan & Shaver, 1987). Bowlby (1973) postulated that these individual differences are rooted in *internal working models* of the self (as worthy or unworthy of love and care) and others (as responsive or unresponsive in times of need), which develop in the context of transactions with early caregivers and other important attachment figures. Working models of attachment are thought to be cognitive–affective–motivational schemas that regulate the attachment system by directing not only feelings and behavior but also attention, memory, and cognition in attachment-relevant contexts (Bowlby, 1973; Bretherton & Munholland, 1999; Collins & Allard, 2001; Collins, Guichard, Ford, & Feeney, 2004; Collins & Read, 1994; Main, Kaplan, & Cassidy, 1985; Shaver, Collins, & Clark, 1996).

Adult attachment researchers typically define four prototypic attachment styles derived from two underlying dimensions (Bartholomew & Horowitz, 1991; Brennan, Clark, & Shaver, 1998; Fraley & Waller, 1998). The first dimension, labeled *anxiety*, reflects the degree to which individuals worry about being rejected, abandoned, or unloved by significant others. The second dimension, labeled *avoidance*, reflects the degree to which individuals limit intimacy and interdependence with others. *Secure* individuals are low in both anxiety and avoidance. They feel valued by others and worthy of affection, and they perceive attachment figures as generally responsive, caring, and reliable. They are comfortable developing close relationships and depending on others when needed. *Preoccupied* individuals are high in anxiety but low in avoidance. They have an exaggerated desire for closeness and dependence but lack confidence in others' availability and responsiveness in times of need. They depend greatly on the approval of others for a sense of personal well-being but have heightened concerns about being rejected or abandoned. *Fearful-avoidant* individuals are high in both anxiety and avoidance. They experience a strong sense of distrust in others coupled with heightened expectations of rejection, which result in discomfort with intimacy and avoidance of close relationships. Finally, *dismissing-avoidant* individuals are low in anxiety but high in avoidance. They view close relationships as relatively unimportant, and they value independence and self-reliance. They perceive attachment figures as generally unreliable and unresponsive but view themselves as confident and invulnerable to negative feelings. They attempt to maintain a positive self-image in the face of potential rejection by minimizing attachment needs, distancing themselves from others, and restricting expressions of emotionality.

These individual differences in attachment style are thought to be rooted in underlying differences in working models of self and others, and they can be understood in terms of rules that regulate the attachment system and guide cognitive, emotional, and behavioral responses to emotionally distressing situations (Fraley & Shaver, 2000; Kobak & Sceery, 1988; Mikulincer & Shaver, 2003). For example, secure attachment is organized by rules that allow acknowledgment of distress and turning to others for comfort and support when needed. In contrast, avoidant attachment is organized by rules that restrict acknowledgment of distress and inhibit dependence on others (a *deactivating* strategy), whereas anxious attachment is organized by rules that direct attention toward distress and attachment figures in a hypervigilant manner that inhibits autonomy and self-reliance (a *hyperactivating* strategy). Consistent with these assumptions, research indicates that secure and insecure adults differ systematically in the way they regulate distress and in their tendency to seek proximity to and support from significant others in response to adversity (Brennan, Wu, & Loev, 1998; Collins & Feeney, 2000; Collins & Feeney, 2005; Collins, Kane, Guichard, Ford, & Feeney, 2005; Florian, Mikulincer, & Bucholtz, 1995; Fraley & Shaver, 1998; Mikulincer & Florian, 1995; Mikulincer, Florian, & Weller, 1993; Ognibene & Collins, 1998; Simpson, Rholes, & Nelligan, 1992). As we discuss in greater detail later, these different strategies for coping with one's *own* distress have important implications for understanding how individuals respond to the emotional distress of *others*.

Exploration

The urge to explore the environment—to work, play, discover, create, and take part in activities with peers—is regarded as another basic component of human nature that is critical to personal adaptation (Bowlby, 1988). For adults, these exploratory activities may take many forms, including pursuing a career (Hazan & Shaver, 1990), engaging in leisure activities (Carnelley & Ruscher, 2000), working toward important personal goals (Brunstein, 1993; Brunstein, Dangelmayer, & Schultheiss, 1996; Feeney, 2004; Ruehlman & Wolchik, 1988), or developing new friendships. From a normative perspective, the attachment and exploratory behavioral systems are thought to be antithetical to each other, such that focused and productive exploration is likely to occur only when attachment needs have been satisfied and the attachment system is deactivated (Bowlby, 1969/1982, 1988). That is, when an individual of any age is feeling secure (free from both physical and psychological threat), he or she is likely to explore away from attachment figures; but when an individual is alarmed or distressed, the attachment system will take priority, and the individual will feel an urge toward proximity.[2]

Because a sense of felt security is necessary for productive exploration, individuals of all ages will be more likely to explore the environment, take on challenges, and make discoveries when they are confident that an attachment figure will be available, accessible, and responsive should the need arise. As Bowlby (1979) observes, "human beings of all ages are happiest and able to deploy their talents to best advantage when they are confident that, standing behind them, there are one or more trusted persons who will come to their aid should difficulties arise" (p. 103). Thus the ability to confidently explore the environment stems in part from having a caregiver who can serve as a *secure base* for exploration—one who both encourages and supports such exploration and has proven him- or herself to be readily available and responsive when comfort, assistance, or protection has been sought. In other words, being able to use a relationship partner as a secure base for exploration depends on the degree to which that partner has proven to be a *safe haven* in times of stress.

Just as children use their parents as a secure base for exploration by keeping note of the parents' whereabouts, exchanging glances, and from time to time returning to the parents to share in enjoyable mutual contact, adults are likely to engage in similar forms of behavior. For example, an adult is likely to keep track of a spouse's whereabouts, maintain phone contact when exploring away from the spouse for an extended period of time, or share details of his or her explorations with the spouse (Feeney, 2004; Feeney & Collins, 2004). Adults may also look to their partners for encouragement, advice, or instrumental aid in achieving their exploratory goals. Although very few empirical investigations of these normative secure-base support-seeking processes appear in the adult attachment literature (or in the broader social support and relationships literatures), several recent studies suggest that the support of personal goal strivings by significant others has important implications for goal achievement, personal well-being, and relationship functioning (Brunstein, 1993; Brunstein et al., 1996; Feeney, 2004; Ruehlman & Wolchik, 1988). Furthermore, because a sense of security is necessary for productive exploration, it is not surprising that individual differences in attachment style have been linked to systematic differences in exploratory behavior in both children (Ainsworth et al., 1978) and adults (Carnelley & Ruscher, 2000; Elliot & Reis, 2003; Feeney, 2005; Hazan & Shaver, 1990; Mikulincer, 1997). As would be expected, secure individuals show more adaptive patterns of exploration and have a healthier balance between attachment behavior and exploratory behavior, compared with their insecure counterparts.

Caregiving

The propensity to care for the needs of others is regarded by attachment theory as another major component of human nature and is the focus of this chapter. Whereas the attachment system is a normative safety-regulating system that reduces the risk of the *self* coming to harm, the caregiving system is a safety-regulating system that reduces the risk of a *close other* coming to harm (Bowlby, 1969/1982; George & Solomon, 1999; Kunce & Shaver, 1994). From a normative perspective, the caregiving system alerts individuals to the needs of others and motivates them to provide protection, comfort, and assistance to (and promote the overall adaptive functioning of) those who are either chronically or situationally dependent on them (Collins & Feeney, 2000; Feeney & Collins, 2001). Thus the caregiving behavioral system will be activated most strongly when a close other is facing adversity or personal challenge. However, the caregiving and attachment behavioral systems (*within* an individual) will be antithetical to each other, such that sensitive and responsive caregiving is likely to occur only when the caregiver's own attachment needs have been satisfied and the attachment system is deactivated (Bowlby, 1969/1982, 1988). That is, when a caregiver is feeling secure, he or she will be able to devote attention and resources to the needs of others; but when the caregiver's own security is threatened and his or her own attachment system has been activated, caregiving behavior (the ability to respond to the attachment and exploratory needs of another) is likely to be impaired to some degree.[3]

Although the caregiving behavioral system is most often discussed in the context of parent–child relationships (see George & Solomon, 1999), Bowlby (1969/1982, 1988) recognized the importance of caregiving in adult intimate relationships, and he suggested that healthy and secure intimate relationships are possible only when relationship partners are aware of their vital role as caregivers to one another (see also Bretherton, 1987). In the sections that follow, we provide an in-depth discussion of the caregiving behavioral system by examining the normative processes that activate and motivate caregiving behavior in close relationships and the ways in which these normative processes are shaped by individual differences in the caregiver's working models of attachment and caregiving.

CAREGIVING: NORMATIVE PROCESSES

In order for attachment bonds to function effectively, the attachment and exploratory behavior of one partner must be coordinated with the caregiving behavior of his or her attachment figure. Indeed, Bowlby (1969/1982) referred to attachment bonds as a "shared dyadic programme" (p. 377) in which careseekers and caregivers play complementary roles and in which the behavior of one partner commonly meshes with that of the other. The caregiving behavioral system is thus an integral component of attachment bonds (Bowlby, 1969/1982; George & Solomon, 1999; Kunce & Shaver, 1994). Just as infants are motivated to remain in close proximity to their primary caregivers, caregivers feel a strong urge to remain close to their infants and young children; they routinely monitor their infant's whereabouts and remain ready to respond on short notice should any threat arise.

Of course, effective caregiving involves more than simply monitoring a partner's whereabouts and remaining alert to signs of distress. In its optimal form, caregiving includes sensitivity and responsiveness to another person's expressed needs and signals, and it should include a broad array of behaviors that complement a partner's attachment and exploratory behavior (George & Solomon, 1999; Kunce & Shaver, 1994; Reis & Patrick, 1996). Thus, according to attachment theory, caregiving serves two major functions: (1) to meet the dependent partner's need for security by responding to signals of distress or potential threat (providing a *safe haven*); and (2) to support the attached person's autonomy and exploration when not distressed (providing a *secure base*). Although the concept of a secure base can be viewed more broadly as an attachment relationship that incorporates both safe-haven and secure-base dynamics (see Crowell et al., 2002; Waters & Cummings, 2000), we find it useful to distinguish between these two forms of support because they have different antecedents, interpersonal dynamics, and consequences (on which we elaborate subsequently).

Safe-Haven and Secure-Base Caregiving Processes

Figure 7.1 illustrates the dynamics of safe-haven and secure-base caregiving in dyadic interaction. For simplicity, the figure refers to the member of the dyad who could potentially provide care in a given situation as the "caregiver" and to the person who could potentially benefit from support as the "care seeker." However, it is important to keep in mind that in adult relationships, the caregiving and care-seeking roles are not exclusively assigned to one member of the couple versus another. Depending on the situation, adults typically move fluidly from one role to the other—sometimes seeking care and sometimes giving care.

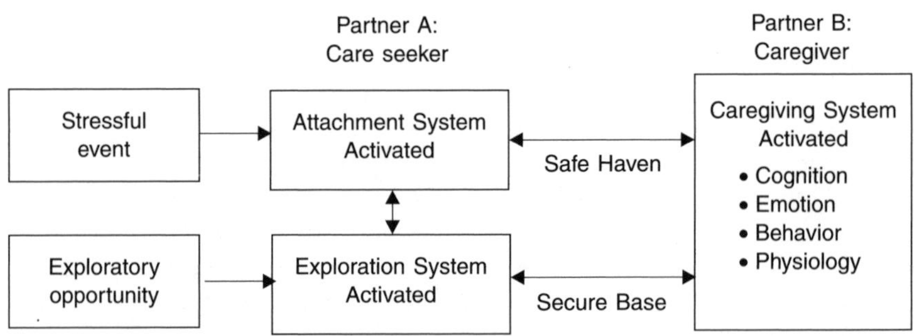

FIGURE 7.1. Illustration of interpersonal safe-haven and secure-base processes.

The top portion of the model depicts the *safe-haven* function of caregiving, which is set into motion when an individual (Partner A) experiences a stressful or threatening life event, which activates the *attachment* system and motivates the individual to seek comfort and support from a caregiver (Partner B).[4] Caregivers provide a *safe haven* for their relationship partners when they respond sensitively and appropriately to their partners' distress and to their resulting need for comfort, reassurance, and/or assistance. It is important to note that although caregiving behavior will typically be activated in response to a partner's expression of distress, it may also be directly triggered by the occurrence of a stressful life event or by the caregiver's awareness of a potential threat to the partner. Thus caregivers will often engage in proactive or preemptive behavior that promotes their partner's health and welfare.

The specific type of care provided in any situation will, of course, depend on the nature of the stressful event and may include a variety of emotional and instrumental support efforts aimed at providing comfort, assistance, or protection. Safe-haven support in adulthood may include (1) encouraging open communication of thoughts and feelings; (2) showing interest in the partner's problems and validating his or her concerns, worries, and fears; (3) conveying a sense of confidence in a partner's ability to handle the stressful situation; (4) affirming the partner's worth and reassuring the partner that he or she is loved and valued; (5) providing physical closeness and affection; (6) providing instrumental assistance as needed (information, advice, problem solving, task assistance, and direct intervention aimed at providing protection or removing sources of danger or threat); and (7) conveying continued availability. Thus effective safe-haven caregiving behaviors are those that restore an attached partner's felt security by soothing emotional distress and supporting his or her own coping efforts, as well as behaviors that convey (and provide) availability and assistance if needed.

The bottom portion of Figure 7.1 depicts the *secure-base* function of caregiving, which is set into motion when an individual (Partner A) experiences an exploratory opportunity, which activates the *exploration* system and motivates the individual to seek support from or share his or her experiences with a caregiver (Partner B).[5] Caregivers provide a secure base for their relationship partners when they respond sensitively and appropriately to their partners' exploratory behavior and to their need for encouragement in their exploratory activity. The provision of secure-base support includes a variety of behaviors that support a relationship partner's goal strivings, personal growth, and exploration. Secure-base support may include (1) encouraging the partner to accept challenges and try new things; (2) showing interest in and validation of the partner's personal goals, plans, and desires for the future; (3) conveying a sense of confidence in a partner's ability to handle challenges and to succeed; (4) providing instrumental assistance as needed (information, advice, assistance in removing obstacles); (5) not interfering with or intruding in the partner's explorations; (6) celebrating the partner's successes and responding sensitively to his or her failures; and (7) balancing an acceptance of the partner's need for self-growth with the conveyance of continued availability if needed (Feeney, 2004; Feeney & Collins, 2004). Thus effective secure-base caregiving behaviors are those that encourage and facilitate a partner's exploratory behavior and personal growth, as well as behaviors that convey (and provide) availability and assistance if needed.

Regardless of the specific type of support being offered, effective caregiving should promote the overall health and welfare of a relationship partner and should lead to better relationship quality (e.g., greater satisfaction, trust, commitment, and intimacy). However, because safe-haven and secure-base caregiving serve different functions, we expect each form of caregiving to have some important unique consequences (immediate and long term) for the support recipient (Feeney, 2004; Feeney & Collins, 2004). For example, some unique consequences of safe-haven care include reduced stress (both psychological and physiological), improved coping capacity, perceived (and actual) safety, and problem resolution. Therefore, long-term improvements in the support recipient's emotional well-being are likely to be an important consequence of safe-haven caregiving. Another important consequence of safe-haven caregiving should be a general perception that one's home base is secure; that is, a general sense of *relationship-specific felt security* (see Collins & Feeney, 2004a, for additional discussion). Some unique consequences of secure-base care for the support recipient include higher levels of self-esteem, perceived (and actual) competency, self-confidence, and self-efficacy and greater willingness and effort to pursue personal goals, accept challenges, take risks, and learn new things. Therefore, long-term improvements in the self (personal growth) are likely to be important consequences of secure-base caregiving.

We have differentiated between safe-haven and secure-base forms of caregiving in order to highlight their unique functions and features. However, it is important to note that care-seeking situations in adulthood often involve aspects of both attachment (in which the care seeker faces a personal threat) and exploration (in which the care seeker faces a personal challenge); hence the resulting caregiving response often requires a combination of safe-haven and secure-base support behaviors. Furthermore, although the specific support behaviors may differ across the two forms of caregiving, effective caregiving of either type shares a core set of features and is likely to involve a common set of skills, resources, and adaptive motivations (on which we elaborate next).

What Are the Key Features of, and Necessary Ingredients for, Effective Caregiving?

Regardless of the specific form of support being offered, we suggest that effective caregiving is characterized by two key features: (1) *sensitivity* to the partner's signals, and (2) interpersonal *responsiveness*. *Sensitivity* reflects the degree to which the caregiver's behavior is in synchrony with, and appropriately contingent on, the partner's needs (Ainsworth et al., 1978; Bowlby, 1969/1982; George & Solomon, 1999). A sensitive caregiver takes his or her cues from and allows his or her interventions to be paced by the care seeker, is attuned to the care seeker's signals, interprets them correctly, and responds promptly and appropriately (providing the type and amount of support that is wanted and needed). Sensitive caregivers recognize the times when they should wait and not interfere or step in and provide guidance or assistance. An insensitive caregiver, on the other hand, may not notice the care seeker's signals, may misinterpret or ignore them when they are noticed, may interfere with activities in an arbitrary way, and may respond late, inappropriately, or not at all to a need for support. Thus insensitive caregivers may be neglectful, overinvolved, intrusive, or otherwise out of synch with their partner's needs.

The second key feature of effective caregiving is *interpersonal responsiveness*, which reflects not the type or amount of support that is provided but the *manner* in which it is provided. Specifically, responsive care is provided in a way that leads the recipient to feel understood, validated, and cared for (Reis & Shaver, 1988). To accomplish this, caregivers must offer support in a way that expresses generous intentions, protects their partner's esteem, validates their partner's feelings and needs, respects their partner's point of view, and conveys love, acceptance, and understanding. Clearly, providing responsive care is not always easy, and even well-intended support efforts can have unintended negative consequences (Dunkel-Schetter, Blasband, Feinstein, & Herbert, 1992; Rini, 2001). For example, when offering help or assistance in response to stress (safe-haven support), caregivers may offer support in a way that makes their partners feel weak, helpless, needy, or inadequate; that induces guilt or indebtedness; or that makes their partners feel like a burden. A caregiver may also minimize or discount his or her partner's problem or may blame or criticize the partner for his or her own misfortune. When offering support in response to challenging or growth-related tasks (secure-base support), a caregiver may offer support or assistance in a way that undermines the partner's confidence, belittles the partner's goals and personal strivings, or fails to respect the partner's desire for autonomy by (explicitly or implicitly) discouraging or impeding pursuit of explorations outside of the relationship.

Given the complexity of providing effective care and the many pitfalls that caregivers may face in the process, it is no wonder that many support attempts fail to provide recipients with the support and encouragement they most need in times of stress or personal challenge (Dunkel-Schetter et al., 1992; Rini, 2001). To be sure, caregivers are not solely responsible for these failed support attempts. Care seekers play an important role in shaping their support interactions (for example, by failing to clearly express their needs or by being resistant to the caregiver's helping efforts), and we do not want to underestimate the importance of dyadic processes in shaping caregiving dynamics in couples (Collins & Feeney, 2000, 2004b). Nevertheless, it is clear that effective caregiving is a difficult process that is likely to be easier for some people than for others, and in some relationships than in others.

To understand systematic differences in patterns of caregiving, we identify three broad types of factors that should be necessary for the provision of sensitive and responsive care. These include (1) skills and abilities, (2) resources, and (3) motivation.

Skills and Abilities

In order for caregivers to provide sensitive and responsive care, they must possess a variety of skills and abilities that enable them to accurately discern the needs of others and respond flexibly to a wide range of needs as they arise. For example, they must have the ability to empathize with and take the perspective of others and the ability to accurately decode verbal and nonverbal signals. Caregivers must also have adequate knowledge about how to provide the appropriate type and amount of support that is needed and a sense of mastery and self-efficacy with regard to helping others. Effective emotion regulation skills are also necessary for responsive caregiving. Individuals who have difficulty regulating their own emotions (especially distress-related emotions) are likely to have difficulty responding to the needs of others, either because they tend to focus on their own distress or because they tend to direct their attention away from distress, which may lead them to distance themselves from the person in need. Although skills and abilities are often conceptualized in terms of individual differences (e.g., general perspective-taking ability), caregiving skills can also vary across relationships (e.g., unique understanding of the needs and preferences of a particular partner) and across situations (e.g., feelings of self-efficacy in certain conditions, such as those that require instrumental support versus those that require emotional support).

Resources

Effective caregiving requires adequate cognitive, emotional, and material resources. In describing the conditions necessary for parents to be sensitive and attentive caregivers, Bowlby (1988) acknowledged that adequate time and a relaxed atmosphere are necessary. These same resources should be necessary for adults to be responsive to one another. For example, if individuals are stressed, overwhelmed with work or personal responsibilities, and experiencing time constraints, it is likely that their caregiving behavior will suffer because they will be self-focused and may temporarily lack the energy and cognitive resources necessary to discern and attend to the needs of others. In addition, if self-regulatory resources are depleted, caregivers may be less able to inhibit unhelpful support behaviors (e.g., criticism) and may lack the patience needed to be cooperative and nonintrusive in their caregiving efforts. It is important to note that this lack of resources can be either chronic (e.g., chronic self-focus or chronic stress, which deplete mental and self-regulatory resources) or situational (e.g., situation-specific self-focus or anxiety).

Motivation

Finally, even if caregivers have appropriate skills and sufficient resources to provide care, they must be motivated to deploy those resources in the service of others. We distinguish between two different aspects of motivation: (1) an individual's overall degree of motivation to provide care (conceptualized as the degree of felt responsibility for responding to another's needs) and (2) the specific form of that motivation (conceptualized in terms of altruistic vs. egoistic motivation). First, because caregiving often involves a good deal of responsibility, as well as a substantial amount of resources (and sometimes personal sacrifice), caregivers must be motivated to accept that responsibility and expend the time and effort required to provide effective support. Thus individuals may differ in the degree to which they experience a sense of felt responsibility for the welfare of another (Clark & Mills, 1993). If caregivers are not sufficiently motivated, they may either provide low levels of care or ineffective forms of care that are out of synch with their partner's needs. Caregiving motivation may differ between people (e.g., a general communal orientation), between relationships (e.g., felt responsibility for, and commitment to, a particular partner), or between situations (e.g., heightened sense of responsibility in response to high need).

Second, even if individuals are equally motivated to care for another in terms of overall felt responsibility, they may differ in the degree to which that motivation is generated by altruistic concerns (the desire to relieve the other's suffering and promote his or her welfare) or egoistic concerns (the desire to gain explicit benefits for the self or to avoid sanctions). Caregivers who are motivated by relatively altruistic concerns will be more likely to provide sensitive and responsive care because their caregiving efforts will be guided by their partner's needs rather than by their own needs. As a result, they should be more attuned to their partner's signals, more willing to expend the effort needed to respond appropriately to these signals, and more likely to provide support in a manner that expresses their benevolent motives. In contrast, caregivers who are motivated by egoistic concerns will be less effective caregivers because they will be focused on their own needs rather than on the needs of their partners. For example, a caregiver who is motivated to provide care in order to reduce his or her own distress or out of a sense of obligation is likely to be controlling rather than cooperative and may provide support in a manner that expresses annoyance or a sense of burden. A caregiver who is motivated to provide care in order to be loved or to satisfy his or her own needs for intimacy is likely to become overinvolved or intrusive in his or her caregiving efforts and may express dissatisfaction if his or her partner fails to show adequate gratitude or appreciation. Motivations for caregiving may be chronic (e.g., a general altruistic motivation for helping others), relationship specific (e.g., altruistic or egoistic motivations with regard to a specific partner), and/or situation specific (e.g., helping out of obligation or to avoid sanctions in a particular situation).

Between- and within-Person Variability in Skills, Resources, and Motivation

Our goal here is not to provide an exhaustive list of skills, resources, and motivations necessary for effective caregiving but to offer a useful framework for identifying the types of factors that might enhance (or inhibit) responsive caregiving—and to specify how these factors vary at the between and within-person levels—so that we can begin to specify more systematically why *some people* are better caregivers than others (e.g., why secure individuals are better caregivers than insecure individuals), why people are better caregivers in *some relationships* than in others (e.g., why people take better care of those to whom they are more strongly committed), and why people are better caregivers on *some occasions* than on others (e.g., why people are better caregivers on their low-stress days than on their high-stress days or on days when they are feeling accepted and secure compared with days when they are feeling rejected or insecure). We now turn our attention to individual differences in the capacity for effective caregiving. In doing so, we discuss how the preceding factors can help us explain why attachment security enhances one's ability to be truly responsive to the needs of others and to serve as an effective safe haven and secure base for relationship partners.

CAREGIVING: INDIVIDUAL DIFFERENCES

Although caring for close others is presumed to be a universal human tendency, and although the caregiving behavioral system is thought to be normatively activated in response to others' needs, individuals clearly differ in the degree to which their caregiving systems are sensitive to (easily triggered by) the needs of others and in the way they express their caregiving behavior. Thus, although caregiving behavior, like attachment behavior, is to some degree preprogrammed (meaning that it is ready to develop along certain lines when certain conditions elicit it), Bowlby (1969/1982, 1988) emphasized that all the detail is learned. These details of caregiving are undoubtedly learned from many different sources, but it is likely that individuals learn a great deal about caregiving from the significant people in their lives who have been responsible for their care (Kunce & Shaver, 1994). Thus, although the caregiving system is theoretically distinct from the attachment system, the two systems are thought be linked both developmentally and behaviorally (George & Solomon, 1999). There are at least two important ways in which the caregiving and attachment systems are linked: (1) working models of caregiving should overlap with working models of attachment and (2) the dynamics of the caregiving system will be shaped by the dynamics of the attachment system.

Working Models of Attachment and Caregiving

If caregiving is organized and regulated by its own behavioral system, then individuals should develop internal working models of caregiving that guide the expression of the caregiving behavioral system by directing cognitive, emotional, and behavioral responses to the needs of others (George & Solomon, 1999). Furthermore, because individuals first learn about *seeking and giving* care in the context of their own experiences of being cared for by attachment figures, it is reasonable to assume that internal working models of attachment (which consist of rules that guide support-seeking behaviors and the regulation of personal distress) will overlap to some degree with internal working models of caregiving (which should consist of rules that guide caregiving behaviors and the regulation of a significant other's distress). This implies that there will be systematic individual differences in caregiving behavior and that these differences will be rooted, at least in part, in one's history of *receiving* care from others (Kunce & Shaver, 1994).

From the perspective advanced here, the quality of care that a person receives from others leaves a complex signature on the developing person's personality and worldview, thereby shaping many of the skills, resources, and motivations necessary for effective caregiving.[6] For example, through interactions with their own caregivers, individuals may develop favorable or unfavorable attitudes about the costs and benefits of providing care to others and about the acceptability or unacceptability of dependence. They are also likely to develop, or fail to develop, a sense of responsibility for the welfare of others and characteristic motives for helping others that are either relatively altruistic or relatively egoistic. Individuals are also likely to acquire a behavioral repertoire of effective or ineffective caregiving strategies and action tendencies. Together, these various components will guide cognition (e.g., attention, memory, and social inference processes), emotion (e.g., empathy, personal distress, anger), and behavior in situations that involve safe-haven or secure-base caregiving.

Adult attachment researchers have only recently begun to examine the caregiving behavioral system in depth, so they have not yet articulated a clear conceptual framework for understanding the content and function of representational models of caregiving or for identifying individual differences in these models.[7] However, they have examined the association between working models of attachment and caregiving behavior, primarily within the context of romantic relationships. These studies (summarized next) have shown that individual differences in attachment style are linked in predictable ways to patterns of caregiving in couples—suggesting that internal working models of caregiving are indeed organized in a manner complementary to, and therefore partially predictable from, attachment models.

The Interrelated Dynamics of Attachment and Caregiving

In adulthood, the caregiving and attachment systems are likely to be interrelated in at least two important ways. First, as noted earlier, Bowlby suggested that it is only when attachment needs have been met and the attachment system is deactivated that individuals can turn their attention and energy to other behavioral systems, such as caregiving. Thus, at the *intra*personal level, the attachment and caregiving behavioral systems will influence one another such that caregiving may be impaired if the caregiver's own feelings of security are threatened. Felt security (either chronic, in a particular relationship, or in a particular situation) should, therefore, facilitate one's ability to be truly sensitive and responsive to the needs of others (Mikulincer et al., 2001; Mikulincer, Shaver, Gillath, & Nitzberg, 2005; Murray, Holmes, & Collins, in press).

Second, because an intimate partner is both a support recipient (a target of one's caregiving) and a support provider (a source of one's own care and security), activation of the caregiving system is likely also to activate the attachment behavioral system. As such, the caregiving system in adult intimate relationships may sometimes operate *in the service* of attachment needs, and these attachment needs are often incompatible with effective caregiving. For example, individuals who are anxious about being rejected or unloved (either chronically or in the context of a specific relationship) may become overinvolved in caregiving behavior in order to create dependence (to make themselves indispensable to their partners) or to satisfy their own need to be close to their partners. In contrast, avoidant caregivers may fail to notice or respond to their partners' distress in the service of their own need to deactivate attachment concerns. In both of these examples, the caregiving behavior of insecure individuals is likely to be ineffective because the caregiver's own attachment needs will impede his or her ability to do what is in the best interest of the partner.

Individual Differences in Patterns of Caregiving

As the preceding discussion makes clear, there are many reasons to expect a close connection between attachment and caregiving dynamics in adulthood and to expect that individual differences in attachment style will be an important factor in understanding effective and ineffective caregiving processes in couples. Secure caregivers—who are confident that they are loved by others, who perceive others as responsive and available, who are comfortable with intimacy and interdependence, and who effectively regulate their emotions—will be better equipped to provide responsive care because they have more of the necessary skills and resources for attending to the signals of close others and responding flexibly to needs as they arise and because their own attachment needs are less likely to interfere with their caregiving activities. In addition, secure individuals are likely to have more adaptive beliefs and attitudes about care seeking and caregiving that increase their sense of responsibility for the welfare of others and motivate them to provide help and support for relatively altruistic reasons. For these and many other reasons, secure individuals will be better able to serve as safe havens for their partners in times of stress and as secure bases for exploration.

In contrast, the caregiving behavior of insecure adults is likely to be impaired in a number of important ways, and different forms of insecurity should be linked to different patterns of unresponsive care and to different underlying dynamics. Individuals who are high in attachment-related anxiety—who are worried about being rejected and unloved, who depend a great deal on others for a sense of personal well-being, who are uncertain of the responsiveness of others, and who have a hyperactivating style of emotion regulation—may have some of the skills necessary for effective caregiving (e.g., compassion for others, comfort with intimacy and emotional expression) but may lack some of the resources and adaptive motivation needed to be truly responsive to the needs of others. Specifically, anxious individuals may be preoccupied with their own attachment needs and highly self-focused, which leaves them with fewer cognitive and emotional resources for understanding and responding to the needs of others. In addition, although they may be highly motivated to provide care to their partners, they may do so for largely egoistic reasons (to satisfy their own attachment needs). Thus they are likely to provide care that is intrusive, overinvolved, controlling, or otherwise out of synch with their partner's needs. Moreover, anxious caregivers may sometimes fail to provide adequate secure-base support—failing to support or encourage their partner's exploration—if they perceive that such exploration may threaten their relationship. For these and many other reasons, the caregiving style of anxious individuals is likely to be relatively ineffective, although not neglecting.

A very different pattern may characterize the caregiving behavior of individuals who are high in attachment-related avoidance. Avoidant individuals—who value independence and self-reliance, who view others as generally unresponsive and unreliable, and who have a deactivating style of emotion regulation—are likely to lack many of the important skills that are necessary for effective caregiving. In addition, avoidant individuals are less likely to develop the deep sense of closeness, commitment, and interdependence that is necessary for understanding another's needs and for creating a sense of felt responsibility for another's welfare. Moreover, their need to minimize attachment concerns will tend to direct their attention away from partners who are in distress and to provide support for relatively egoistic reasons (to avoid sanctions, to eliminate a source of annoyance). As a result, they are likely to discount or minimize their partners' worries and needs and, when they do provide support, they are less likely to do so in a manner that makes their partners feel loved, valued, and cared for. For example, because they are apt to provide support with reluctance or annoyance, they may deliver support in a manner that makes their partners feel weak or needy, inadequate or incompetent, or like a burden. For these and many other reasons, avoidant individuals are likely to be relatively neglecting, and when they do provide support it is likely to be insensitive (out of sync with their partners' needs) and unresponsive (given in a manner that is relatively unhelpful).

In the following sections, we review empirical evidence relevant to normative processes and individual differences in safe-haven and secure-base caregiving behavior. We present highlights of our own program of research on caregiving in adult intimate relationships, but we also summarize research by other scholars in this area. In each section, we begin by describing studies relevant to normative processes, followed by a review of studies on attachment style differences in caregiving behavior. Within each section, we organize our review by research methodology in order to highlight the strengths and weakness of each approach and to identify trends that converge, or fail to converge, across different methodologies.

EMPIRICAL EVIDENCE FOR SAFE-HAVEN PROCESSES

Normative Processes

Observational Studies

We began our research on safe-haven caregiving processes by conducting an observational study in which we videotaped dating couples while one member of the couple (the "care seeker") disclosed a stressful problem (a recent personal concern or worry) to his or her partner (Collins & Feeney, 2000). Caregivers in this study showed evidence of sensitivity by matching their overall support effort and specific support behaviors to the needs expressed by their partners. For example, when care seekers' needs were greater and more clearly expressed (as evidenced by higher levels of emotional and instrumental disclosure), caregivers responded with greater support effort and more helpful forms of support (more behavioral responsiveness and more emotional and instrumental support). Care seeking and caregiving behaviors were also coordinated, such that the type of help offered (emotional or instrumental support) was matched to the type of help sought. Normatively, the provision of safe-haven support should lead to reduced distress for the support recipient, and one useful index of this stress reduction is improvements in mood from before to after the discussion. Results of this study provided some evidence for this process in that care seekers whose partners provided more responsive support during their interaction felt better after their interaction than they did before their interaction. Finally, couples who engaged in more supportive interactions (as judged by both members of the couple and by independent observers) had happier and more secure relationships. This finding is consistent with the idea that effective caregiving is a critical feature of secure relationships in adulthood.

Evidence for the normative activation of caregiving behavior was also provided in an interesting field study by Fraley and Shaver (1998), who observed couples waiting to depart in a public airport. Couples were identified as either separating from each other (one member of the couple was about to depart without his or her partner) or not separating (both members of the couple were traveling together). Because couples who are separating from each should be more likely to have their attachment and caregiving systems activated, they should evidence more spontaneous care-seeking and caregiving behavior. Consistent with this assumption, and relative to couples who were not separating, couples who were separating from each other engaged in more care-seeking (seeking and maintaining contact with one another) and caregiving behavior toward one another.

A Diary Study

We obtained further evidence for normative safe-haven processes by investigating *within-person* variability in support-seeking and caregiving behavior in a daily diary study of couples (Collins & Feeney, 2005). In this study, we asked both members of romantic couples to complete a nightly diary for 3 weeks in which they recorded stressful life events, support-seeking and caregiving behavior, mood and personal well-being, and thoughts and feelings about their relationship each day. Results indicated that individuals sought more social support from their partners on days when they experienced more stressful life events (normative activation of the attachment system), and their partners responded by providing more support on days when care seekers expressed greater need (normative activation of the caregiving system). Moreover, on days when support recipients perceived that their partners had been more supportive and responsive to their needs, they felt more loved and valued by their partners and more secure in their relationships (these effects were independent of daily conflict). Thus variability in feelings of relationship security was linked to evidence of a partner's responsiveness to one's needs.

Experimental Studies

The preceding studies provide initial evidence for the normative activation and operation of the caregiving behavioral system by showing that caregivers tend to increase their support efforts in response to greater need expressed by their partners. To provide more definitive evidence of responsiveness to need, we brought couples into the lab and created a stressful event (a speech task) for one member of the couple (the care seeker) and then manipulated the caregiver's perception that his or her partner was either extremely distressed about the upcoming speech task (the high-need condition) or not at all distressed (the low-need condition; Feeney & Collins, 2001). The caregiver was then given an opportunity to write a private note to his or her partner, which provided a behavioral measure of support and caregiving. From a normative perspective, the caregiving behavioral system should be activated with greater intensity when the partner is perceived to be in greater distress. Consistent with this assumption, caregivers wrote notes that were rated as more supportive (by both independent observers and by the recipients of the notes) in the high-need condition than in the low-need condition. Thus caregivers adjusted their degree of support in line with the perceived needs of their partners. Moreover, caregivers in this study increased their support efforts in the absence of any explicit support-seeking behavior by their partners; the awareness that their partners were facing adversity was enough to increase their support efforts.

We extended and replicated these findings in a recent study using a similar laboratory paradigm but a broader range of outcome variables that included cognitive, emotional, and behavioral responses to a partner's needs (Collins, Ford, Guichard, & Feeney, 2005). Results showed that caregivers in the high-need condition, relative to those in the low-need condition, wrote notes that were rated (by independent raters and by the note recipients) as more emotionally supportive, experienced greater empathy (sympathy and concern for their partners' well-being), and were more mentally focused on their partners (e.g., they were more likely to report that they were distracted by thoughts of their partners while they were working on their own puzzle task). These results provide clear evidence that caregivers modulated their caregiving efforts in line with their partner's needs by deploying greater cognitive, emotional, and behavioral resources when their partners needed them most.

Individual Differences: Attachment Style and Patterns of Caregiving

The studies reviewed thus far provide convergent evidence that caregiving behavior is normatively activated when a romantic partner is facing adversity and that caregivers regulate their behavior so that it meshes with the behavior and needs of the person being cared for. We now turn to studies that reveal that these normative patterns are often moderated by individual differences in attachment style and that adults with different attachment styles show substantially different patterns of caregiving behavior.

Self-Report Studies

The first study to explore the links between attachment style and caregiving in intimate relationships was conducted by Kunce and Shaver (1994). Based on an extensive review of the literature describing caregiving behaviors associated with infant attachment styles, these researchers developed an adult Caregiving Questionnaire that assesses four relationship-specific caregiving dimensions. These caregiving dimensions include (1) proximity versus distance (e.g., "When my partner seems to want or need a hug, I'm glad to provide it"); (2) sensitivity versus insensitivity (e.g., "I'm very good at recognizing my partner's needs and feelings, even when they're different from my own"); (3) cooperation versus control (e.g., "I tend to be too domineering when trying to help my partner"); and (4) compulsive caregiving (e.g., "I tend to get overinvolved in my partner's problems and difficulties"). In a series of studies, these researchers found that each attachment style was associated with a unique pattern of caregiving. Specifically, individuals with a secure attachment style reported relatively low levels of compulsive (overinvolved) and controlling caregiving and relatively high levels of proximity (physical forms of comfort) and sensitivity. In contrast, preoccupied individuals reported relatively high levels of proximity and compulsive caregiving but relatively low levels of sensitivity and cooperation—suggesting that although they are capable of providing affectionate caregiving, their caregiving may be somewhat intrusive and out of synch with their partner's needs. Dismissing-avoidant individuals reported the lowest levels of compulsive caregiving and provision of proximity, and they also reported relatively low levels of sensitivity. Finally, fearful-avoidant individuals reported relatively low levels of proximity and sensitivity, while simultaneously reporting relatively high levels of compulsive caregiving.

This basic pattern of findings has been replicated in several other studies. For example, in a large sample of committed couples, we found that, relative to secure individuals (those low in avoidance and anxiety), individuals who were high in attachment-related avoidance were less responsive and more controlling and that individuals who were high in attachment-related anxiety were more compulsive and more controlling (Feeney & Collins, 2001). Likewise, in a sample of married couples, Feeney (1996) found that secure spouses reported the most favorable style of caregiving, marked by high responsiveness (sensitivity, proximity, and cooperation) and low compulsiveness. In contrast, fearful spouses reported relatively low responsiveness and a more compulsive caregiving style, whereas dismissing spouses reported low responsiveness and low compulsiveness. Preoccupied spouses generally fell in between secure and fearful individuals in their caregiving characteristics. Finally, Carnelley, Pietromonaco, and Jaffe (1996) found that both married and dating individuals who were characterized by a fearful-avoidant attachment style (high anxiety and high avoidance) reported less overall caregiving activity (measured by an index that reflected low engagement, low reciprocity, and high neglect). Among married (but not dating) couples, preoccupied respondents also reported less caregiving activity.

Taken together, these studies reveal that secure attachment is associated with more effective caregiving behavior in intimate relationships. Secure adults are sensitive to their partner's cues, willing to provide physical proximity and comfort when needed; they are more cooperative than controlling in their caregiving style and less likely to be overinvolved in their caregiving efforts. In contrast, insecure attachment is associated with less effective caregiving behavior, but, as expected, the particular pattern of ineffective care depends on the particular type of insecurity. Avoidant individuals are relatively neglectful and controlling, whereas anxious individuals are relatively intrusive, overinvolved, and controlling.

Observational Studies

Observational studies provide converging evidence for attachment differences in patterns of caregiving. The first investigation in this regard is that of Simpson, Rholes, and Nelligan (1992). They introduced a stressor to the female members of romantic couples by telling them that they would be participating in a frightening but ambiguous laboratory procedure (which was designed to evoke distress, thereby activating the attachment system). Couples were then unobtrusively videotaped as they interacted during a waiting period. Results indicated that men who were low in avoidance were more responsive to their partners' needs in that they provided greater support (more reassurance and emotional support and more supportive comments) when their partners showed higher levels of distress, whereas those who were higher in avoidance provided *less* support when their partners were more distressed. This study provided the first behavioral evidence that attachment-related avoidance is associated with decreased responsiveness to need. (Caregivers' attachment anxiety scores were unrelated to observed caregiving behavior in this study.)

In an important follow-up investigation, Rholes, Simpson, and Orina (1999) coded additional behavioral responses from this same sample of couples. Specifically, they examined expressions of anger during the stress period and during a poststress recovery period. Avoidant men in the caregiving role expressed more anger toward their partners during the stress period, especially when their partners were more distressed. In addition, during the recovery period, they interacted less positively with their partners if their partners had sought more support from them during the stress period. (Caregivers' anxiety scores were unrelated to observed expressions of anger.) Coupled with the support findings described previously, these findings indicate that avoidant men find their partners' expressions of need to be aversive and that they respond by distancing themselves from their partners (by providing less support and by interacting with their partners in less positive ways, even after the stressful episode was concluded).

Simpson, Rholes, Orina, and Grich (2002) replicated this study but focused on female caregivers. In this study, avoidant women provided less support to their partners during the waiting period regardless of their partners' levels of distress. In addition, women who had more secure representations of their parents—as measured by the Adult Attachment Interview (George, Kaplan, & Main, 1984)—provided more support in response to increased need. Once again, attachment anxiety did not predict caregiving behavior.

Further evidence for the link between avoidance and poor caregiving was provided in Fraley and Shaver's (1998) observational field study of airport separations. Results revealed that, among those who were separating from their partners (and, hence, had a greater need to seek and/or provide care), avoidant women (but not men) displayed less contact seeking, less caregiving, and more distancing behavior. Anxiety was not related to caregiving behavior in either women or men who were separating (although anxious women reported more emotional distress, and anxious men showed less contact maintenance and more distancing behavior).

We also examined individual differences in safe-haven caregiving processes in the observational study described previously (Collins & Feeney, 2000). In that study we videotaped couples while one member of the couple described a personal stressor or worry to his or her partner. Contrary to expectations, and to other observational research, avoidant attachment was not significantly related to caregiving behavior in this investigation. However, we found that individuals who were higher in attachment-related anxiety were less effective caregivers; they provided less instrumental support, were less responsive to their partners during the conversation, and exhibited more negative caregiving behavior, and this was especially true when their partners' needs were less clear (i.e., when their partners engaged in less direct support-seeking behavior). These findings provided the first behavioral evidence that attachment anxiety limits one's ability to be a good caregiver.

Finally, Westmaas and Silver (2001) provided evidence that insecure attachment impedes effective support in peer interactions. In this study, women were videotaped while they interacted with another young woman whom, they were led to believe, had just been diagnosed with cancer. Avoidant women were rated by observers as less verbally and nonverbally supportive and as having less eye contact during the interaction. Avoidant women also rated their own interactions as less warm and supportive. Anxiety was unrelated to behavioral support, but anxious women reported feeling more anxious during their interaction, and they were much more likely to report self-critical thoughts after the interaction (as measured in a free-response thought listing). This latter finding suggests that, even after interacting with a person who had disclosed an important personal crisis, anxious women were relatively self-focused—occupied with thoughts about their own interpersonal performance.

Experimental Studies

The observational studies reviewed here provide converging evidence that attachment-related avoidance is associated with poor caregiving. However, the evidence for attachment anxiety is much more mixed. Unlike self-report studies, which show that anxiety is associated with ineffective care, the observational studies reveal less evidence of impaired caregiving. One reason for this inconsistency may be that the particular type of caregiving deficiencies shown by anxious individuals (overinvolved, intrusive, and controlling care) may be less visible in certain types of laboratory interactions. Fortunately, our recent experimental studies provide a much clearer picture of the unique deficiencies of anxious and avoidant caregivers.

As described earlier, we created a laboratory paradigm that would enable us to clearly identify patterns of responsive and unresponsive care by manipulating the caregiver's belief that his or her partner was either extremely distressed (high need) or not at all distressed (low need) about an upcoming speech task (Feeney & Collins, 2001). From an attachment theoretical perspective, responsive caregiving should be appropriately contingent on the partner's needs. Thus caregivers should show increased support effort in response to greater need. As described previously, we found evidence for this normative process in that caregivers, on average, wrote notes that were more supportive when they believed that their partners were more distressed. However, this normative increase in support was not true for all caregivers. Avoidant caregivers tended to provide low levels of emotional support in both the high- and low-need conditions and to provide more instrumental support in the low-need condition than in the high-need condition. Thus avoidant caregivers not only showed no evidence of responding to their partners' needs for support, but they even showed a tendency to provide less support in the condition in which their partners needed it the most. In contrast to avoidant caregivers, anxious caregivers showed some evidence of responsiveness, although they were not always in synch with their partner's needs; they provided more instrumental support to their partners in the high-need condition than in the low-need condition, but they provided the same level of emotional support regardless of their partners' levels of need. Taken together, these findings indicate that secure caregivers (those low in avoidance and anxiety) provided the most responsive support to their partners, whereas avoidant and anxious caregivers were, in various ways, out of synch with their partner's needs.

We extended these findings in a recent study in which we used the same paradigm but examined a more diverse set of caregiving outcomes, including cognitive, emotional, and behavioral responses to partner need (Collins, Ford, et al., 2005). In this study, secure caregivers (those low in both chronic and relationship-specific anxiety and avoidance) showed clear evidence of responsiveness—they provided more behavioral support in the high- than in the low-need condition, as evidenced by an increase in the number of times they checked a computer monitor for messages from their partners and by an increased willingness to switch tasks with their partners. They also reported greater empathy, more partner focus, and greater mental distraction in the high-need condition than in the low-need condition. In addition, relative to insecure caregivers, secure caregivers wrote notes that were judged to be more supportive in both conditions. In contrast, anxious caregivers showed clear evidence of being out of synch with their partners' needs. Caregivers high in anxiety failed to increase their support in response to their partners' needs and showed high levels of empathy, cognitive rumination, and partner focus regardless of their partners' levels of distress, indicating a clear lack of sensitivity to their partners' emotional cues and ineffective use of their cognitive-emotional resources. Anxious individuals were also less willing to switch tasks in the high-need condition than in the low-need condition and wrote notes that were judged to be less supportive in both need conditions. Thus, unlike secure caregivers, anxious caregivers failed to modulate their cognitive, emotional, and behavioral responses in accordance with their partner's needs. Interestingly, anxious caregivers also made more negative dispositional attributions (perceiving their partners as weaker and more emotionally unstable) in the high-need condition (when they were led to believe that their partners were extremely distressed about the upcoming stressful task). One reason for this effect may be that anxious caregivers, who depend on their partners as critical sources of their own safety, felt frustrated or threatened when they perceived that their partners were not "stronger and wiser." Finally, avoidant caregivers showed a pattern of relative neglect. Regardless of partner need, they wrote notes that were judged to be less supportive and were less willing to switch tasks with their partners. They also reported less empathy, less partner focus, and less mental distraction during their puzzle task. In summary, this study provides the clearest evidence to date concerning the effective regulation of caregiving behavior by secure individuals and the unique patterns of ineffective care associated with attachment anxiety and avoidance.

Taken together, our laboratory findings provide converging evidence that attachment-related avoidance and anxiety interfere with one's ability to be truly responsive to the needs of others. One limitation of these studies, however, is our inability to draw causal inferences about the effect of attachment security on caregiving behavior. Fortunately, recent studies by Mikulincer and his colleagues provide experimental evidence that a sense of attachment security increases empathy and prosocial responses. In a series of studies, Mikulincer et al. (2001) primed a sense of attachment security using both supraliminal and subliminal procedures and then measured empathy and personal distress in response to vignettes describing a person in need. Across all studies, activation of attachment security increased empathic reactions (compassion, sympathy) and decreased personal distress. In another series of studies, Mikulincer, Shaver, Gillath, and Nitzberg (2005) found that subliminal and supraliminal priming of attachment security increased compassion, willingness to help, and actual agreement to help a stranger in a laboratory context in which the stranger was (ostensibly) undergoing a very stressful series of tasks. Finally, Mikulincer and his colleagues have shown that secure-base priming decreases hostile reactions toward outgroup members (Mikulincer & Shaver, 2001) and increases the endorsement of self-transcendence (prosocial) values (Mikulincer et al., 2003). Taken together, these investigations provide evidence for a causal link between feeling secure and prosocial tendencies; and, although these studies did not involve romantic couples, they have clear implications for behavior in such contexts.

Mechanisms Explaining Individual Differences in Caregiving

In addition to identifying individual differences in patterns of caregiving, we have also been interested in identifying the specific factors and mechanisms that explain these differences (Feeney & Collins, 2001). We began by investigating a variety of chronic skills (empathic abilities, knowledge about how to support other people), resources (chronic self-focus), and motivational factors (communal and exchange orientation toward others, relationship commitment, closeness, and trust, and particular motivations for taking care of their partners).

First, which variables explained the tendency for avoidant individuals to be unresponsive and controlling caregivers? Mediation analyses suggested that avoidant adults tend to be unresponsive because they lack knowledge about how to support others, lack a prosocial orientation toward others, and lack relationship interdependence. In addition, avoidant adults' tendency to be controlling caregivers was mediated by their lack of prosocial orientation and their lack of relationship trust. Next, which variables explained the tendency for anxious adults to be compulsive and controlling caregivers? Anxious individuals tend to be compulsive caregivers because they have a high sense of relationship interdependence coupled with a lack of relationship trust and relatively selfish motives for caring for their partners. In addition, the tendency of anxious adults to be controlling caregivers appears to be mediated by their lack of relationship trust and their relatively selfish motives. These findings provide an initial step in identifying the unique patterns of skills, resources, and motives that help us understand why people with different attachment styles care for their partners in the particular ways that they do. Compatible findings have emerged in recent studies of attachment differences in volunteering (Gillath et al., 2005) and altruism (Mikulincer et al., 2005) in nonromantic domains.

Motivations for Caregiving

Another question that we have been addressing in our research concerns the degree to which specific motivations for providing support to one's partner influences caregiving behavior. We conducted a study that focused explicitly on caregiving motivations as important mechanisms that might underlie the provision of responsive or unresponsive support. Here we present a few highlights from this study (see Feeney & Collins, 2003, for more details).

We began by developing a Motivations for Caregiving Questionnaire that measures reasons for providing care (and reasons for *not* providing care) to a romantic partner. We included items that reflect specific types of selfish or egoistic motives—such as helping a partner in order to avoid negative consequences—and items that reflect more altruistic motives, such as helping out of concern for one's partner or to reduce a partner's suffering. We also included items based on hypotheses about the types of motives that we thought would be characteristic of people with different attachment styles. Based on factor analyses, we identified a series of specific motivations that activate and inhibit caregiving behavior. We then examined whether these motivations are associated with a variety of personal and relationship characteristics, including the caregivers' attachment style and caregiving history.

With respect to attachment style, we found that secure individuals (those low in avoidance and anxiety) were more likely to help their partners for altruistic reasons and less likely to help them for egoistic reasons. In contrast, avoidant caregivers were more likely to endorse egoistic motives and less likely to endorse altruistic ones. For example, they were more likely to help their partners because they felt obligated to help (and wanted to avoid sanctions for not helping) and because they expected to get something explicit in return; and they were less likely to help their partners because they felt love, concern, and responsibility for their partners or because they enjoyed it. When asked why they sometimes chose *not* to help their partners, avoidant caregivers reported that they disliked distress, lacked concern or a sense of responsibility for their partner, and perceived their partner to be difficult and too dependent. Avoidant caregivers were also more likely to report that they sometimes failed to help their partners because they lacked the skills and resources needed for doing so.

Anxious caregivers, on the other hand, reported helping for both egoistic and altruistic reasons—although they enjoyed helping and were motivated by feelings of love and concern for their partners, they also helped because they felt obligated (and wanted to avoid sanctions for not helping) and because they hoped to get something in return. In addition, anxious individuals reported helping their partners for relatively egoistic relationship purposes—to create closeness and interdependence, to gain love and acceptance, and to increase the likelihood that their partners would remain in their relationship. Thus, although anxious caregivers may be heavily engaged in caregiving behavior, their caregiving efforts are often in the service of their own attachment needs. Finally, when asked why they sometime chose *not* to help their partners, anxious caregivers reported that they sometimes lacked the skills needed to help and that their partners were difficult and unappreciative.

In addition to these links between caregiving motivations and adult attachment style, we also found associations between caregiving motivations and attachment *history* with parents. Specifically, people who reported having had an unsupportive caregiving history with their parents when they were growing up were more likely to report that they helped their partners for selfish reasons. For example, they were more likely to say that they helped in order to receive a specific benefit in return, to make their partners dependent on them, or because they felt obligated and wanted to avoid sanctions. In addition, when asked why they sometimes chose *not* to help their partners, those with an unsupportive caregiving history were more likely to say that they disliked distress, lacked concern or a sense of responsibility for their partners' well-being, or that their partners were difficult and unappreciative. These findings are consistent with the hypothesis that working models of caregiving are rooted, at least in part, in one's history of receiving care from important attachment figures, and they suggest that individuals who have received unresponsive care from their own attachment figures are more likely to develop maladaptive motives for approaching or avoiding caregiving toward others. Of course, because these findings are based on retrospective reports of relationships with parents, they must be interpreted with caution.

The next major question we addressed in this study was whether specific motivations for providing support influence caregiving behavior in couples. Again, the reason we think it is important to study caregiving motivations is that they should influence the quality of care that is provided within a relationship (and may help explain why secure and insecure individuals differ in the type of care they provide to their romantic partners). Consistent with expectations, responsive caregivers were those who reported helping their partners because they felt love and concern for them, because they were good at helping, and because they enjoyed helping. In contrast, the less responsive and more overinvolved and controlling caregivers were those who reported helping because they felt obligated, because they wanted to get something in return, or because their partners were perceived to be needy and incapable. Interestingly, overinvolved caregivers were also more likely to say that they helped their partners in order to increase their partners' dependence on them and to keep their partners in the relationship. This latter finding suggests that high levels of care are often motivated by egoistic concerns. Taken together, these results suggest that the underlying motives that people have for caregiving play a vital role in determining the quality of care that is provided.

EMPIRICAL EVIDENCE FOR SECURE-BASE PROCESSES

Empirical investigations of secure-base caregiving processes have been rare in the adult attachment literature and in the broader social support and relationship literatures. This seems particularly surprising given that individuals routinely assign credit for their accomplishments and successes to the support of the significant people in their lives—people who have encouraged them to grow as individuals and strive to reach their full potentials. A few studies have examined links between adult attachment and exploratory behavior (Carnelley & Ruscher, 2000; Elliot & Reis, 2003; Hazan & Shaver, 1990; Mikulincer, 1997). However, there have been no empirical investigations of secure-base caregiving processes in adulthood—processes that support or hinder a relationship partner's exploration. In response to this important gap, Feeney (2004, 2005) has begun a program of research examining secure-base caregiving processes in adult intimate relationships, exploring both normative processes (Feeney, 2004) and individual differences (Feeney, 2005).

Normative Processes

Feeney (2004) conducted a first in-depth investigation of normative secure-base caregiving processes in a sample of couples who were in committed romantic relationships (married, engaged, or dating seriously). This investigation included both an observational and an experimental session.

Observational Session

First, secure-base caregiving processes were examined in the context of discussions that couple members had about one member's personal goals and exploratory opportunities. The goal discussions were videotaped, and caregiver and care-recipient behaviors were coded by independent observers.

After the discussion, couple members completed questionnaires assessing their perceptions of the interaction, their mood, state self-esteem, and the care recipient's perceived likelihood of achieving his or her goals.

In addressing the question of the specific ways in which caregiving and care-seeking behaviors influence one another in dyadic interaction, findings revealed that the behaviors of caregivers and care recipients were meshed in complementary ways. For example, caregivers who were coded by observers as being supportive of and comfortable with their partners' goals had partners who discussed their goals openly, confidently explored various avenues for achieving their goals, and were receptive to support attempts. Interestingly, caregivers who were coded by observers as being intrusive and controlling during the discussion had partners who tended to modify their goals during the course of the discussion.

This investigation also permitted the examination of some immediate outcomes of secure-base caregiving for the recipient. Interestingly, when recipients felt that their goals were supported by their partners during the discussion, they experienced increases in self-esteem and positive mood after the discussion (controlling for global self-esteem and mood before the discussion) and rated their likelihood of achieving their goals to be greater after the discussion than before the discussion. Thus this investigation revealed that supporting a partner's goal strivings and exploration had important implications for his or her happiness and self-esteem and for his or her perceptions of the likelihood of achieving specific goals, at least in the short term.

Experimental Session

A second phase of the investigation was conducted in order to experimentally examine some immediate consequences of secure-base caregiving behavior (and lack thereof) for recipients. As one member of the couple (the care receiver) worked on a computer puzzle game, secure-base caregiving behavior was manipulated through the use of an instant messaging system. Care receivers were randomly assigned to one of four experimental conditions: (1) *intrusive/controlling*—the care receiver received frequent messages, ostensibly from the caregiver, that either provided answers to the puzzle or told them what to do next; (2) *intrusive/supportive*—the care receiver received frequent messages that communicated encouragement and emotional support (e.g., "good job," "hard one"); (3) *nonintrusive/supportive*—the care receiver received two encouraging and emotionally supportive messages during the course of the game (e.g., "good luck, "good job"); (4) *control*—the care receiver received no messages during the game. After the game, care receivers reported their perceptions of partner support, their own moods, and their stated self-esteem. Puzzle performance was assessed, and responses to the caregivers' messages were also coded for those who responded. The general pattern of results is highlighted here (see Feeney, 2004, for details).

How did care recipients construe their partner's support messages? Care receivers in the intrusive conditions (especially those in the intrusive/controlling condition) viewed their partners' messages as more frustrating and insensitive than those in the nonintrusive supportive condition. Moreover, care receivers in both of the supportive conditions viewed their partners' messages as more helpful than those in the intrusive/controlling condition.

With regard to immediate outcomes of manipulated secure-base caregiving behavior (and perceptions of manipulated caregiving), results indicated that care receivers who perceived their partners' messages to be supportive (as opposed to intrusive and insensitive) experienced increases in state self-esteem and positive mood after the puzzle activity. With regard to performance on the puzzle, care receivers in both intrusive conditions scored lower than care receivers in the control condition. This is especially interesting given that participants in the intrusive/controlling condition were actually given some of the answers to the puzzle. Although poor performance in the intrusive conditions could simply reflect the fact that participants were interrupted more frequently in these conditions, participants in this condition may have actively rejected their partners' intrusive support. Consistent with this speculation, care receivers in the intrusive conditions who responded to their partners' instant messages were more rejecting of the support than care receivers who responded to nonintrusive messages.

Individual Differences in the Provision of Secure-Base Support

In addition to evidence of normative secure-base processes, there is also evidence of important individual differences in the provision of secure-base support. Feeney (2005) conducted two studies examining attachment style differences in the provision of secure-base support and in motivations for providing secure-base support. Study 1 utilized the same sample described previously (Feeney, 2004), and Study 2 utilized a new sample of married couples. Results were highly consistent across the two samples and provided clear evidence that secure individuals are better able to serve as a secure base for their romantic partners.

In Study 1, self-reported caregiving measures revealed that avoidant caregivers were less available during their partner's explorations and goal pursuits, whereas anxious caregivers were more intrusive in their partners' exploratory activities. In addition, during the future goals and plans discussion, avoidant caregivers were observed to be less available and less encouraging to their partners. In Study 2, avoidance (especially dismissing avoidance) was also associated with less observed availability during the partners' discussion of his or her goals.

This investigation also examined motives for secure-base support using a new measure that parallels the measure we designed for safe-haven support (Feeney & Collins, 2003). Anxious and avoidant caregivers reported that they support their spouse's exploratory efforts in order to avoid pursuing their own goals, to avoid negative partner responses, and to get something in return (all of which are relatively egoistic motives). Anxious providers also reported supporting their spouses as a way of staying connected and keeping their partners committed. With regard to motives for *not* helping, anxious and avoidant caregivers reported that they sometimes fail to support their spouses' exploration because they perceive their spouses as difficult, feel jealous of their spouses' activities, lack skills, lack a sense of responsibility, perceive their partners' goals as unimportant, and desire to punish their partners. In addition, anxious caregivers reported that they sometimes fail to support their spouses' explorations because they worry that their partners' goal pursuits will harm or threaten their relationship. These findings help explain *why* insecure individuals may be less willing and able to serve as secure bases for their romantic partners; more broadly, they provide important insights into the many different factors that may enhance or inhibit effective secure-base caregiving in couples.

CONCLUSION AND DIRECTIONS FOR FUTURE WORK

As the preceding review makes clear, attachment theory provides an excellent framework for understanding social support and caregiving processes in couples, and the current body of empirical work is impressive both in terms of its theoretical depth and in terms of its use of novel and innovative research methods. Nevertheless, the systematic study of caregiving in intimate relationships is still in its early stages, and many important research questions await future investigation. Here we highlight several topics that we view as high research priorities.

One important topic for future research is to develop a more detailed theoretical account of working models of caregiving and a greater understanding of the ways in which these models are similar to and different from working models of attachment. Adult-attachment researchers have not yet developed a clear framework for understanding the content and function of representational models of caregiving or for identifying individual differences in these models (other than linking them to individual differences in attachment style). To facilitate this effort, it may be useful to begin with a conceptual framework similar to one that has been used to understand the content and function of working models of attachment (Collins & Read,

1994; Collins & Allard, 2001; Collins et al., 2004). For example, it may be useful to conceptualize working models of caregiving in terms of four interrelated components: (1) memories of caregiving experience (receiving as well as giving care); (2) beliefs, attitudes, and expectations about caregiving; (3) goals and motives related to caregiving; and (4) a behavioral repertoire of caregiving plans and strategies. A framework such as this would enable us to develop a more detailed understanding of the internal working models that underlie caregiving dynamics and to identify systematic individual differences in caregiving styles. This framework also raises a number of important theoretical questions that have not yet been considered in the literature. For example, do individuals possess a hierarchy of caregiving models that differ in their level of specificity—*general* working models, working models of particular *types of relationships* (e.g., caring for intimate partners versus caring for children), and working models of *specific relationships*? If so, how do these various models work together to guide the caregiver's cognitive, emotional, and behavioral responses to the needs of others? To answer such questions, researchers will need to develop new methods for assessing the conscious and nonconscious elements of working models and for investigating their role in shaping caregiving outcomes in situations that require safe-haven or secure-base support. We also need studies that compare caregiving dynamics across different types of relationships (e.g., caring for a child, a spouse, or an aging parent) to uncover the features that are common and unique to each caregiving context.

Another important avenue for future research is to examine a broader range of caregiving responses. Most of the current empirical work on caregiving in couples has focused on observed or self-reported caregiving *behavior*—and this is a clear strength of this body of work. However, as implied by the model shown in Figure 7.1, a complete understanding of caregiving dynamics must include not only the behavioral responses of caregivers but also their cognitive, affective, and physiological responses to a partner in need. These outcomes are important in their own right, but they also offer important clues concerning the specific mechanisms that underlie good and poor caregiving behavior. A small number of studies have examined *emotional* responses (anger, sympathy, compassion) to the needs of others (Collins, Ford, et al., 2005; Mikulincer et al., 2001; Mikulincer et al., 2005; Rholes, Simpson, & Orina, 1999), and only one study of which we are aware has investigated *cognitive* reactions to a partner in need (Collins, Ford, et al., 2005). We are not aware of any research that has investigated a caregiver's physiological responses to a partner in distress. If certain physiological systems of attached partners are coregulated in adulthood, as some attachment scholars have suggested (Diamond & Hicks, 2004; Hazan, Gur-Yaish, & Campa, 2004), then the physiology of a caregiver should be responsive to threats that are posed to the well-being of his or her partner. Two potential avenues for future research in this area include the study of neuroendocrine (e.g., cortisol and oxytocin) and cardiovascular responses to an intimate partner who is undergoing a stressful or challenging life event. Studies such as these would enable us to understand the psychobiological underpinnings of normative caregiving processes, as well as individual differences in these processes. We are currently developing methods for examining these processes in the laboratory, and much exciting research lies ahead.

With few exceptions, most of the existing work on caregiving in couples has examined chronic individual differences in attachment style. Thus an important endeavor for future research is to expand our knowledge of *normative* and *relationship-specific* caregiving dynamics in couples. For example, we know very little about the unique role of caregiving in the development and maintenance of secure intimate relationships, or how chronic differences in attachment style interact with relationship characteristics (e.g., satisfaction, commitment, trust) to shape caregiving responses. In addition, although a few studies have investigated the mutual influence of care seekers and caregivers in dyadic interaction (e.g., Collins & Feeney, 2000; Feeney, 2004, 2005; Kobak & Hazan, 1991; Simpson, et al., 1992), we have much to learn about the ways in which a caregiver's behavior is shaped by features of his or her partner (e.g., the partner's attachment style, tendency to seek support directly or indirectly, receptiveness to support efforts, or general coping style). We believe that experimental work will be extremely useful for understanding the normative factors that trigger the caregiving behavioral system and for uncovering the situational, contextual, and dyadic factors that enhance or inhibit responsive caregiving.

Longitudinal investigations examining the long-term outcomes of safe-haven and secure-base caregiving are also important endeavors for future work. We have suggested that safe-haven and secure-base support will have some important unique consequences for care *recipients*, and many of these assumptions await empirical investigation. However, research on the long-term outcomes of caregiving dynamics should also include an investigation of the personal and relationship outcomes for care *providers*. There are likely to be many important direct and indirect benefits to *serving* as a secure base and safe haven, and we suspect that individuals who provide sensitive and responsive support to their partners in times of adversity and who support their partner's personal growth will themselves experience better health and emotional adjustment, as well as better social functioning. We view this as an important and overlooked topic in the field.

In conclusion, the purpose of this chapter was to review and extend the exciting work that is being done on caregiving processes in adult close relationships—and to lay a foundation for the development of future work in this area. Although attachment scholars have made tremendous progress in understanding caregiving dynamics in adulthood, much remains to be discovered about the factors that promote or interfere with effective caregiving processes in couples and about the unique role of caregiving in promoting the health and well-being of both members of a couple. Many of the ideas presented in this chapter are speculative and await future investigation. We hope that this chapter will contribute to this effort by inspiring thoughtful research and by stimulating the development of more refined theoretical models.

ACKNOWLEDGMENTS

Preparation of this chapter was supported by National Science Foundation Grant No. SBR-0096506 to Nancy L. Collins, a National Science Foundation Predoctoral Fellowship to Máire B. Ford, and National Institute of Mental Health Grant No. MH-066119 to Brooke C. Feeney.

NOTES

1. See Collins and Feeney (2000), Feeney (2004), and Feeney and Collins (2004) for a description of our integrative model that incorporates both care *seeking* and care *giving*.
2. It is important to note that exploration may also be used as a strategy for *deactivating* the attachment system. That is, children and adults may turn toward exploratory behavior as a means of regulating their attachment needs. For example, a key marker of avoidant attachment in children is their tendency to actively direct attention away from their caregiver following a separation and to attend almost exclusively to the environment (Ainsworth et al., 1978). There is some evidence that avoidant adults , who are motivated to inhibit their attachment needs, may also use exploratory behavior as a means of deactivating attachment-related thoughts and feelings (Hazan & Shaver, 1990).
3. We do not mean to imply that individuals will always place their own security above the safety and security of others. Parents routinely sacrifice their own well-being for the welfare of their children, and so, too, do intimate partners routinely sacrifice for one another. However, our point (and, we believe, Bowlby's point) is not that one's own needs are given priority over the needs of others but that the ability to effectively respond to the needs of others will be impaired , to some degree, when an individual is also concerned with his or her own attachment needs.
4. Of course, not every personal stressor will require support or assistance from others. Individuals will be more likely to seek support when they perceive events to be more threatening and when they need additional coping resources. See Collins and Feeney (2000; Feeney & Collins, 2004) for a more extended discussion of safe-haven support-seeking behavior.
5. Of course, not every personal goal or challenge will require support or assistance from others. Thus it is expected that challenges and goals that are perceived to be more daunting and difficult to obtain will increase one's desire for support from a significant other and lead one to solicit more active forms of secure-base

caregiving (e.g., assistance, encouragement). In other cases, simply the perception that one's home base is secure and available *if needed* should suffice. See Feeney (2004; Feeney & Collins, 2004) for a more extended discussion of secure-base support-seeking behavior.

6. Empirical support for this assumption is provided in a variety of different literatures. First, research on the development of prosocial behavior in children finds that children who come from secure and loving homes show more empathic concern for others, behave in more sympathetic ways toward peers in distress, and are more prosocially oriented (Eisenberg & Fabes, 1998; Kestenbaum, Farber, & Sroufe, 1989). Second, research on caregiving in adult intimate relationships shows that individuals who recall their parents as having been warm and responsive toward them show evidence of more responsive caregiving behavior toward their romantic partners and report more adaptive caregiving motivations (Carnelley, Pietromonaco, & Jaffe, 1996; Feeney, 1996; Feeney, B. & Collins, 2003). Finally, research on parenting behavior shows that parents' memories of their attachment experiences with their own parents (as assessed in the Adult Attachment Interview) predict the quality of their caregiving behavior toward their children. Although causal inferences cannot be drawn in any of these lines of work, these findings provide converging evidence for an important association between receiving care and giving care, and they are consistent with the idea that individuals learn about both care-seeking and caregiving roles in their childhood relationships and apply some of this learning to their relationships with peers, romantic partners, and their own children.
7. See George and Solomon (1999) for an in-depth discussion of these issues in the context of *maternal–infant* caregiving. These researchers have launched an important program of research in an effort to provide theoretical and empirical elaboration of maternal–infant caregiving dynamics. In doing so, they present a framework for conceptualizing and studying maternal caregiving in which parents are viewed as developing adults who possess an organized caregiving system and an accompanying set of representational models that are linked developmentally and behaviorally to attachment, yet are still distinct from it. They have also developed a semistructured interview for identifying individual differences in maternal caregiving styles and the internal working models that underlie them.

REFERENCES

Ainsworth, M., Blehar, M., Waters, E., & Wall, S. (1978). *Patterns of attachment: A psychological study of the Strange Situation*. Hillsdale, NJ: Erlbaum.

Bartholomew, K., Cobb, R. J., & Poole, J. (1997). Adult attachment patterns and social support processes. In G. R. Pierce, B. Lakey, I. Sarason, & B. Sarason (Eds.), *Sourcebook of social support and personality* (pp. 359–378). New York: Plenum Press.

Bartholomew, K., & Horowitz, L. M. (1991). Attachment styles among young adults: A test of a four-category model. *Journal of Personality and Social Psychology, 61*, 226–244.

Bowlby, J. (1973). *Attachment and loss: Vol. 2. Separation*. New York: Basic Books.

Bowlby, J. (1979). *The making and breaking of affectional bonds*. London: Tavistock.
Bowlby, J. (1980). *Attachment and loss: Vol. 3. Loss: Sadness and depression*. New York: Basic Books
Bowlby, J. (1982). *Attachment and loss: Vol. 1. Attachment* (2nd ed.). New York: Basic Books. (Original edition published 1969)
Bowlby, J. (1988). *A secure base*. New York: Basic Books.
Brennan, K. A., Clark, C. L., & Shaver, P. R. (1998). Self-report measurement of adult attachment: An integrative overview. In J. A. Simpson & W. S. Rholes (Eds.), *Attachment theory and close relationships* (pp. 46–76). New York: Guilford Press.
Brennan, K. A., Wu, S., & Loev, J. (1998). Adult romantic attachment and individual differences in attitudes toward physical contact in the context of adult romantic relationships. In J. A. Simpson & W. S. Rholes (Eds.), *Attachment theory and close relationships* (pp. 394–428). New York: Guilford Press.
Bretherton, I. (1985). Attachment theory: Retrospect and prospect. *Monographs of the Society for Research in Child Development, 50*, 3–35.
Bretherton, I. (1987). New perspectives on attachment relations: Security, communication, and internal working models. In J. D. Osofsky (Ed.), *Handbook of infant development* (2nd ed., pp. 1061–1100). New York: Wiley.
Bretherton, I., & Munholland, C. (1999). Internal working models in attachment relationships: A construct revisited. In J. Cassidy & P. R. Shaver (Eds.), *Handbook of attachment: Theory, research, and clinical applications* (pp. 89–111). New York: Guilford Press.
Brunstein, J. C. (1993). Personal goals and subjective well-being: A longitudinal study. *Journal of Personality and Social Psychology, 65*, 1061–1070.
Brunstein, J. C., Dangelmayer, G., & Schultheiss, O. C. (1996). Personal goals and social support in close relationships: Effects on relationship mood and marital satisfaction. *Journal of Personality and Social Psychology, 71*, 1006–1019.
Carnelley, K., & Ruscher, J. (2000). Adult attachment and exploratory behavior in leisure. *Journal of Social Behavior and Personality, 15*, 153–165.
Carnelley, K. B., Pietromonaco, P. R., & Jaffe, K. (1996). Attachment, caregiving, and relationship functioning in couples: Effects of self and partner. *Personal Relationships, 3*, 257–278.
Clark, M. S., & Mills, J. (1993). The difference between communal and exchange relationships: What it is and is not. *Personality and Social Psychology Bulletin, 19*, 684–691.
Collins, N. L., & Allard, L. M. (2001). Cognitive representations of attachment: The content and function of working models. In G. J. O. Fletcher & M. S. Clark (Eds.), *Blackwell handbook of social psychology: Vol. 2. Interpersonal processes* (pp. 60–85). Oxford, UK: Blackwell.
Collins, N. L., & Feeney, B. C. (2000). A safe haven: An attachment theory perspective on support-seeking and caregiving in intimate relationships. *Journal of Personality and Social Psychology, 78*, 1053–1073.
Collins, N. L., & Feeney, B. C. (2004a). An attachment theory perspective on closeness and intimacy. In D. Mashek & A. Aron (Eds.), *Handbook of closeness and intimacy* (pp. 163–187). Mahwah, NJ: Erlbaum.
Collins, N. L., & Feeney, B. C. (2004b). Working models of attachment shape perceptions of social support: Evidence from experimental and observational studies. *Journal of Personality and Social Psychology, 87*, 363–383.

Collins, N. L., & Feeney, B. C. (2005). *Attachment processes in daily interaction: Feeling supported and feeling secure.* Unpublished manuscript, University of California, Santa Barbara.

Collins, N. L., Ford, M. B., Guichard, A. C., & Feeney, B. C. (2005). *Responding to need in intimate relationships: The role of attachment security.* Unpublished manuscript, University of California, Santa Barbara.

Collins, N. L., Guichard, A. C., Ford, M. B., & Feeney, B. C. (2004). Working models of attachment: New developments and emerging themes. In W. S. Rholes & J. A. Simpson (Eds.), *Adult attachment: Theory, research, and clinical implications* (pp. 196–239). New York: Guilford Press.

Collins, N. L., Kane, H., Guichard, A. C., & Ford, M. B., & Feeney, B. C. (2005). *Support-seeking behavior and motivations in intimate relationships: The role of attachment security.* Unpublished manuscript, University of California, Santa Barbara.

Collins, N. L., & Read, S. J. (1994). Cognitive representations of attachment: The structure and function of working models. In K. Bartholomew & D. Perlman (Eds.), *Advances in personal relationships: Vol. 5. Attachment processes in adulthood* (pp. 53–90). London: Kingsley.

Crowell, J., Treboux, D., Gao, Y., Fyffe, C., Pan, H., & Waters, E. (2002). Assessing secure base behavior in adulthood: Development of a measure, links to adult attachment representations and relations to couples' communication and reports of relationships. *Developmental Psychology, 38*, 679–693.

Diamond, L. M., & Hicks, A. M. (2004). Psychobiological perspectives on attachment: Implications for health over the lifespan. In W. S. Rholes & J. A. Simpson (Eds.), *Adult attachment: Theory, research, and clinical implications* (pp. 240–263). New York: Guilford Press.

Dunkel-Schetter, C., Blasband, D. E., Feinstein, L. G., & Herbert, T. B. (1992). Elements of supportive interactions: When are attempts to help effective? In S. Spacapan & S. Oskamp (Eds.), *Helping and being helped: Naturalistic studies: The Claremont symposium on applied psychology* (pp. 83–114). Newbury Park, CA: Sage.

Eisenberg, N., & Fabes, R. A. (1998). Prosocial development. In W. Damon & N. Eisenberg (Eds.), *Social, emotional, and personality development* (pp. 701–778). New York: Wiley.

Elliot, A. J., & Reis, H. T. (2003). Attachment and exploration in adulthood. *Journal of Personality and Social Psychology, 85*, 317–331.

Feeney, B. C. (2004). A secure base: Responsive support of goal strivings and exploration in adult intimate relationships. *Journal of Personality and Social Psychology, 87*, 631–648.

Feeney, B. C. (2005). *Individual differences in secure base support provision: The role of attachment style, relationship characteristics, and underlying motivations.* Unpublished manuscript, Carnegie Mellon University, Pittsburgh, PA.

Feeney, B. C., & Collins, N. L. (2001). Predictors of caregiving in adult intimate relationships: An attachment theoretical perspective. *Journal of Personality and Social Psychology, 80*, 972–994.

Feeney, B. C., & Collins, N. L. (2003). Motivations for caregiving in adult intimate relationships: Influences on caregiving behavior and relationship functioning. *Personality and Social Psychology Bulletin, 29*, 950–968.

Feeney, B. C., & Collins, N. L. (2004). Interpersonal safe haven and secure base caregiving processes in adulthood. In W. S. Rholes & J. A. Simpson (Eds.), *Adult attachment: Theory, research, and clinical implications* (pp. 300–338). New York: Guilford Press.

Feeney, J. A. (1996). Attachment, caregiving, and marital satisfaction. *Personal Relationships, 3*, 401–416.

Florian, V., Mikulincer, M., & Bucholtz, I. (1995). Effects of adult attachment style on the perception and search for social support. *Journal of Psychology, 129*, 665–679.

Fraley, R. C., & Shaver, P. R. (1998). Airport separations: A naturalistic study of adult attachment dynamics in separating couples. *Journal of Personality and Social Psychology, 75*, 1198–1212.

Fraley, R. C., & Shaver, P. R. (2000). Adult romantic attachment: Theoretical developments, emerging controversies, and unanswered questions. *Review of General Psychology, 4*, 132–154.

Fraley, R. C., & Waller, N. G. (1998). Adult attachment patterns: A test of the typological model. In J. A. Simpson & W. S. Rholes (Eds.), *Attachment theory and close relationships* (pp. 77–114). New York: Guilford Press.

George, C., Kaplan, N., & Main, M. (1984). *Attachment interview for adults*. Unpublished manuscript, University of California at Berkeley.

George, C., & Solomon, J. (1999). Attachment and caregiving: The caregiving behavioral system. In J. Cassidy & P. R. Shaver (Eds.), *Handbook of attachment: Theory, research, and clinical applications* (pp. 649–670). New York: Guilford Press.

Gillath, O., Shaver, P. R., Mikulincer, M., Nitzberg, R. E., Erez, A., & van IJzendoorn, M. H. (2005). Attachment, caregiving, and volunteering: Placing volunteerism in an attachment-theoretical framework. *Personal Relationships, 12*, 425–446.

Hazan, C., Gur-Yaish, & Campa, M. (2004). What does it mean to be attached? In W. S. Rholes & J. A. Simpson (Eds.), *Adult attachment: Theory, research, and clinical implications* (pp. 55–85). New York: Guilford Press.

Hazan, C., & Shaver, P. R. (1987). Romantic love conceptualized as an attachment process. *Journal of Personality and Social Psychology, 52*, 511–524.

Hazan, C., & Shaver, P. R. (1990). Love and work: An attachment-theoretical perspective. *Journal of Personality and Social Psychology, 59*, 270–280.

Kestenbaum, R., Farber, E. A., & Sroufe, L. A. (1989). Individual differences in empathy among preschoolers: Relation to attachment history. *New Directions for Child Development, 44*, 51–64.

Kobak, R. R., & Hazan, C. (1991). Attachment in marriage: Effects of security and accuracy of working models. *Journal of Personality and Social Psychology, 60*, 861–869.

Kobak, R. R., & Sceery, A. (1988). Attachment in late adolescence: Working models, affect regulation, and perception of self and others. *Child Development, 59*, 135–146.

Kunce, L. J., & Shaver, P. R. (1994). An attachment-theoretical approach to caregiving in romantic relationships. In K. Bartholomew & D. Perlman (Eds.), *Advances in personal relationships: Vol. 5. Attachment processes in adulthood* (pp. 205–237). London: Kingsley.

Main, M., Kaplan, N., & Cassidy, J. (1985). Security in infancy, childhood, and adulthood: A move to the level of representation. *Monographs of the Society for Research in Child Development, 50*, 66–104.

Mikulincer, M. (1997). Adult attachment style and information processing: Individual differences in curiosity and cognitive closure. *Journal of Personality and Social Psychology, 72*, 1217–1230.

Mikulincer, M., & Florian, V. (1995). Appraisal of and coping with a real-life stressful situation: The contribution of attachment styles. *Personality and Social Psychology Bulletin, 21*, 406–414.

Mikulincer, M., Florian, V., & Weller, A. (1993). Attachment styles, coping strategies, and posttraumatic psychological distress: The impact of the Gulf War in Israel. *Journal of Personality and Social Psychology, 64*, 817–826.

Mikulincer, M., Gillath, O., Halevy, V., Avihou, N., Avidan, S., & Eshkoli, N. (2001). Attachment theory and reactions to others' needs: Evidence that activation of the sense of attachment security promotes empathic responses. *Journal of Personality and Social Psychology, 81*, 1205–1224.

Mikulincer, M., Gillath, O., Sapir-Lavid, Y., Yaakobi, E., Arias, K., Tal-Aloni, L., & Bor, G. (2003). Attachment theory and concern for others' welfare: Evidence that activation of the sense of secure base promotes endorsement of self-transcendence values. *Basic and Applied Social Psychology, 25*, 299–312.

Mikulincer, M., & Shaver, P. R. (2001). Attachment theory and intergroup bias: Evidence that priming the secure base schema attenuates negative reactions to out-groups. *Journal of Personality and Social Psychology, 81*, 97–115.

Mikulincer, M., & Shaver, P. R. (2003). The attachment behavioral system in adulthood: Activation, psychodynamics, and interpersonal processes. In M. P. Zanna (Ed.), *Advances in experimental social psychology* (Vol. 35, pp. 53–152). San Diego: Academic Press.

Mikulincer, M., Shaver, P. R., Gillath, O., & Nitzberg, R. E. (2005). Attachment, caregiving, and altruism: Boosting attachment security increases compassion and helping. *Journal of Personality and Social Psychology, 89*, 817–839.

Murray, S. L., Holmes, J. G., & Collins, N. L. (in press). Optimizing assurance: The risk regulation system in close relationship. *Psychological Bulletin.*

Ognibene, T. C., & Collins, N. L. (1998). Adult attachment styles, perceived social support, and coping strategies. *Journal of Social and Personal Relationships, 15*, 323–345.

Reis, H. T., & Patrick, B. C. (1996). Attachment and intimacy: Component processes. In E. T. Higgins & A. W. Kruglanski (Eds.), *Social psychology: Handbook of basic principles* (pp. 523–563). New York: Guilford Press.

Reis, H. T., & Shaver, P. (1988). Intimacy as an interpersonal process. In S. Duck & D. F. Hay (Eds.), *Handbook of personal relationships: Theory, research, and interventions* (pp. 367–389). Chichester, UK: Wiley.

Rholes, W. S., Simpson, J. A., & Orina, M. M. (1999). Attachment and anger in an anxiety-provoking situation. *Journal of Personality and Social Psychology, 76*, 940–957.

Rini, C. M. (2001). Social support effectiveness: Measurement, prediction, and relation to psychological health during pregnancy. *Dissertation Abstracts International, 62*(2-B), 1144.

Ruehlman, L. S., & Wolchik, S. A. (1988). Personal goals and interpersonal support and hindrance as factors in psychological distress and well-being. *Journal of Personality and Social Psychology, 55*, 293–301.

Shaver, P. R., Collins, N. L., & Clark, C. L. (1996). Attachment styles and internal working models of self and relationship partners. In G. J. O. Fletcher & J. Fitness (Eds.), *Knowledge structures in close relationships: A social psychological approach* (pp. 25–61). Mahwah, NJ: Erlbaum.

Simpson, J. A., Rholes, W. S., & Nelligan, J. S. (1992). Support seeking and support giving within couples in an anxiety-provoking situation: The role of attachment styles. *Journal of Personality and Social Psychology, 62*, 434–446.

Simpson, J. A., Rholes, W. S., Orina, M. M., & Grich, J. (2002). Working models of attachment, support giving, and support seeking in a stressful situation. *Personality and Social Psychology Bulletin, 28*, 598–608.

Waters, E., & Cummings, E. (2000). A secure base from which to explore close relationships. *Child Development, 71*, 164–172.

Westmaas, J. L., & Silver, R. C. (2001). The role of attachment in responses to victims of life crises. *Journal of Personality and Social Psychology, 80*, 425–438.

8

Attachment, Mental Representations of Others, and Gratitude and Forgiveness in Romantic Relationships

MARIO MIKULINCER, PHILLIP R. SHAVER,
and KEREN SLAV

According to attachment theory (Bowlby, 1969/1982, 1973, 1980), adults' behavior in close relationships and their subjective construal of these relationships are shaped by mental representations (*working models*) whose origins lie in early childhood relationships with primary caregivers and that continue to evolve as people develop new relationships throughout life. In other words, theoretically speaking, people construe person–environment transactions subjectively, store representations of typical transactions in an associative memory network, and use these representations to understand new interpersonal transactions and to organize action plans. In Bowlby's (1980) words, "Every situation we meet in life is constructed in terms of representational models we have of the world about us and of ourselves. Information reaching us through our sense organs is selected and interpreted in terms of those models, its significance for us and for those we care for is evaluated in terms of them, and plans of action are conceived and executed with those models in mind" (p. 229).

Bowlby (1969/1982) imagined that a person's history of significant social experiences is stored in at least two kinds of working models: representations of relationship partners' responses to one's own proximity-seeking bids (*working models of others*) and representations of one's own lovability and competence (*working models of self*). Thus attachment working models include representations of the availability, responsiveness, sensitivity, and goodwill of others, as well as representations of the self's own capabilities for mobilizing others' support and one's feelings of being loved and valued by others. In this chapter, we focus mainly on a person's working models of others and their influence on attitudes and behaviors toward close relationship partners. These working models of others seem to underlie attachment-style differences in caregiving behavior (see Collins, Guichard, Ford, & Feeney, Chapter 7, this volume) and the appraisals people make of conflicts that inevitably arise in close relationships (see Simpson, Campbell, & Weisberg, Chapter 9, this volume). They frequently affect one's appraisals of relationship partners, expectations concerning how they will behave, and interpretations of their actions (see Shaver & Clark, 1994; Shaver & Hazan, 1993; Shaver & Mikulincer, 2002, for reviews of relevant studies). In this chapter, we extend existing research on working models of others by focusing on the way they moderate two important kinds of reactions to close relationship partners—gratitude toward a generous, caring partner and forgiveness toward a partner who has been disloyal, inconsiderate, or hurtful.

We begin by briefly reviewing the parts of attachment theory that deal with the nature and development of working models (Bowlby, 1969/1982, 1973, 1980). We then specify how the two major dimensions of attachment insecurity, avoidance and anxiety—as well as their prototypical underlying strategies of distress regulation (deactivation and hyperactivation of the attachment system)—affect working models of others. Next, we provide a detailed review of empirical work on the manifestations of working models of others in a person's beliefs and attitudes toward relationship partners. Following this, we present new ideas and report new evidence on attachment-style differences in the intensity and subjective construal of gratitude and forgiveness. We also review new data from a diary study, which indicate that working models of others influence daily fluctuations in gratitude and forgiveness, sometimes even overriding the effects of partner behaviors on a particular day. At the end we place these new findings in a broader array of recent findings concerning the interplay of the attachment, caregiving, and sexual behavioral systems.

ATTACHMENT STYLE AND MENTAL REPRESENTATIONS OF OTHERS

As explained throughout this book, there are now hundreds of studies testing ideas and hypotheses derived from Bowlby's (1969/1982, 1973, 1980) theory over the past three decades. According to Bowlby (1969/1982), proximity-seeking behavior, beginning in early infancy, is regulated by an innate *attachment behavioral system* that evolved biologically to protect a person from danger by ensuring that he or she maintains proximity to caring and supportive others (*attachment figures*). The parameters of this system are affected by social experiences (Bowlby, 1973), especially with early caregivers, resulting in measurable individual differences in *attachment style* (secure, anxious, avoidant)—the systematic pattern of relational expectations, emotions, and behaviors that results from the internalization of a particular history of attachment experiences (Fraley & Shaver, 2000). Attachment theory views these relational styles as core personality characteristics that are regularly applied to new situations and relationships, guiding interpersonal cognitions, emotions, behaviors, and coping or affect-regulation strategies (e.g., Collins & Read, 1994; Mikulincer & Shaver, 2003).

Attachment styles are conceptualized as regions in a two-dimensional space (e.g., Ainsworth, Blehar, Waters, & Wall, 1978; Brennan, Clark, & Shaver, 1998). The first dimension, typically called attachment *avoidance*, reflects the extent to which a person distrusts relationship partners' goodwill and strives to maintain autonomy and emotional distance from partners. The second dimension, typically called attachment *anxiety*, reflects the degree to which a person worries that a partner will not be available in times of need. People who score low on both dimensions are said to be secure, or securely attached. The two dimensions can be measured with reliable and valid self-report scales, such as the Experience in Close Relationships scale (ECR; Brennan et al., 1998), and they are associated in theoretically predictable ways with interpersonal functioning, affect regulation, and relationship quality (see Shaver & Clark, 1994; Shaver & Hazan, 1993; Shaver & Mikulincer, 2002, for reviews).

Recently, Mikulincer and Shaver (2003) proposed that variations along the dimensions of attachment anxiety and avoidance reflect both a person's sense of attachment security and the ways in which he or she deals with distress. According to Mikulincer and Shaver (2003), people who score low on these dimensions hold internalized representations of comforting attachment figures, which create a continuing sense of attachment security, positive self-regard, and reliance on constructive strategies of affect regulation. Those who score high on either attachment avoidance or attachment anxiety possess internalized representations of frustrating or unavailable attachment figures and hence suffer from a continuing sense of attachment insecurity. These insecure individuals rely on what Cassidy and Kobak (1988) called *secondary attachment strategies* (contrasted with the primary strategy of seeking proximity to an attachment figure in times of need), which involve either deactivating or hyperactivating the attachment system in an attempt to regulate distress. Whereas high scores on the attachment avoidance dimension indicate reliance on deactivating strategies—inhibition of proximity seeking, denial of attachment needs, maintenance of emotional and cognitive distance from others, and compulsive reliance on self as the sole source of protection—high scores on the attachment anxiety dimension reflect hyperactivating strategies: energetic attempts to attain greater proximity, support, and love combined with a lack of confidence that it will be provided (Mikulincer & Shaver, 2003).

Variations in attachment anxiety and avoidance are important reflections of a person's working models of others (Bowlby, 1973; Shaver & Hazan, 1993; Shaver & Mikulincer, 2002). According to Bowlby (1973), social experiences with attachment figures beginning in infancy form a foundation for the development of models of others (beliefs about others' availability, goodwill, supportiveness, and trustworthiness). Whereas a security-enhancing interaction with an available and responsive relationship partner promotes positive representations of the partner, a negative interaction with a cold, unavailable, or rejecting partner damages one's sense of security and strengthens negative mental representations. These cognitive products can be generalized across recurrent interactions with an attachment figure. Moreover, they can be generalized across relationships via top-down schematic processing of new partners and relationships, creating central building blocks of a person's working models of others.

Bowlby's (1973) reasoning about the formation of working models of others implies that insecurely attached people, who score high on either or both attachment insecurity dimensions, hold negative beliefs about others' intentions and traits. This does not mean, however, that anxious and avoidant people—although both are conceptualized in attachment theory as insecure—have similar working models of others. According to Bowlby (1980), working models of others do not consist only of directly internalized experiences with attachment figures but also reflect the operation of regulatory strategies that can defensively bias the appraisal of these figures. That is, hyperactivating and deactivating strategies can systematically bias insecure people's working models of others and shape systematic differences between anxious and avoidant individuals in the ways they appraise others' traits and behaviors.

Avoidant, or deactivating, strategies can exacerbate negative views of others and preserve them in the face of disconfirming evidence. According to Mikulincer and Shaver (2003), these biases result from two psychological processes. First, deactivating strategies divert attention away from any attachment-related information, including information about others' positive traits, intentions, and behaviors (Mikulincer & Shaver, 2003). As a result, genuine signals of a partner's support and love can be missed and, even when noted, can be processed mentally in a shallow manner, be easily forgotten, and remain inaccessible when later appraisals of relationship partners are made. This dismissal of positive information about relationship partners sustains avoidant people's negative and rigid images of others. Second, deactivating strategies involve suppression of negative self-aspects from consciousness and overemphasis on self–other dissimilarity and self-uniqueness (Mikulincer & Shaver, 2003). These maneuvers encourage projection of the suppressed material onto relationship partners (in a process that Freud, 1915/1957, called "defensive projection"), thereby further reinforcing negative views of others. In other words, avoidant individuals' negative appraisals of relationship partners are guided, in part, by a defensive preference for distance and a desire to view themselves as stronger and better than other people. These now well-documented psychodynamic, defensive processes are one of the hallmarks of attachment theory that make it different from other currently popular theories of personality and relationship-related cognition (Shaver & Mikulincer, 2005).

Anxious, or hyperactivating, strategies often influence the formation of complex and ambivalent appraisals of others. Although anxiously attached people have a history of negative interactions with attachment figures (Shaver & Hazan, 1993), they still believe that, if they intensify their proximity-seeking bids to a sufficient degree, they may get a relationship partner, viewed as unreliable or insufficiently available, to pay attention and provide adequate support (Cassidy & Kobak, 1988). This hopeful attitude seems to stem from previous relationships in which parents or other relationship partners were sometimes responsive and sometimes not, thereby placing anxiously attached people on a partial reinforcement schedule that seems to reward intensity and persistence in proximity-seeking attempts (Shaver & Hazan, 1993). As a result, anxiously attached people do not form a simple, strong negative view of others, because such a view would imply that proximity seeking is hopeless (the avoidant person's view). Rather, the anxious person, although often angry as well as frightened, tends to take some of the blame for a partner's unreliable attention and care, thus causing a lowering of self-confidence and self-esteem ("Something is wrong with me; I don't have what it takes to gain his loyal attention and regard"; Mikulincer & Shaver, 2003). These mental gyrations lead to ambivalent views of others, which include appraisals of others' simultaneous great potential value and frequent unavailability or lack of support. They sustain both hope for true love and security and doubts about the self's ability to attain and hold onto them.

According to Mikulincer and Shaver (2003), three additional cognitive processes exacerbate the negative side of this ambivalence. First, anxious, hyperactivating strategies intensify the vigilant monitoring of relationship partners' behaviors and slant perceptions in the direction of noticing or imagining insufficient availability and responsiveness. Hence the likelihood of negative views of partners as rejecting and distant is increased, because partners cannot always be available or at one's beck and call. Second, hyperactivating strategies involve mental rumination on real or imagined signs of a partner's lack of immediate availability, which heightens the mental availability of negative views of a partner and causes them to be more accessible in social perception. Third, hyperactivating strategies intensify the pursuit of close proximity and fusion with relationship partners, which in turn encourages anxious people to project their negative self-views onto relationship partners in order to create an illusory sense of similarity and union (a process that the psychoanalyst Klein, writing in 1940, called "projective identification"). In this way, paradoxically, a negative view of others is guided in part by the anxious person's negative self-views combined with an intense longing for social connectedness.

There is extensive evidence that attachment anxiety and avoidance in adulthood are associated with negative appraisals of parents (who were often our research participants' primary caregivers). In their pioneering study of adult attachment, Hazan and Shaver (1987) found that adults who endorsed a secure style of romantic attachment described their parents as more respectful, responsive, caring, accepting, and undemanding, as compared with the parent descriptions of anxious and avoidant adults. These findings have been conceptually replicated by several other investigators who used different self-report scales for rating parents' traits and behaviors (e.g., Brennan & Shaver, 1998; Mickelson, Kessler, & Shaver, 1997; Rothbard & Shaver, 1994). In two other attachment studies (Levy, Blatt, & Shaver, 1998; Priel & Besser, 2001), participants' open-ended descriptions of their parents were content analyzed, and it was found that parent descriptions provided by insecurely attached adults were characterized by less benevolence, acceptance, differentiation, and elaboration and more ambivalence than the descriptions provided by secure participants.

There is also extensive evidence concerning insecurely attached people's negative appraisals of their romantic partners. Several studies have found that attachment insecurities are associated with lower ratings of a romantic partner's emotional involvement, intimacy, commitment, and love (e.g., Collins & Read, 1990; Feeney & Noller, 1990; Kirkpatrick & Davis, 1994; Mikulincer & Erev, 1991; Shaver & Brennan, 1992; Simpson, 1990) and with a more negative appraisal of a partner's personal traits (e.g., Mikulincer & Arad, 1999; Young & Acitelli, 1998). Interestingly, Pietromonaco and Feldman-Barret (1997) found attachment-style differences in appraisals of a romantic partner only during daily interpersonal conflicts (as recorded with the Rochester Interaction Record during a week-long daily diary study). On these occasions, anxiously attached participants appraised their partners more positively and avoidant participants appraised their partners more negatively than did secure participants. However, following the discussion of a major unresolved problem in the laboratory, Simpson, Rholes, and Phillips (1996) found that anxious persons' appraisals of their partners became more negative than those of securely attached persons (see Simpson et al., Chapter 9, in this volume for conceptually similar findings). This complex pattern of reactions provides an example of anxiously attached people's ambivalent and fluctuating representations of their relationship partners.

Attachment insecurity is also related to perceptions of a relationship partner's supportiveness. Using a variety of perceived support scales, dozens of studies have documented that attachment anxiety and avoidance are associated with views of family members, friends, and romantic partners as being inadequately supportive (e.g., Blain, Thompson, & Whiffen, 1993; Davis, Morris, & Kraus, 1998; Priel, Mitrany, & Shahar, 1998; Volling, Notaro, & Larsen, 1998; Ognibene & Collins, 1998). Other studies have found that attachment anxiety and avoidance are inversely related to the number of persons listed as support providers (i.e., perceived size of the support network) and the degree of satisfaction with the support received (e.g., Markiewicz, Reis, & Gold, 1997; Priel & Shamai, 1995; Trinke & Bartholomew, 1997). In a recent laboratory study, Collins and Feeney (2004) found that anxious and avoidant participants who received standardized low-support messages from their romantic partners perceived the partners as less supportive in a prior interaction than securely attached participants perceived their partners to be. That is, insecure people seem predisposed to exacerbate negative appraisals of actual examples of their partners' lack of adequate support in accordance with their chronic negative working models.

Insecure people's negative appraisals of others are manifested even in their views of human nature in general, especially with regard to other people's trustworthiness. For example, Collins and Read (1990) reported that insecure participants in their studies were less likely to believe that human beings are altruistic, willing to stand up for their beliefs, and able to control their lives, and Luke, Maio, and Carnelley (2004) found that attachment avoidance was associated with more negative evaluations of humanity in general (i.e., less satisfaction with humanity and its evolution). Furthermore, Collins and Read (1990) found that attachment insecurity was associated with lower ratings of romantic partners' predictability, dependability, and faith. This pattern of associations has been conceptually replicated in subsequent studies by other investigators (e.g., Cozzarelli, Hoekstra, & Bylsma, 2000; Mikulincer, 1998; Simpson, 1990). In a series of five studies, Mikulincer (1998) provided further evidence of links between attachment style and the sense of trust. Insecure study participants exhibited faster access to memories of trust betrayal and slower access to memories of trust validation; they also reported fewer trust validation episodes in their current romantic relationships. Interestingly, however, avoidant people dismissed the importance of trust-betrayal episodes, whereas anxious people ruminated on them and reacted to them with strong negative emotions.

Similar attachment-style differences have been found in the ways people explain a relationship partner's negative behavior (e.g., Collins, 1996; Sumer & Cozzarelli, 2004; Whisman & Allan, 1996). For example, Collins

(1996) asked people to think about six hypothetical negative partner behaviors, write an open-ended explanation of each one, and complete an attribution questionnaire. She found that more anxious and avoidant people provided more explanations that implied lack of confidence in their partner's love, attributed the partner's negative behavior to more stable and global causes, and were more likely to view these behaviors as negatively motivated. Similarly, Whisman and Allan (1996) reported that attachment anxiety was associated with attributing greater responsibility to their partners for ambiguously caused negative behaviors. And in a study of married couples, Gallo and Smith (2001) found that both wives' and husbands' attachment anxiety and husbands' attachment avoidance were associated with damaging patterns of causal attributions for spousal behavior (viewing a spouse's hurtful behavior as due to more intentional, stable, and global causes).

Attachment insecurity is also associated with negative expectations concerning a romantic partner's future behavior (e.g., Baldwin, Fehr, Keedian, Seidel, & Thompson, 1993; Baldwin, Keelan, Fehr, Enns, & Koh Rangarajoo, 1996; Mikulincer & Arad, 1999). These negative expectations have been documented not only with explicit self-report scales but also by using cognitive tasks that tap implicit mental processes. For example, Baldwin et al. (1993) used a lexical-decision task in which participants read sentences that established either an attachment-related interpersonal context ("If I depend on my partner then my partner will . . . ") or an attachment-unrelated context ("If I wash the dishes then my partner will . . . "), as well as target strings of letters that represented positive outcome words ("support"), negative outcome words ("leave"), neutral words ("read"), or nonwords. Participants were asked to determine as quickly as possible whether each target string of letters formed a word. Reaction times (RTs) served as a measure of the accessibility of thoughts related to the target words—the quicker the RT, the higher the inferred accessibility. Findings revealed that insecurely attached people reacted with relatively short lexical decision times (indicating heightened accessibility) to words connoting negative partner behaviors within an attachment-related context.

Recently, Zayas, Shoda, and Ayduk (2002) studied cognitive processes related to attachment style using the Implicit Association Task (IAT; Greenwald, McGhee, & Schwartz, 1998), a categorization task designed to measure the strength of automatic associations between a target concept (e.g., romantic partner) and an attribute (e.g., positive or negative traits). In this task, the measured presence of a strong automatic association between a target concept and an attribute implies that activation of the target concept automatically and effortlessly activates the attribute (indicated by a faster RT to the attribute in the presence of the target concept than in the presence of a different concept). Zayas and colleagues (2002) found that self-reports of attachment avoidance were related to stronger automatic associations between, on the one hand, two target concepts—current romantic partner and mother—and, on the other hand, negative personal attributes. That is, self-reports of attachment avoidance were associated with implicit negative mental representations of significant others.

There is also empirical evidence concerning the hypothesized biases in perceived self–other similarity and projective tendencies of insecurely attached persons. In a series of studies, Mikulincer, Orbach, and Iavnieli (1998) found that anxious people were more likely than secure people to perceive others as similar to themselves and to show a false-consensus bias in both trait and opinion descriptions, whereas avoidant individuals were more likely to perceive other people as dissimilar to themselves and to exhibit a false-distinctiveness bias. In a subsequent study, Mikulincer and Horesh (1999) examined attachment-style differences in the projection of self-relevant traits onto another person and found that avoidant individuals were likely to perceive others as having the self's own unwanted traits, could more easily retrieve an example of a known person whose traits included the ones they disliked in themselves, and made more faulty inferences that their own unwanted traits were among the ones they had seen associated with another person. Anxious individuals were more likely to perceive in an unknown person traits that defined their actual selves, could more easily retrieve an example of a known person whose traits resembled their actual–self traits, and made faulty inferences that their own actual traits had been mentioned among those associated with another person they read about.

In summary, there is a great deal of evidence documenting attachment-style variations in working models of others and their manifestations in a person's appraisals, beliefs, expectations, and interpretations of a relationship partner's traits and behaviors. We believe that these attachment-related variations in working models can also shape a person's responses to a partner's positive or negative behaviors and thus affect the intensity and quality of experiences of gratitude and forgiveness within close relationships. In the following sections, we present ideas and review our new research findings concerning attachment-related variations in gratitude and forgiveness.

ATTACHMENT AND GRATITUDE

Gratitude has recently received a great deal of attention in both the scientific and popular literature on psychology, where it is viewed as a potential remedy for many of life's hardships, as well as a means to achieve peace of mind, happiness, physical health, and more fulfilling relationships (Emmons & McCullough, 2003). It is also an essential theme in the sacred writings of the three major monotheistic faiths (Judaism, Christianity, and Islam) and in Buddhist and Hindi thinking (Emmons & Crumple, 2000). Gratitude has also played an important role in philosophy, dividing philosophers into those who glorify gratitude and those who believe that behind expressions of gratitude lie hidden egoistic motives and feelings of commitment or obligation (McCullough, Emmons, & Tsang, 2002).

In psychology, gratitude has been viewed diversely as an emotion, a personality characteristic, an attitude, an ethical virtue, or an adaptive response (Emmons & McCullough, 2003). However, despite these many perspectives, theorists generally agree that gratitude can be defined or conceptualized in terms of three definitional components. First, the object of gratitude is always the "other," whether another human being, a nonhuman natural being (e.g., an animal), or a superhuman (e.g., God; Teigen, 1997). Second, gratitude stems from the perception of a positive personal consequence (e.g., a material, emotional, or spiritual gain) of the actions of the "other," which has not necessarily been earned or deserved (Emmons & McCullough, 2003). Third, gratitude involves the appraisal of the other's actions as intentionally constructed around the goal of benefiting the person (Heider, 1958; Weiner, 1985). According to Lazarus and Lazarus (1994), gratitude results from recognizing the other's goodwill and appreciating his or her generous action as an altruistic gift.

From a psychoanalytic perspective, Klein (1957) focused on the sources of gratitude during infants' interactions with a primary caregiver and equated the ability to feel gratitude and the ability to love. Essentially, Klein (1957), like Bowlby (1973), proposed that pleasurable interactions with a sensitive and responsive caregiver lead to the formation of positive mental representations of others. In her view, these positive representations subdue destructive emotions, such as greed and envy, and lead infants to feel that they have received from their caregiver a unique gift that they wish to keep, thereby laying the foundation for feeling gratitude toward any generous other. Furthermore, according to Klein (1957), the development of gratitude, which means assimilation of a "good object" that has enriched the self, goes together with the parallel development of generosity—the wish to benefit others and share with them the gift one has received. Klein (1957) also viewed gratitude as an inner resource that helps us to withstand hardship and mental pain and to accept the tragedies of life without bitterness.

The view of gratitude as an inner resource has recently reemerged in a more actualization-oriented approach to psychology—the "positive psychology" movement (Seligman, 2002). In this approach, happiness and satisfaction with life are not consequences of luck or genetics, but rather the result of personality strengths—characteristics that may be shaped and fostered by social experiences and deliberate personal effort (Seligman, 2002). Gratitude is one of these strengths, and it is viewed as aiding people to live better within society, contributing to societal harmony, and advancing people's health and well-being (Snyder & McCullough, 2000). In support of this view, Emmons and McCullough (2003) found that priming thoughts of gratitude on a daily basis led to subsequent positive changes in their research participants' well-being.

In a recent study, McCullough et al. (2002) formulated a personality-focused conceptualization of gratitude and constructed a self-report scale to measure individual differences in the disposition to feel gratitude (the Gratitude Questionnaire-6, or GQ-6). In their view, the "grateful disposition" is a general tendency to recognize the contribution made by the generosity of others to one's own positive achievements and to feel thankful. People who are high in the grateful disposition are expected to feel more intense gratitude in response to positive events and to feel grateful for more aspects of and more people in their lives. In an empirical study of the grateful disposition, Watkins, Woodward, Stone, and Kolts (2003) found that more grateful individuals tend not to feel deprived in their lives but rather to experience abundance, feel gratitude for the contributions of others to their personal well-being, and appreciate the small pleasures in life that are available to most people.

From an attachment perspective, the experience of gratitude during positive interactions with others should go hand in hand with the feelings of being protected, accepted, and valued and the formation of positive working models of others as available, responsive, supportive, and loving (Bowlby, 1973; Shaver & Hazan, 1993). As a result, attachment security should be closely associated with the disposition to feel gratitude. In contrast, avoidant individuals can be expected to react with less gratitude to others' generous behavior. They tend not to believe in others' goodwill and do not wish to depend on or be supported by them (Mikulincer & Shaver, 2003). Moreover, expression of gratitude toward a relationship partner can be interpreted as a sign of closeness, which is incongruent with an avoidant person's preference for emotional distance.

People who score high on attachment anxiety can be expected to show ambivalent reactions to others' generous behavior. Anxiously attached people tend not to believe they deserve others' kindness and so may worry that they will not be able to reciprocate fully or meet a partner's needs and expectations, which in turn may dilute gratitude with strong doses of fear and anxiety. In addition, for anxiously attached people, positive interpersonal experiences may be reminiscent of previous experiences that began well but ended painfully. Once attuned to negative memories, the anxious mind may suffer from a spread of negative affect that interferes with the experience of gratitude.

In two recent studies, we began to test the hypothesized links between attachment style dimensions and gratitude while assessing both dispositional manifestations of gratitude and its daily expressions toward a particular romantic partner. In the first study, we examined relations between attachment anxiety and avoidance, on the one hand, and the grateful disposition, as well as the ways in which people subjectively experience episodes of gratitude, on the other. The subjective experiences included thoughts, feelings, and wishes that emerged when people felt grateful toward another person. In addition, we explored whether associations between attachment-style dimensions and gratitude variables could be explained by alternative variables related to working models of self and others (e.g., self-esteem and interpersonal trust).

We asked 142 Israeli undergraduates (83 women and 59 men) to complete the Experience in Close Relationships scale (ECR; Brennan et al., 1998), a measure of attachment-related attachment anxiety and avoidance; the GQ-6 scale (McCullough et al., 2002) as a measure of dispositional gratitude; the Rosenberg (1979) self-esteem scale, and the Rotter (1967) interpersonal trust scale. In addition, study participants completed the Gratitude Experience Scale (GES)—a 29-item scale created specifically for this study to assess the subjective experience of gratitude episodes. Participants were asked to recall a specific situation in which they felt grateful to someone and to rate the extent to which they experienced each of the feelings, thoughts, and wishes described in the scale. The 29 items were generated in a pilot study, in which 60 Israeli undergraduates freely described, in an open-ended format, their subjective experiences of gratitude in particular situations.

A preliminary principal-components analysis with Varimax rotation revealed that the 29 GES items could be summarized in terms of seven main factors (with eigenvalues greater than 1), which together accounted for 69.4% of the item variance. Factor 1 (28.8% of the explained variance) included five items (loading > .40) tapping what in attachment theory are called secure-base feelings (e.g., "I felt there is someone who cares for me"; "I felt secure"). Factor 2 (15.9%) included five items tapping feelings of happiness and love (e.g., "I felt happy and satisfied"; "I felt love for the person I was grateful to"). Factor 3 (6.1%) included four items tapping the experience of narcissistic threats (e.g., "I felt I was risking my personal freedom"; "I thought I was giving up my dignity"). Factor 4 (5.5%) included five items reflecting generosity and a positive outlook on life (e.g., "I felt appreciative of the good things in my life"; "I felt the need to do good deeds"). Factor 5 (5.1%) contained three items tapping a sense of distrust in the other's goodwill (e.g., "I doubted that person's motives"; "I feared that this person would take advantage of me in the future"). Factor 6 (4.4%) was based on four items reflecting a sense of inferiority and vulnerability (e.g., "I felt weak and needy"; "I felt vulnerable"). Factor 7 (3.6%) included three items tapping feelings of obligation toward the other person (e.g., "I felt a need to find a way to repay that person"; "I felt obliged to that person").

As can be seen, the subjective experience of gratitude is not monolithic and not simply affectively positive. Rather, it is a multifaceted, complex experience that includes positive feelings of happiness, love, security, and a positive outlook on life together (in some cases) with self-focused fears, feelings of vulnerability and obligation, and distrust of a benefactor's intentions. Cronbach alphas for the seven factors were acceptable (ranging from .68 to .89). We therefore computed seven scores for each participant by averaging the items loading higher than .40 on each factor.

Analyses revealed that the two attachment dimensions, avoidance and anxiety, contributed uniquely to the grateful disposition and the experience of gratitude beyond their associations with self-esteem and trust (see Table 8.1). Specifically, avoidant attachment was inversely associated with the grateful disposition (GQ-6 total score) and the experience of secure-base feelings, happiness and love, and generosity feelings; it was positively associated with the experience of narcissistic threats and distrust. Attachment anxiety was not significantly associated with the grateful disposition, but it was related significantly and uniquely to secure-base feelings, happiness and love, and generosity on the positive side of the ledger and to narcissistic threats and feelings of inferiority and obligation on the negative side.

These findings correspond with avoidant and anxious individuals' models of others. On the one hand, avoidant attachment, which includes negative models of others, is associated with lower dispositional gratitude and a more negative experience of gratitude episodes (more narcissistic threats and distrust, fewer secure-base feelings, and less happiness and love). On the other hand, attachment anxiety, which includes ambivalent models of others, is not significantly associated with the disposition toward gratitude, but it is associated with a more ambivalent experience of grati-

TABLE 8.1. Pearson Correlations and Standardized Regression Coefficients Examining the Attachment–Gratitude Link (after Controlling for Self-Esteem and Interpersonal Trust)

	Attachment avoidance		Attachment anxiety	
Gratitude variable	*r*	Beta	*r*	Beta
GQ-6 total score	–.38**	–.36**	.07	.10
GES factors				
Secure-base feelings	–.41**	–.41**	.36**	.37**
Happiness/love	–.32**	–.33**	.27**	.28**
Narcissistic threats	.49**	.49**	.20*	.22*
Positive outlook on life	–.21*	–.22*	.24**	.26**
Distrust in other's goodwill	.32**	.31**	.14	.09
Inferiority feelings	.16	.14	.35**	.30**
Obligation feelings	.01	–.02	.26**	.27**

* $p < .05$; ** $p < .01$.

tude episodes (happiness, love, security, and generosity feelings together with narcissistic threats and inferiority feelings). These associations cannot be explained by variations in self-esteem or trust.

In the second study, we examined whether the observed attachment–gratitude links are relevant to marital relationships and can be observed in the daily experiences of gratitude in response to specific partner behaviors. For this purpose, we asked 55 newlywed couples (both husbands and wives) who had lived together from 1 to 5 years to complete the ECR scale, the GQ-6, and the GES (our gratitude experiences measure). In addition, they completed a daily questionnaire every evening for a period of 21 days. When completing this questionnaire, each spouse independently marked positive and negative behaviors the partner had exhibited that day and rated the extent to which he or she felt grateful to the spouse during that day. Based on these responses, we computed two daily scores for each participant: (1) the difference between the number of perceived positive partner behaviors and the number of perceived negative partner behaviors on a given day and (2) the degree of gratitude toward the partner on that day.

The results for the GQ-6 and the GES replicated the findings of the first study, documenting avoidant people's generally aversive characterization of gratitude episodes and anxious people's ambivalent experience of these episodes. More important, hierarchical linear models revealed significant contributions of dispositional attachment orientations and daily fluctuations in partner's positive behaviors to daily feelings of gratitude toward the partner (see Table 8.2). For both husbands and wives, perceived positive behavior on the part of one's spouse on a given day was significantly associated with greater gratitude toward the partner on that day. Beyond this dyadic effect, dispositional attachment avoidance, but not anxious attachment, significantly predicted lower levels of gratitude toward one's partner across the 21 days. This effect was significant for both husbands and wives. Interestingly, a significant interaction was observed between husbands' avoidance and daily perceptions of wives' behavior as determinants of daily feelings of gratitude (see Table 8.2). Whereas less avoidant husbands reported more gratitude on days when they perceived more positive spousal behavior, more avoidant husbands reported relatively low levels of gratitude even on days when they noticed their wives' positive behavior.

The findings indicate that avoidant attachment is associated with inhibition of daily feelings of gratitude toward one's spouse. This inhibitory effect was observed on the part of both husbands and wives. In addition, husbands' (but not wives') avoidance moderated the extent to which a spouse's positive behavior elicited gratitude. In other words, a husband's avoidant attachment not only inhibits the daily experience of gratitude but also interferes with the ability of a wife's good behavior to elicit gratitude.

TABLE 8.2. Hierarchical Linear Model Coefficients for the Effects of Dispositional Attachment Orientations and Daily Partner Positive Behaviors on Daily Feelings of Gratitude

Effect	Husbands' gratitude	Wives' gratitude
Daily partner positive behavior	.31*	.32*
Dispositional attachment avoidance	–.41*	–.35*
Dispositional attachment anxiety	.02	.01
Avoidance × partner's positive behavior	–.29*	.02
Anxiety × partner's positive behavior	.01	.01

* $p < .01$.

ATTACHMENT AND FORGIVENESS

Conflicts, offenses, and transgressions are unavoidable in close relationships, because no two people's interests, attitudes, and behaviors are perfectly in synch all the time. Eventually, everyone is bound to feel frustrated, offended, "let down," betrayed, or wronged by his or her perhaps otherwise supportive relationship partner. Conflicts and interpersonal transgressions are obviously a major source of negative feelings that have the potential to disrupt a relationship (e.g., Fincham, 2000; Gottman, 1993; Lazarus, 1991). The most common responses to such transgressions are seeking distance from one's partner (avoidance), seeking to harm him or her in return (revenge), or regulating anger and hostility constructively and forgiving the offending partner (e.g., Fincham, 2000; McCullough, 2000). Whereas avoidance and revenge can exacerbate relational tensions, erode affectional bonds, and lead eventually to relationship dissolution, forgiveness can result in more benevolent interpersonal interactions and the restoration of relational harmony (e.g., Fincham, 2000; McCullough, 2000). Because forgiveness is often a key to maintaining a mutually satisfying romantic relationship, we focus in this section on associations between the attachment insecurity dimensions and forgiveness.

Forgiveness requires a transformation (or what Rusbult, Verette, Whitney, Slonk, & Lipkus, 1991, called "accommodation") of interpersonal motives—inhibition of angry feelings and the impulse to act destructively against a relationship partner and promotion of more constructive actions to overcome an impasse created by the partner's hurtful behavior (e.g., Fincham, 2000; McCullough, 2000). McCullough, Worthington, and Rachal (1997a) defined forgiveness as "a set of motivational changes, whereby one becomes decreasingly motivated to retaliate against and maintain estrangement from an offending relationship partner and increasingly motivated by conciliation and goodwill for the offender, despite the offender's hurtful actions" (pp. 321–322). Forgiveness is a prosocial emotional stance aimed at benefiting the relationship partner and the relationship, and it can be distinguished from related constructs, such as condoning a partner's behavior (justifying a transgression and thus removing the need for forgiveness), pardoning the partner (which is more appropriate in the legal realm), forgetting (which removes the offense from consciousness), and denial (being unable or unwilling even to see the offense; see Enright, 1991; Enright, Gassin, & Wu, 1992; and McCullough, 2000, for a more complete discussion of these distinctions.)

There is good evidence for the beneficial role of forgiveness in close relationships. Several studies have yielded documented positive associations between dispositional forgiveness and marital satisfaction (e.g., Fincham & Beach, 2001; Fincham, Paleari, & Regalia, 2002). In addition, forgiveness has been positively associated with relational commitment, intimacy, trust, and the effective resolution of conflicts (e.g., Fincham, Beach, & Davila, 2004). Studies indicate that forgiveness benefits not only a person's relationship but also his or her own health and well-being (e.g., Coyle & Enright, 1997).

Research has also begun to reveal the psychological processes that underlie forgiveness and the personality traits that characterize people who are inclined to forgive. For example, several studies have shown that forgiveness is facilitated by empathy for a transgressor and generous attributions and appraisals concerning the transgressor's traits and hurtful actions (e.g., Bradfield & Aquino, 1999; Fincham, 2000; McCullough et al., 1997b; Worthington et al., 2000). Specifically, people who were more inclined to forgive a specific transgressor felt more empathy for him or her, appraised the person as more likable, and attributed less responsibility to the person for the hurtful behavior. Another way of saying this is that the tendency to forgive is associated with positive mental representations of relationship partners. Research has also revealed that rumination about the transgression and the intrusive recurrence of transgression-related thoughts and images tends to interfere with forgiveness (McCullough, Bellah, Kilpatrick, & Johnson, 2001). In addition, the disposition to forgive is associated with higher levels of agreeableness, moral responsibility, and humility and lower levels of neuroticism, negative affectivity, and narcissism (e.g., Ashton, Paunonen, Helmes, & Jackson, 1998; Exline, Baumeister, Bushman, Campbell, & Finkel, 2004; McCullough et al., 2001).

From an attachment perspective, the motivational transformation involved in forgiving a relationship partner is likely to be facilitated by attachment security. As documented earlier, securely attached people are confident of others' availability and love, view others as generally trustworthy and dependable, and interpret their interpersonal behaviors as being aimed at maintaining and fostering intimacy and relational harmony (Shaver & Hazan, 1993). As a result, secure people can be expected to provide more benign explanations for a partner's hurtful actions and to attribute them to less intentional and less stable causes and hence be more inclined to forgive the partner. In contrast, avoidant individuals should be less forgiving because they possess negative models of others and hostile attitudes toward relationship partners and tend to attribute a partner's negative behavior to his or her bad intentions and untrustworthy personality. In support of this view, a recent study reported a significant association between avoidant attachment and the tendency to forgive relationship partners in both dating and marital relationships (Kachadourian, Fincham, & Davila, 2004).

In the case of anxiously attached individuals, reactions to a partner's negative behavior tend to be influenced by two conflicting forces. On the one hand, their inclination to intensify negative emotions and ruminate on threats should fuel intense and prolonged bouts of anger toward a relationship partner, thereby interfering with forgiveness. Indeed, Kachadourian et al. (2004) found evidence for such interference in married couples, although not in dating couples. On the another hand, anxiously attached people's separation anxiety, desperate need for a partner's love, and overly dependent attitude might lead them to suppress resentment and anger and incline them toward self-protective forgiveness. This kind of forgiveness might be accompanied by recurrent intrusive thoughts about the transgression and heightened doubts about the partner's availability, responsiveness, and dependability; about their own self-worth; and about the stability and longevity of their relationship. In other words, although attachment anxiety might not preclude forgiveness, it might engender ambivalence about forgiveness and thus reduce its relational and personal benefits.

Following Kachadourian et al.'s (2004) initial examination of the attachment–forgiveness link, we conducted two studies in which we assessed the subjective experience of forgiveness and daily expressions of forgiveness toward one's relationship partner. In the first study, a new sample of 140 Israeli undergraduates (71 women and 69 men) completed the ECR scale (Brennan et al., 1998); the Forgiving Scale (McCullough et al., 1997a), which measures the disposition to forgive; the Transgression-Related Interpersonal Motivations Inventory (TRIM; McCullough et al., 2001), which assesses dispositions toward revenge and avoidance following an offending partner's hurtful actions; the Rosenberg (1979) self-esteem scale, and the Rotter (1967) interpersonal trust scale. In addition, study participants completed the Forgiveness Experience Scale (FES)—a 25-item scale created specifically for this study to reveal the subjective experience of forgiveness. Participants were asked to recall a specific situation in which they forgave a relationship partner who had hurt them and to rate the extent to which they experienced each of the feelings, thoughts, and wishes described in the scale. The 25 items were generated in a preliminary study, in which 50 Israeli undergraduates freely described in an open-ended format their subjective experiences of forgiveness.

A preliminary principal-components analysis with Varimax rotation revealed that the 25 FES items formed five main factors (with eigenvalues greater than 1), which accounted for 58.3% of the item variance. Factor 1 (accounting for 25.8% of the variance) included seven items (with loadings > .40) related to narcissistic wounds (e.g., "I felt vulnerable"; "I felt I gave up my principles"; "I felt humiliated"). Factor 2 (13.9%) consisted of five items tapping a sense of relationship deterioration (e.g., "I lost trust in that person"; "I felt that my relationship with that person was damaged"). Factor 3 (7.1%) included five items measuring feelings of relief and being cleansed (e.g., "I felt that my anger gradually subsided"; "I felt emotionally cleansed"). Factor 4 (5.9%) was defined by five items reflecting a sense of relationship enhancement (e.g., "I felt that the offending person would not repeat his or her actions"; "I felt that my relationship with this person grew stronger"). Factor 5 (5.4%) contained four items tapping empathy and understanding of the partner's actions (e.g., "I understood that the person didn't intend to hurt me"; "I put myself in his or her position and was able to understand"). Cronbach alphas for the five factors were acceptable (ranging from .83 to .88), so we computed five scores for each participant by averaging the items that loaded higher than .40 on each factor.

Pearson correlations and multiple regression analyses revealed that the two attachment dimensions made unique contributions to the disposition to forgive and the experience of forgiveness, beyond their associations with self-esteem and trust (see Table 8.3). As expected, avoidant attachment was inversely associated with the disposition to forgive and positively associated with dispositions toward revenge and avoidance following an offending partner's hurtful actions. In addition, more avoidant people reported more severe narcissistic wounds, a higher sense of relationship deterioration, a lower sense of relationship enhancement, and less empathy and understanding associated with "forgiving" an offending partner. Attachment anxiety was not significantly associated with dispositions toward forgiveness, avoidance, or revenge, but it made a significant unique contribution to the experience of narcissistic wounds associated with "forgiveness" (which we place in quotation marks because the genuineness of the forgiveness is in doubt).

Overall, avoidant attachment, which involves negative models of others, is associated with lower dispositional forgiveness and a more negative experience of forgiveness episodes (deeper narcissistic wounds, less empathy, and a sense of relationship deterioration). Anxious attachment, which involves ambivalent models of others, is not significantly associated with the disposition to forgive, but it is associated with experiencing "forgiveness" in conjunction with lowered self-worth. As with gratitude, these findings cannot be explained simply by self-esteem or trust.

In a second study of forgiveness, we examined the attachment–forgiveness link in the context of marriage and assessed daily fluctuations in the tendency to forgive one's spouse. Each evening for 21 consecutive days, we

TABLE 8.3. Pearson Correlations and Standardized Regression Coefficients Examining the Attachment–Forgiveness Link (after Controlling for Self-Esteem and Interpersonal Trust)

	Attachment avoidance		Attachment anxiety	
Forgiveness variable	*r*	Beta	*r*	Beta
Disposition to forgive	–.34**	–.35**	.08	.06
TRIM revenge score	.48**	.49**	.10	.07
TRIM avoidance score	.37**	.36**	–.04	–.04
FES factors				
Narcissistic wounds	.31**	.29**	.30**	.32**
Relationship deterioration	.32**	.30**	.19*	.11
Relief/cleansing	–.09	–.14	.16	.15
Relationship enhancement	–.28**	–.28**	.10	.09
Empathy for partner's actions	–.21*	–.23*	–.07	–.08

* $p < .05$; ** $p < .01$.

asked both members of the 55 newlywed couples described earlier (see the section titled "Attachment and Gratitude") to rate the extent to which they forgave their spouses on that day, after marking the positive and negative behaviors exhibited by the spouse on that day. Hierarchical linear models revealed significant contributions of dispositional attachment orientations and daily fluctuations in partner's positive behaviors to the daily tendency to forgive (see Table 8.4). For both husbands and wives, higher scores reflecting partner's positive behaviors on a given day were significantly associated with higher levels of forgiveness on that day. Beyond this dyadic effect, both attachment anxiety and attachment avoidance significantly predicted lower levels of forgiveness across the 21 days. Interestingly, both attachment anxiety and avoidance significantly interacted with perception of the partner's behavior on a given day in determining the tendency to forgive on that day (see Table 8.4). All of these effects were significant for both husbands and wives.

Regression analyses examining the source of the significant interactions revealed similar patterns of effects for both attachment anxiety and attachment avoidance. On the one hand, participants (either husbands or wives) who scored relatively low on attachment anxiety or avoidance were more inclined to forgive their spouses on days when they perceived more positive spousal behavior. On the other hand, participants (either husbands or wives) who scored relatively high on attachment anxiety or avoidance displayed relatively little inclination to forgive their spouses regardless of their positive behavior on a given day. That is, anxious and avoidant people showed little forgiveness even on days when they perceived their spouses to be available, attentive, and supportive.

TABLE 8.4. Hierarchical Linear Model Coefficients for the Effects of Dispositional Attachment Orientations and Daily Partner Positive Behaviors on Daily Forgiveness

Effect	Husbands' forgiveness	Wives' forgiveness
Daily partner positive behavior	.32**	.34**
Dispositional avoidant attachment	–.40**	–.28**
Dispositional anxious attachment	–.23**	–.27**
Avoidance × partner's positive behavior	–.27**	–.29**
Anxiety × partner's positive behavior	–.23**	–.26**

** $p < .01$.

CONCLUDING REMARKS

The findings from our studies of gratitude and forgiveness indicate that both major forms of attachment insecurity, anxiety and avoidance, are related to reductions in or distortions of these two social virtues, virtues which, when not distorted, contribute strength and longevity to romantic and marital relationships. In general, avoidant attachment is related to lower levels of gratitude and forgiveness, even in relational contexts that might make these feelings seem natural. Anxious attachment has a more complex signature: It does not necessarily eliminate gratitude and forgiveness, but it sullies them with conflicting feelings that almost certainly erode their good effects. Our findings survive controls for self-esteem and interpersonal trust, so the subtlety of attachment theory is needed to explain them. Avoidant attachment includes negative models of relationship partners and deactivating strategies of affect regulation designed to maintain a safe distance from others. Anxious attachment involves mixed models of others, portraying relationship partners both as necessary for safety and self-completion and as inadequate to guarantee those benefits. These forms of insecure attachment do not preclude "love" and "commitment," because they are compatible with people's involvement in long-term relationships, including marriage. But they certainly color the experience of love and commitment, along with gratitude and forgiveness, and render long-term relationships vulnerable to disruption and dissatisfaction.

Our findings regarding attachment style dimensions, gratitude, and forgiveness can be placed in a broader context. In other recent studies (summarized in Gillath, Shaver, & Mikulincer, 2005, and Mikulincer & Shaver, 2005), we discovered that attachment security, both dispositional and experimentally enhanced, is associated with reductions in prejudices and an increase in tolerance for outgroup members; with greater empathy, compassion, and altruism toward others, including strangers in need; and with more universalistic and humanitarian values. In several of these studies, avoidant attachment was associated with reduced empathy, compassion, and kindness, whereas anxious attachment was related to forms of these emotions that were tinged with self-preoccupation and personal distress, which is likely to interfere with unconflicted and maximally effective generosity, just as, in the studies we described here, it cast a negative or ambivalent shadow on gratitude and forgiveness. Nevertheless, in several of our other studies, experimental augmentation of security had beneficial effects on both relatively secure and relatively insecure people, suggesting that insecure defenses can be circumvented or softened by security augmentation. The same optimistic suggestion might be extended to marital or couple therapy that increases attachment security (e.g., Johnson, 2003).

We have interpreted the findings of our security augmentation studies in terms of the effects of the attachment system on the caregiving system, just as Bowlby (1969/1982) and Ainsworth et al. (1978) interpreted some of their observations and findings as effects of the attachment system on the exploratory system (in childhood). When considered within the context of adult romantic relationships, attachment theory's account of the interplay between attachment and caregiving helps explain how a person suffering from dispositional (and perhaps situational) attachment insecurity might lack the capacity for unconflicted empathy, compassion, gratitude, and forgiveness. In Chapter 13 of this volume, Gillath and Schachner consider the interplay between the attachment and sexual systems. In all of these cases, the attachment- theoretical conception of romantic love provided by Hazan and Shaver in the late 1980s (e.g., Hazan & Shaver, 1987; Shaver, Hazan, & Bradshaw, 1988) provides a way to think about the complexity of "love," which can take many forms depending on a person's attachment, caregiving, and sexual histories. These three behavioral systems are complexly interrelated, making it possible for emotional bonds and relational behaviors to be colored by complex patterns of motivation, conflict, and defense that require careful analysis to be fully understood.

REFERENCES

Ainsworth, M. D. S., Blehar, M. C., Waters, E., & Wall, S. (1978). *Patterns of attachment: A psychological study of the Strange Situation*. Hillsdale, NJ: Erlbaum.

Ashton, M. C., Paunonen, S. V., Helmes, E., & Jackson, D. N. (1998). Kin altruism, reciprocal altruism, and the Big Five personality factors. *Evolution and Human Behavior, 19*, 243–255.

Baldwin, M. W., Fehr, B., Keedian, E., Seidel, M., & Thomson, D. W. (1993). An exploration of the relational schemata underlying attachment styles: Self-report and lexical decision approaches. *Personality and Social Psychology Bulletin, 19*, 746–754.

Baldwin, M. W., Keelan, J. P. R., Fehr, B., Enns, V., & Koh Rangarajoo, E. (1996). Social-cognitive conceptualization of attachment working models: Availability and accessibility effects. *Journal of Personality and Social Psychology, 71*, 94–109.

Blain, M. D., Thompson, J. M., & Whiffen, V. E. (1993). Attachment and perceived social support in late adolescence: The interaction between working models of self and others. *Journal of Adolescent Research, 8*, 226–241.

Bowlby, J. (1973). *Attachment and loss: Vol. 2. Separation: Anxiety and anger.* New York: Basic Books.

Bowlby, J. (1980). *Attachment and loss: Vol. 3. Loss: Sadness and depression.* New York: Basic Books.

Bowlby, J. (1982). *Attachment and loss: Vol. 1. Attachment* (2nd ed.). New York: Basic Books. (Original work published 1969)

Bradfield, M., & Aquino, K. (1999). The effects of blame attributions and offender likeableness on forgiveness and revenge in the workplace. *Journal of Management, 25*, 607–631.

Brennan, K. A., Clark, C. L., & Shaver, P. R. (1998). Self-report measurement of adult attachment: An integrative overview. In J. A. Simpson & W. S. Rholes (Eds.), *Attachment theory and close relationships* (pp. 46–76). New York: Guilford Press.

Brennan, K. A., & Shaver, P. R. (1998). Attachment styles and personality disorders: Their connections to each other and to parental divorce, parental death, and perceptions of parental caregiving. *Journal of Personality, 66*, 835–878.

Cassidy, J., & Kobak, R. R. (1988). Avoidance and its relationship with other defensive processes. In J. Belsky & T. Nezworski (Eds.), *Clinical implications of attachment* (pp. 300–323). Hillsdale, NJ: Erlbaum.

Collins, N., & Feeney, B. C. (2004). Working models of attachment shape perceptions of social support: Evidence from experimental and observational studies. *Journal of Personality and Social Psychology, 87*, 363–383.

Collins, N. L. (1996). Working models of attachment: Implications for explanation, emotion, and behavior. *Journal of Personality and Social Psychology, 71*, 810–832.

Collins, N. L., & Read, S. J. (1990). Adult attachment, working models, and relationship quality in dating couples. *Journal of Personality and Social Psychology, 58*, 644–663.

Collins, N. L., & Read, S. J. (1994). Cognitive representations of attachment: The structure and function of working models. In K. Bartholomew & D. Perlman (Eds.), *Attachment processes in adulthood* (pp. 53–92). London: Kingsley.

Coyle, C. T., & Enright, R. D. (1997). Forgiveness intervention with post-abortion men. *Journal of Consulting and Clinical Psychology, 65*, 1042–1046.

Cozzarelli, C., Hoekstra, S. J., & Bylsma, W. H. (2000). General versus specific mental models of attachment: Are they associated with different outcomes? *Personality and Social Psychology Bulletin, 26*, 605–618.

Davis, M. H., Morris, M. M., & Kraus, L. A. (1998). Relationship-specific and global perceptions of social support: Associations with well-being and attachment. *Journal of Personality and Social Psychology, 74*, 468–481.

Emmons, A. E., & Crumple, C. H. (2000). Gratitude as a human strength: Appraising the evidence. *Journal of Social and Clinical Psychology, 19*, 56–69.

Emmons, A. E., & McCullough, M. E. (2003). Counting blessings versus burdens: An experimental investigation of gratitude and subjective well-being in daily life. *Journal of Personality and Social Psychology, 84*, 377–389.

Enright, R. D. (1991). The moral development of forgiveness. In W. M. Kurtines & J.

L. Gewirtz (Eds.), *Handbook of moral behavior and development* (pp. 123–152). Hillsdale, NJ: Erlbaum.

Enright, R. D., Gassin, E. A., & Wu, C. (1992). Forgiveness: A developmental view. *Journal of Moral Education, 21*, 99–114.

Exline, J. J., Baumeister, R. F., Bushman, B. J., Campbell, W. K., & Finkel, E. J. (2004). Too proud to let go: Narcissistic entitlement as a barrier to forgiveness. *Journal of Personality and Social Psychology, 87*, 894–912.

Feeney, J. A., & Noller, P. (1990). Attachment style as a predictor of adult romantic relationships. *Journal of Personality and Social Psychology, 58*, 281–291.

Fincham, F. D. (2000). The kiss of the porcupines: From attributing responsibility to forgiving. *Personal Relationships, 7*, 1–23.

Fincham, F. D., & Beach, S. R. H. (2001). Forgiving in close relationships. In F. Columbus (Ed.), *Advances in psychological research* (Vol. 7, pp. 163–197). Huntington, NY: Nova Science.

Fincham, F. D., Beach, S. R. H., & Davila, J. (2004). Forgiveness and conflict resolution in marriage. *Journal of Family Psychology, 18*, 72–81.

Fincham, F. D., Paleari, F. G., & Regalia, C. (2002). Forgiveness in marriage: The role of relationship quality, attributions, and empathy. *Personal Relationships, 9*, 27–37.

Fraley, R. C., & Shaver, P. R. (2000). Adult romantic attachment: Theoretical developments, emerging controversies, and unanswered questions. *Review of General Psychology, 4*, 132–154.

Freud, S. (1957). Instincts and their vicissitudes. In J. Strachey (Ed. & Trans.), *The standard edition of the complete psychological works of Sigmund Freud* (Vol. 3, pp. 157–186). London: Hogarth Press. (Original work published 1915)

Gallo, L. C., & Smith, T. W. (2001). Attachment style in marriage: Adjustment and response to interaction. *Journal of Social and Personal Relationships, 18*, 263–289.

Gillath, O., Shaver, P. R., & Mikulincer, M. (2005). An attachment-theoretical approach to compassion and altruism. In P. Gilbert (Ed.), *Compassion: Its nature and use in psychotherapy* (pp. 121–147). London: Brunner-Routledge.

Gottman, J. M. (1993). *What predicts divorce? The relationship between marital processes and marital outcomes*. Hillsdale, NJ: Erlbaum.

Greenwald, A. G., McGhee, D. E., & Schwartz, J. L. K. (1998). Measuring individual differences in implicit cognition: The Implicit Association Test. *Journal of Personality and Social Psychology, 74*, 1464–1480.

Hazan, C., & Shaver, P. R. (1987). Romantic love conceptualized as an attachment process. *Journal of Personality and Social Psychology, 52*, 511–524.

Heider, F. (1958). *The psychology of interpersonal relations*. New York: Wiley.

Johnson, S. M. (2003). Attachment theory: A guide for couple therapy. In S. M. Johnson & V. E. Whiffen (Eds.), *Attachment processes in couple and family therapy* (pp. 103–123). New York: Guilford Press.

Kachadourian, L. K., Fincham, F., & Davila, J. (2004). The tendency to forgive in dating and married couples: The role of attachment and relationship satisfaction. *Personal Relationships, 11*, 373–393.

Kirkpatrick, L. A., & Davis, K. E. (1994). Attachment style, gender, and relationship stability: A longitudinal analysis. *Journal of Personality and Social Psychology, 66*, 502–512.

Klein, M. (1940). Mourning and its relationship with manic-depressive states. *International Journal of Psychoanalysis, 12*, 47–82.

Klein, M. (1957). *Envy and gratitude*. London: Free Press.

Lazarus, R. S. (1991). *Emotion and adaptation*. New York: Oxford University Press.

Lazarus, R. S., & Lazarus, B. N. (1994). *Passion and reason: Making sense of our emotions*. New York: Oxford University Press.

Levy, K. N., Blatt, S. J., & Shaver, P. R. (1998). Attachment styles and parental representations. *Journal of Personality and Social Psychology, 74*, 407–419.

Luke, M. A., Maio, G. R., & Carnelley, K. B. (2004). Attachment models of self and others: Relations with self-esteem, humanity-esteem, and parental treatment. *Personal Relationships, 11*, 281–303.

Markiewicz, D., Reis, M., & Gold, D. P. (1997). An exploration of attachment styles and personality traits in caregiving for dementia patients. *International Journal of Aging and Human Development, 45*, 111–132.

McCullough, M. E. (2000). Forgiveness as a human strength: Theory, measurement, and links to well-being. *Journal of Social and Clinical Psychology, 19*, 43–55.

McCullough, M. E., Bellah, C. G., Kilpatrick, S. D., & Johnson, J. L. (2001). Vengefulness: Relationships with forgiveness, rumination, well-being, and the big five. *Personality and Social Psychology Bulletin, 27*, 601–610.

McCullough, M. E., Emmons, R. A., & Tsang, J. (2002). The grateful disposition: A conceptual and empirical topography. *Journal of Personality and Social Psychology, 82*, 112–127.

McCullough, M. E., Worthington, E. L., & Rachal, K. C. (1997a). Interpersonal forgiving in close relationships. *Journal of Personality and Social Psychology, 73*, 321–336.

McCullough, M. E., Worthington, E. L., & Rachal, K. C. (1997b). Interpersonal forgiving in close relationships: II. Theoretical elaboration and measurement. *Journal of Personality and Social Psychology, 75*, 1586–1603.

Mickelson, K. D., Kessler, R. C., & Shaver, P. R. (1997). Adult attachment in a nationally representative sample. *Journal of Personality and Social Psychology, 73*, 1092–1106.

Mikulincer, M. (1998). Attachment working models and the sense of trust: An exploration of interaction goals and affect regulation. *Journal of Personality and Social Psychology, 74*, 1209–1224.

Mikulincer, M., & Arad, D. (1999). Attachment working models and cognitive openness in close relationships: A test of chronic and temporary accessibility effects. *Journal of Personality and Social Psychology, 77*, 710–725.

Mikulincer, M., & Erev, I. (1991). Attachment style and the structure of romantic love. *British Journal of Social Psychology, 30*, 273–291.

Mikulincer, M., & Horesh, N. (1999). Adult attachment style and the perception of others: The role of projective mechanisms. *Journal of Personality and Social Psychology, 76*, 1022–1034.

Mikulincer, M., Orbach, I., & Iavnieli, D. (1998). Adult attachment style and affect regulation: Strategic variations in subjective self–other similarity. *Journal of Personality and Social Psychology, 75*, 436–448.

Mikulincer, M., & Shaver, P. R. (2003). The attachment behavioral system in adulthood: Activation, psychodynamics, and interpersonal processes. In M. P. Zanna

(Ed.), *Advances in experimental social psychology* (Vol. 35, pp. 53–152). New York: Academic Press.

Mikulincer, M., & Shaver, P. R. (2005). Mental representations of attachment security: Theoretical foundation for a positive social psychology. In M. W. Baldwin (Ed.), *Interpersonal cognition* (pp. 233–266). New York: Guilford Press.

Ognibene, T. C., & Collins, N. L. (1998). Adult attachment styles, perceived social support, and coping strategies. *Journal of Social and Personal Relationships, 15*, 323–345.

Pietromonaco, P. R., & Feldman Barrett, L. (1997). Working models of attachment and daily social interactions. *Journal of Personality and Social Psychology, 73*, 1409–1423.

Priel, B., & Besser, A. (2001). Bridging the gap between attachment and object relations theories: A study of the transition to motherhood. *British Journal of Medical Psychology, 74*, 85–100.

Priel, B., Mitrany, D., & Shahar, G. (1998). Closeness, support, and reciprocity: A study of attachment styles in adolescence. *Personality and Individual Differences, 25*, 1183–1197.

Priel, B., & Shamai, D. (1995). Attachment style and perceived social support: Effects on affect regulation. *Personality and Individual Differences, 19*, 235–241.

Rosenberg, M. (1979). *Conceiving the self*. New York: Basic Books.

Rothbard, J. C., & Shaver, P. R. (1994). Continuity of attachment across the life span. In M. B. Sperling & W. H. Berman (Eds.), *Attachment in adults: Clinical and developmental perspectives* (pp. 31–71). New York: Guilford Press.

Rotter, J. (1967). A new scale for the measurement of interpersonal trust. *Journal of Personality, 35*, 651–665.

Rusbult, C. E., Verette, J., Whitney, G. A., Slovik, L. F., & Lipkus, I. (1991). Accommodation processes in close relationships: Theory and preliminary empirical evidence. *Journal of Personality and Social Psychology, 60*, 53–78.

Seligman, M. E. P. (2002). *Authentic happiness: Using the new positive psychology to realize your potential for lasting fulfillment*. New York: Simon & Schuster.

Shaver, P. R., & Brennan, K. A. (1992). Attachment styles and the "big five" personality traits: Their connections with each other and with romantic relationship outcomes. *Personality and Social Psychology Bulletin, 18*, 536–545.

Shaver, P. R., & Clark, C. L. (1994). The psychodynamics of adult romantic attachment. In J. M. Masling & R. F. Bornstein (Eds.), *Empirical studies of psychoanalytic theories: Vol. 5. Empirical perspectives on object relations theory* (pp. 105–156). Washington, DC: American Psychological Association.

Shaver, P. R., & Hazan, C. (1993). Adult romantic attachment: Theory and evidence. In D. Perlman & W. Jones (Eds.), *Advances in personal relationships* (Vol. 4, pp. 29–70). London: Kingsley.

Shaver, P. R., Hazan, C., & Bradshaw, D. (1988). Love as attachment: The integration of three behavioral systems. In R. J. Sternberg & M. Barnes (Eds.), *The psychology of love* (pp. 68–99). New Haven, CT: Yale University Press.

Shaver, P. R., & Mikulincer, M. (2002). Attachment-related psychodynamics. *Attachment and Human Development, 4*, 133–161.

Shaver, P. R., & Mikulincer, M. (2005). Attachment theory and research: Resurrection of the psychodynamic approach to personality. *Journal of Research in Personality, 39*, 22–45.

Simpson, J. A. (1990). Influence of attachment styles on romantic relationships. *Journal of Personality and Social Psychology, 59*, 971–980.

Simpson, J. A., Rholes, W. S., & Phillips, D. (1996). Conflict in close relationships: An attachment perspective. *Journal of Personality and Social Psychology, 71*, 899–914.

Snyder, C. R., & McCullough, M. E. (2000). A positive psychology field of dreams: "If you build it, they will come. . . . " *Journal of Social and Clinical Psychology, 19*, 151–160.

Sumer, N., & Cozzarelli, C. (2004). The impact of adult attachment on partner and self-attribution and relationship quality. *Personal Relationships, 11*, 355–371.

Teigen, H. K. (1997). Luck, envy, and gratitude: It could have been different. *Scandinavian Journal of Psychology, 38*, 313–323.

Trinke, S. J., & Bartholomew, K. (1997). Hierarchies of attachment relationships in young adulthood. *Journal of Social and Personal Relationships, 14*, 603–625.

Volling, B. L., Notaro, P. C., & Larsen, J. J. (1998). Adult attachment styles: Relations with emotional well-being, marriage, and parenting. *Family Relations, 47*, 355–367.

Watkins, P. C., Woodward, K., Stone, T., & Kolts, R. L. (2003). Gratitude and happiness: Development of a measure of gratitude, and relationships with subjective well-being. *Social Behavior and Personality, 31*, 431–452.

Weiner, B. (1985). An attributional theory of achievement motivation and emotion. *Psychological Review, 92*, 548–573.

Whisman, M. A., & Allan, L. E. (1996). Attachment and social cognition theories of romantic relationships: Convergent or complementary perspectives? *Journal of Social and Personal Relationships, 13*, 263–278.

Worthington, E. L., Kurusu, T. A., Collins, W., Berry, J. W., Ripley, J. S., & Baier, S. N. (2000). Forgiving usually takes time: A lesson learned by studying interventions to promote forgiveness. *Journal of Psychology and Theology, 28*, 3–20.

Young, A. M., & Acitelli, L. K. (1998). The role of attachment style and relationship status of the perceiver in the perceptions of romantic partner. *Journal of Social and Personal Relationships, 15*, 161–173.

Zayas, V., Shoda, Y., & Ayduk, O. N. (2002). Personality in context: An interpersonal systems perspective. *Journal of Personality, 70*, 851–900.

9

Daily Perceptions of Conflict and Support in Romantic Relationships

The Ups and Downs of Anxiously Attached Individuals

JEFFRY A. SIMPSON, LORNE CAMPBELL,
and YANNA J. WEISBERG

At times, romantic relationships are similar to emotional roller coasters in which partners experience euphoric emotional highs that are rapidly followed by dejecting lows. For many people, these contrasting moments of joy and despair are experienced infrequently. For others, tumultuous emotional ups and downs are a habitual part of life. Attachment theory offers a coherent framework for understanding why certain people are prone to experiencing sharp emotional swings and how these perceptions might then influence how romantic partners and relationships are viewed. Bowlby (1973, 1980), in fact, conjectured that the working models of highly anxious people should strongly color and sometimes jade how these individuals perceive and evaluate their partners and relationships from day to day.

In this chapter, which is a tribute to the life and work of Phil Shaver, we first review principles from attachment theory (Bowlby, 1973, 1980) and from Fraley and Shaver's (2000) model of attachment anxiety that might bear on these processes. Following this, we review empirical evidence on the working models and interpersonal proclivities of people who score high in attachment anxiety. We then report new evidence from a daily diary and social interaction study that indicates that more anxiously attached people tend to perceive more frequent and severe daily conflict in their romantic relationships than do less anxious persons, that they report feeling more hurt by these conflicts, and that they believe that conflicts forecast a more negative future for their relationships. This new evidence also reveals that highly anxious individuals typically weigh daily relationship events more heavily when judging the daily quality of their relationships than do their less anxious counterparts. We also present a set of conceptually parallel findings from the social interaction portion of the study, which reveals that when highly anxious individuals actually discuss important relationship conflicts with their partners, they appear more distressed (rated by observers) and report feeling greater distress relative to less anxious people. Moreover, they remain more distressed, even when their partners are rated as behaving more positively toward them. We conclude the chapter by integrating these findings and considering their broader theoretical implications.

THEORETICAL FOUNDATIONS

Attachment Theory

Bowlby (1969, 1973, 1980) believed that early interactions with significant others instill expectations and beliefs that subsequently shape social perceptions and behavior about what relationships and relationship partners should be like during adulthood. These beliefs, which form a core component of working models, ostensibly involve "if–then" propositions that specify the behaviors and responses expected from attachment figures in attachment-relevant situations (e.g., *if* I am upset, *then* I can rely on my partner for comfort and attention). Research has revealed multiple ways in which working models influence information processing in close relationships. Working models can, for instance, influence whether and how individuals selectively attend to and perceive their partners, how they arrive at inferences and judgments about their partners' actions, and how they preferentially remember—or fail to remember—critical behaviors enacted by their partners (see Collins & Allard, 2001).

Two relatively orthogonal dimensions define individual differences in adult attachment (see Brennan, Clark, & Shaver, 1998). The first dimension, labeled *avoidance*, reflects the degree to which individuals feel comfortable with closeness and emotional intimacy in relationships. People who score higher on avoidance tend to be less invested in their relationships and strive to remain psychologically and emotionally independent of their partners (Hazan & Shaver, 1994). The second dimension, termed *anxiety*, taps the degree to which individuals worry and ruminate about being rejected or abandoned by their partners. Prototypically secure people typically score lower on both attachment dimensions.

Fraley and Shaver (2000) have recently introduced a model that specifies the major interpersonal functions that could be served by each attachment dimension. They conjecture that the avoidance dimension primarily regulates attachment-relevant behavior, especially in anxiety-provoking situations (e.g., seeking support vs. retracting from attachment figures in distressing situations). The anxiety dimension, by comparison, entails an appraisal/monitoring system that gauges the degree to which individuals are maintaining sufficient physical, psychological, or emotional closeness to their attachment figures. Fraley and Shaver (2000) claim that the appraisal/monitoring system should be particularly sensitive to cues (inputs) that connote changes in the level of rejection and support from attachment figures (e.g., romantic partners). This should be particularly true for highly anxious individuals, whose appraisal/monitoring systems are likely to be set at lower activation thresholds and, hence, are more easily triggered by relationship threats (see Simpson & Rholes, 1994). Given the greater importance of identifying potentially negative events (Gaelick, Bodenhausen, & Wyer, 1985), however, highly anxious individuals might notice and place slightly greater weight on cues of rejection than on cues of support. One of the principal outputs of the anxiety system should be the level of felt security, which can range from extreme anxiety when rejection is perceived as high and support as low to extreme contentment when rejection is viewed as low and support as high.

Attachment Anxiety

Several lines of research have examined how the working models of highly anxious individuals guide perceptions of romantic partners and relationships and the strong impact that perceptions of relationship-based conflict and support exert on highly anxious people.

Working Models and Relationship Perceptions

In general, highly anxious individuals worry about being abandoned (Hazan & Shaver, 1987) and crave emotional support, closeness, and reassurance from their romantic partners (Collins & Read, 1990). These desires and worries motivate highly anxious persons to monitor their partners and relationships closely for signs of deficient or declining availability and emotional proximity (Cassidy & Berlin, 1994). Recent research has, in fact, documented that attachment figures tend to be more chronically accessible in the minds of highly anxious people (e.g., Mikulincer, Gillath, & Shaver, 2002).

The working models of highly anxious individuals also appear to bias how romantic partners and relationships are perceived. When asked to imagine their partners behaving negatively toward them, for example, highly anxious people typically make more negative attributions about their partners' behavior, believe that their partners are selfish and deliberately unresponsive to their needs, question their partners' love, feel less secure about the relationship, and feel greater anger toward their partners compared with less anxious people (Collins, 1996).

These results imply that the hypervigilance of anxiously attached individuals should elevate the monitoring and appraisal of relationship-threatening cues in particular, perhaps motivating them to interpret information in a way that typically confirms their negative expectations of attachment figures (Shaver & Mikulincer, 2002). These proclivities could make highly anxious individuals even more vulnerable to experiencing distress and expressing concerns about the future stability of their relationships. To compound matters, highly anxious individuals typically rely on emotion-focused coping strategies when they are distressed, strategies that frequently amplify distress (Mikulincer & Florian, 1995, 1998). This tendency, in turn, might impel highly anxious individuals to perceive their partners and relationships even less positively.

Many of these conjectures have been supported by cross-sectional studies revealing that highly anxious persons tend to experience stronger feelings and more variable "highs and lows" in their relationships than other people (e.g., Collins & Read, 1990; Hazan & Shaver, 1987). They also report greater distress, anxiety, and impulsiveness in their social interactions (Shaver & Brennan, 1992); experience stronger negative emotions in their romantic relationships (Simpson, 1990); and tend to have stable but very dissatisfying relationships (Kirkpatrick & Davis, 1994). Much less is known, however, about the day-to-day proximal variables that make the relationships of highly anxious individuals so rocky.

Perceptions of Conflict and Support

Bowlby (1973, 1980) claimed that perceptions of conflict and support in relationships should be central to how highly anxious individuals view themselves, their partners, and their relationships. Although highly anxious individuals crave comfort and support, they are unhappy with the degree of support available from significant others (Rholes, Simpson, Campbell, & Grich, 2001), and they tend to mistrust support providers (Bartholomew, Cobb, & Poole, 1997). Moreover, during social interactions, highly anxious individuals who are distressed perceive more hurtful intent when their partners provide "ambiguous" support. As a result, they remember their partners as behaving in a less supportive manner in a prior, unrelated videotaped interaction than neutral observers rated the partners (Collins & Feeney, 2004). Similar results have been discovered across chronically stressful life transitions. Prior to childbirth, for example, highly anxious women not only perceive less available emotional support from their husbands than do less anxious women, but they also perceive appreciably less support than their husbands report providing (Rholes et al., 2001). When they believe that support is being offered, however, highly anxious individuals are inclined to acknowledge it, and their romantic relationships do *not* decline in satisfaction across time (Rholes et al., 2001). In addition, when providing support to their romantic partners, highly anxious individuals perceive that their interactions are less warm and less supportive, and they presume that their partners are less satisfied with the support that they have provided than their partners truly are (Collins & Feeney, 2000).

With respect to relationship-based conflicts, highly anxious people are aware of the negative as well as the positive opportunities that conflict can offer (Fishtein, Pietromonaco, & Feldman Barrett, 1999). Nevertheless, when conflicts arise, highly anxious individuals resort to emotion-focused coping strategies to regulate their negative affect (Mikulincer & Florian, 1998; Pistole, 1989), display dominating or coercive behaviors (Feeney, Noller, & Callan, 1994; Levy & Davis, 1988), and exhibit greater hostility and more relationship-damaging behaviors, especially when dealing with possible relationship threats (Simpson, Rholes, & Phillips, 1996). Ironically, these coercive and distrusting actions may produce what highly anxious individuals dread the most—alienation of their partners and eventual relationship loss.

Prior Diary Studies

To date, only a few adult attachment diary studies have been conducted. Tidwell, Reis, and Shaver (1996) tested relations between adult attachment styles, daily patterns of social interaction, and emotional variability in social interactions involving same-sex peers, opposite-sex peers, mixed-sex peers, and larger groups across 1 week. They found that more anxiously attached individuals varied more than did either secure or avoidant persons in the amount of positive emotions and promotive interactions reported, but *not* in the amount of negative emotions or intimacy. It is important to note that Tidwell et al. (1996) did not focus on social interactions between individuals and their romantic partners, that is, persons more likely to be bona fide attachment figures.

Pietromonaco and Feldman Barrett (1997) examined links between interaction quality, emotional reactions, and views of self and others for all social interactions lasting at least 10 minutes in a week-long diary study. Although highly preoccupied (anxious) individuals did not display more extreme emotional responses across different types of relationship partners (e.g., strangers, friends, romantic partners), they did report more positive emotions, greater satisfaction, and more positive views of others, especially after high-conflict interactions. As noted earlier, high-conflict situations may provide these individuals with special opportunities to achieve two cherished goals—gaining their partners' attention and promoting greater intimacy and felt security.

Finally, Bradford, Feeney, and Campbell (2002) explored interactions between romantic partners, focusing on their daily disclosures during 7 consecutive days. More anxious individuals were less satisfied with the disclosures they had with their partners, and more anxious women reported that their interactions were more negative. The partners of more anxiously attached individuals also reported disclosing less to them, and these partners also reported that their disclosures tended to be less intimate, more negative, and less satisfying.

The Current Predictions

These theoretical considerations and empirical findings led us to derive three sets of hypotheses structured around perceptions of daily conflict in relationships, perceptions of daily conflict and support in relation to assessments of daily relationship quality, and perceptions of daily conflict and support in relation to judgments of one's *partner's* daily relationship quality.

Perceptions of Relationship Conflict

If, as Fraley and Shaver (2000) suggest, the appraisal/monitoring system is designed to detect whether attachment figures are withdrawing, highly anxious individuals should be more inclined than other people to perceive heightened relationship conflict on a daily basis. In particular, given that highly anxious individuals rely more heavily on emotion-focused coping (Mikulincer & Florian, 1998), attribute less positive intentions to their partners in ambiguous situations (Collins, 1996), and display less functional behaviors when trying to settle serious relationship conflicts (Simpson et al., 1996), they should perceive more frequent and more severe daily relationship conflicts than less anxious individuals. To the extent that their working models bias perceptions of daily conflict, more anxious people should also perceive greater daily relationship-based conflict in their relationships than would be expected based on their *partner's* perceptions of daily relationship-based conflict. In addition, they should report that their daily conflicts are more likely to escalate or expand beyond the original source and, if so, their dating partners should confirm these perceptions.

Perceptions of Conflict and Support in Relation to Assessments of Relationship Quality

According to Fraley and Shaver (2000), highly anxious people should rely more heavily on immediate cues of relationship conflict and support when making judgments of the daily quality and future well-being of their relationships, and their partners should also be aware of these stronger contingencies. Accordingly, highly anxious individuals and their romantic partners should both perceive that relationship-based conflicts are likely to have more deleterious effects on the future of their relationships. On the flip side, both might also perceive that supportive behaviors could have more positive long-term effects on their relationships. Effects involving perceptions of support, however, might be weaker than those involving conflict, given the greater importance and diagnostic value of negative events in most relationships.

Finally, even though highly anxious individuals typically are involved in less satisfying relationships (Feeney, 1999), their level of relationship quality should be moderated by their perceptions of daily conflict and daily support. More specifically, on days when highly anxious individuals perceive greater daily conflict, they should report less relationship quality. However, on days when they perceive greater support, they should report greater relationship quality.

Perceptions of Conflict and Support in Relation to Perceptions of Partners' Relationship Quality

More anxious individuals may also be more reactive to conflict than less anxious individuals when estimating how their *partners* feel about the relationship. Highly anxious individuals tend to project their own relationship feelings, insecurities, and worries onto their partners (Mikulincer & Horesh, 1999). Consequently, they should be more tempted to presume that their partners are experiencing lower relationship quality on days when they (i.e., highly anxious individuals) perceive greater relationship conflict. By the same token, they may also presume that their partners are experiencing higher relationship quality on days when they perceive heightened relationship support. In view of the biasing effects of their working models (Collins & Allard, 2001), highly anxious individuals should also perceive that their partners are experiencing less relationship quality than should be expected according to their partners' actual reports of daily relationship quality.

Finally, highly anxious individuals should be less confident about the future of their relationships, especially if they perceive greater relationship conflict in their daily interactions. The same basic pattern should hold when they perceive (or infer) their partners' amount of confidence regarding the future of the relationship. And highly anxious individuals should also perceive (or infer) that their partners hold a dimmer view about the future of the relationship than should be expected from their partners' own daily reports of the relationship's future.

A DAILY DIARY AND SOCIAL INTERACTION STUDY

To test these sets of predictions, we conducted a two-part study (see Campbell, Simpson, Boldry, & Kashy, 2005, for details). In the first part of the study, both partners in a large sample of long-term dating couples independently completed daily diaries for 14 consecutive days. In the second part, the same couples returned to the lab and were videotaped while trying to resolve the most important unresolved conflict that surfaced in the diary period.

The Diary Phase of the Study

In the diary phase of the study, both members of 103 dating couples (mean length of relationship = 17.45 months) first completed background questionnaires and then kept daily diaries for 14 consecutive days. The background questionnaires assessed each participant's attachment orientations on the anxiety and avoidance dimensions (using the Adult Attachment Questionnaire; Simpson et al., 1996), perceptions of the quality of the current relationship (using the Perceived Relationship Quality Components Scale; Fletcher, Simpson, & Thomas, 2000), global self-esteem (using Rosenberg's, 1965, self-esteem measure), and neuroticism (using the Neuroticism subscale from the Big Five Inventory; John & Srivastava, 1999).

Participants were then instructed how to complete the daily diaries, which partners completed independently and privately each evening for 14 straight days. Answering a series of face-valid items on 7-point scales, each participant reported his or her daily relationship closeness and satisfaction, his or her daily perceptions of the future happiness and stability of the relationship, and his or her daily perceptions of conflict and support associated with the partner or relationship. Each participant also reported the degree to which each daily conflict escalated or expanded beyond the original topic or issue that instigated the conflict.

Because the data were hierarchically nested, a multilevel modeling approach guided by the actor–partner interdependence model (APIM; Kashy & Kenny, 2000) was used to analyze the diary data. The APIM recognizes that, because individuals are nested within different relationships, their responses and reactions depend on both their own and their *partners'* unique characteristics and inputs. The findings summarized herein capture most of the major results. It is important to note at the outset that only one effect emerged for the avoidance attachment dimension and that few interactions with gender emerged. As anticipated, virtually all of the effects involved the attachment anxiety dimension.

Perceptions of Daily Conflict

According to attachment theory (Bowlby, 1973, 1980), individuals who scored higher in attachment anxiety should perceive more conflict in their relationships on a daily basis, and their perceptions of the severity of conflict should differ from those of persons who score lower in anxiety. Indeed, more anxiously attached individuals did perceive greater relationship conflict on average across the 2-week diary period. They also reported slightly more conflict episodes during the diary period, and they perceived greater conflict than would be expected from their partners' perceptions of the same conflict episodes. In addition, highly anxious individuals reported that their daily conflicts were more likely to expand beyond the original, agreed-on discussion topic or issue than were the conflicts of less anxious individuals. Interestingly, the partners of more anxiously attached individuals also reported (confirmed) that their relationship conflicts were more likely to expand and escalate beyond the confines of the original topic or issue. Although women generally reported being more hurt by conflicts than men did, individuals perceived that their partners were more hurt by conflicts if their partners happened to be more anxiously attached. Finally, analyses that examined the attachment scores of both relationship partners revealed that daily conflicts had more pernicious effects on relationships (reported by *both* partners) when at least one partner was fairly anxious.

Perceptions of Daily Support

Because the appraisal/monitoring system might be more sensitive to detecting conflict than support in relationships, we were uncertain whether effects for anxious attachment would be evident on measures of daily perceived support. Indeed, neither an individual's own level of attachment anxiety nor his or her partner's level was associated with the amount of support perceived on a daily basis. However, women generally perceived more support and more frequent supportive events over the diary period than did men. More anxious individuals believed that supportive events (on days when they occurred) would have more positive implications for future relationship stability, and their partners reported similar perceptions. Finally, consistent with past research showing that highly avoidant people dislike giving or receiving support (Mikulincer & Florian, 1998), more avoidant individuals reported that supportive events in their relationships were a *less* positive experience for them than was true of less avoidant individuals. This, however, was the only avoidance effect that emerged in the entire study.

Links between Conflict and Relationship Quality

According to Fraley and Shaver (2000), more anxiously attached individuals should be more sensitive and reactive to conflicts, as revealed in daily judgments of relationship quality. On days when individuals in general reported more conflict, they also felt less relationship satisfaction and closeness. As displayed in Figure 9.1, however, the predicted interaction revealed that this effect was stronger for highly anxious people. In addition, individuals who perceived greater daily conflict also held less optimistic views about the future of their relationships, with women being slightly more optimistic than men. Nevertheless, as shown in Figure 9.2, the predicted interaction indicated that more anxious individuals were appreciably less optimistic about the future stability of their relationships on days when they perceived greater relationship conflict. In the full sample, people who perceived greater conflict also inferred that their partners were less satisfied or close. Importantly, however, highly anxious individuals believed that their partners were significantly less satisfied and less close on days when their own (i.e., anxious individuals') perceptions of conflict were higher. They also presumed that their partners were less satisfied and less close than would be expected from their partner's actual daily reports of satisfaction and closeness.

In general, individuals who perceived greater relationship conflict also perceived (or inferred) that their partners were less optimistic. As depicted in Figure 9.3, however, the predicted interaction indicated that more anx-

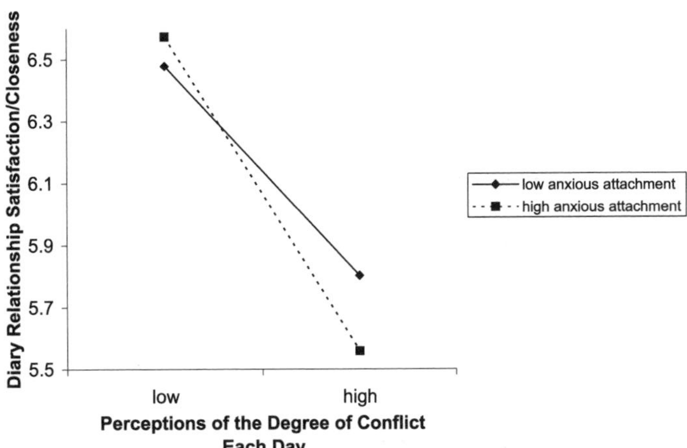

FIGURE 9.1. The interaction of individuals' anxious attachment and overall perceptions of conflict across the diary period predicting daily relationship satisfaction/closeness. Regression lines are plotted for individuals scoring 1 *SD* above and 1 *SD* below the sample means on anxious attachment and daily perceived conflict. The scale on the *y*-axis ranged from 1 to 7.

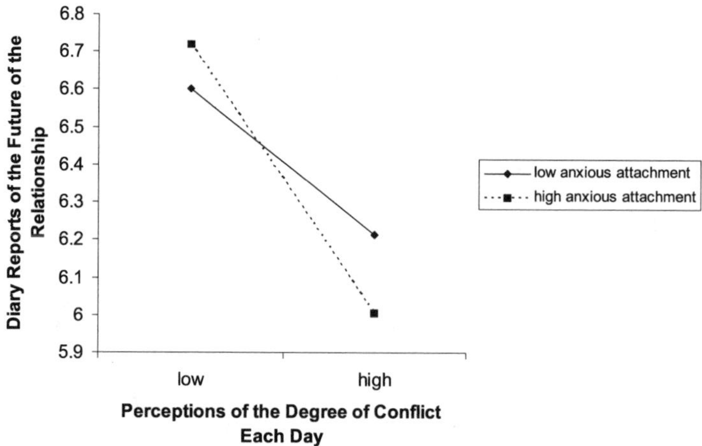

FIGURE 9.2. The interaction of individuals' anxious attachment and overall perceptions of conflict across the diary period predicting daily reports of the future stability of the relationship. Regression lines are plotted for individuals scoring 1 *SD* above and 1 *SD* below the sample means on anxious attachment and daily perceived conflict. The scale on the *y*-axis ranged from 1 to 7.

ious individuals perceived that their partners were less optimistic about the future of the relationship than was true of less anxious persons on days when their own (i.e., anxious individuals') perceptions of daily conflict were higher. More anxiously attached individuals also believed that their partners held a dimmer view about the future of the relationship than would be expected on the basis of their partners' actual reports.

Links between Support and Relationship Quality

On average, on days when individuals perceived greater support, they also reported being more satisfied or close, believed that their partners were more satisfied or close, were more optimistic about the future of the relationship, and presumed that their partners were more optimistic about the future of the relationship. In addition, more anxiously attached individuals were slightly more satisfied than less anxious persons on days when they perceived greater support. From a theoretical standpoint, this finding is important because it suggests that the appraisal/monitoring system may be attuned to both negative *and* positive relationship cues.

The Impact of Positive Behavior

We also explored whether behaving in a more positive, supportive manner toward one's partner during conflicts attenuated the negative effects of daily

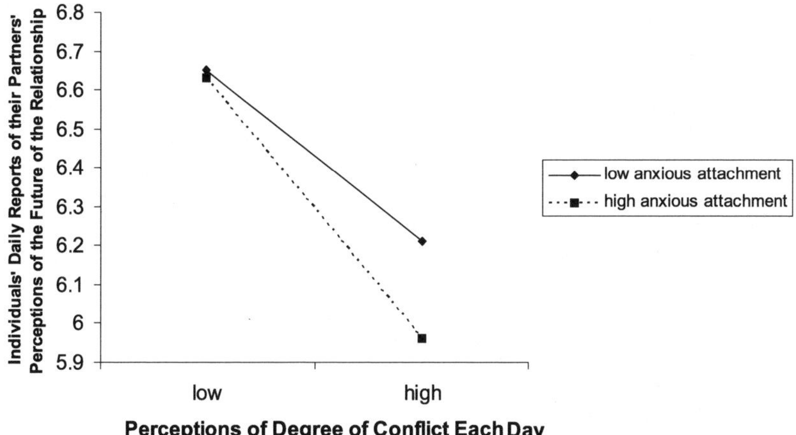

FIGURE 9.3. The interaction of individuals' anxious attachment and overall perceptions of conflict across the diary period predicting daily reports of their partners' perceptions of the future of the relationship. Regression lines are plotted for individuals scoring 1 *SD* above and 1 *SD* below the sample means on anxious attachment and daily perceived conflict. The scale on the *y*-axis ranged from 1 to 7.

conflicts for people in general and for highly anxious people in particular. Overall, individuals felt less hurt during the diary period when their partners reported behaving more positively toward them during daily conflicts. In addition, individuals felt more comforted by their partners' positive behaviors during daily conflict episodes. As shown in Figure 9.4, however, more anxiously attached individuals thought that conflicts would have more damaging long-term consequences for their relationships, *regardless* of how positively their partners reported behaving toward them during daily conflicts. Less anxious individuals, on the other hand, were more comforted by their partner's more positive behaviors.

The Social Interaction Phase of the Study

Once the diary phase of the study had been completed, we invited each couple to our lab to discuss and try to resolve the most important conflict they encountered during the 14-day diary period. Ninety-eight of the original 103 couples returned. When each couple arrived at the lab, they were instructed to "choose the most serious or prominent conflict that occurred during the 14-day diary period that *wasn't* completely resolved." After choosing a specific topic or issue, the partners were told that they had 7 minutes to discuss the conflict while being videotaped with their consent. Immediately after each discussion, both partners reported on 7-point scales how distressed and upset they felt during their discussion. Each discussion

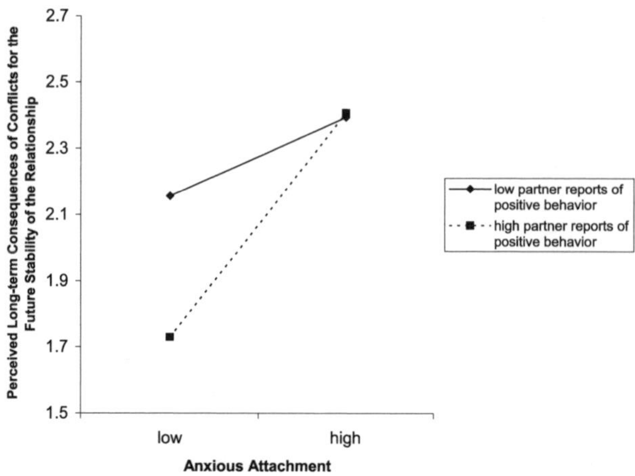

FIGURE 9.4. The interaction of individuals' anxious attachment and how positively their partners reported behaving during conflicts during the diary period predicting perceived long-term consequences of conflict for the future stability of the relationship. Regression lines are plotted for individuals scoring 1 *SD* above and 1 *SD* below the sample means on anxious attachment and partner-reported positive behavior during conflicts. The scale on the *y*-axis ranged from 1 to 7.

was then rated on several theoretically relevant dimensions by sets of trained coders. In addition to attempting to replicate the major findings in the diary data, we also wanted to confirm that highly anxious individuals would remain more distressed even when their partners actually behaved in a conciliatory and sympathetic manner (as evaluated by trained raters).

General Findings

On average, women were rated by the trained observers as overreacting to and escalating the conflict more than men. Replicating the conflict escalation results found in the diary data, more anxious individuals were rated as overreacting to and escalating the conflict more than their less anxious counterparts. As a group, women were rated as appearing more distressed during the discussion than men, and both more anxiously attached individuals *and* their partners were also rated as more visibly distressed or upset. These results also replicate findings from the diary data, which revealed that more anxiously attached people felt more hurt by daily conflicts and that both they and their partners believed the daily conflicts would have more negative consequences for the future stability of their relationships. Women on average also reported being more distressed than men during the discussions, and highly anxious individuals and their partners *both* reported feeling more distressed relative to other individuals.

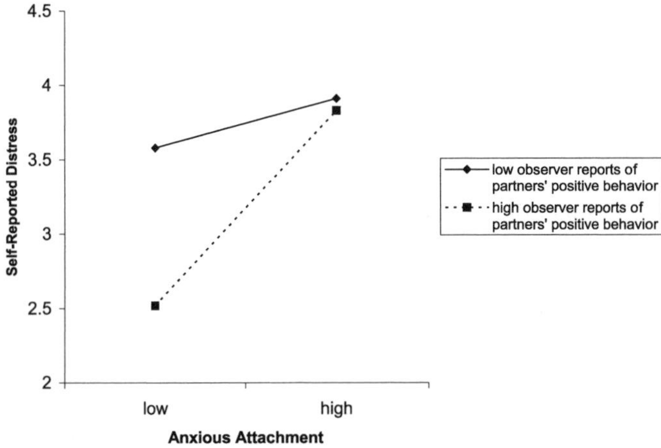

FIGURE 9.5. The interaction of individuals' anxious attachment and how positively their partners were observed to behave during the lab discussion predicting their self-reported distress. Regression lines are plotted for individuals scoring 1 *SD* above and 1 *SD* below the sample means on anxious attachment and observer-rated reports of the partner's positive behavior during the discussion. The scale on the *y*-axis ranged from 1 to 7.

Positive Behaviors and Self-Reported Distress

During the conflict resolution discussions, individuals generally felt less distressed if their partners behaved more positively toward them (rated by observers). However, as predicted, more anxious individuals reported higher levels of distress *regardless* of how positively their partners actually behaved toward them during the discussion (see Figure 9.5). Less anxious individuals, in contrast, felt more distressed if their partners behaved less positively but significantly less distressed if their partners behaved more positively.

BROADER THEORETICAL AND EMPIRICAL IMPLICATIONS

How can this rich and diverse set of new findings be integrated and understood? Fraley and Shaver (2000) have proposed that the appraisal/monitoring system might be a barometer of the degree to which individuals are maintaining sufficient psychological and emotional closeness to their attachment figures. This system should also be calibrated based on an individual's past attachment experiences. Given their history of receiving unpredictable or deficient support, highly anxious individuals ought to have relatively lower thresholds for perceiving threats to proximity maintenance (Simpson & Rholes, 1994). Given the nature of their working models, they should also be hypervigilant to cues of potential loss or rejection (Cassidy & Berlin, 1994), leading them at times to perceive and overestimate relationship conflicts when they may not truly exist.

The diary phase of the research just reviewed confirmed that, during daily interactions with their romantic partners, more anxiously attached individuals perceived greater conflict in their relationships, greater than even their own partners did. They also thought that conflict was comparatively more detrimental to both the current and future quality of their relationships. Moreover, on days when they perceived greater relationship-based conflict, highly anxious individuals inferred that their romantic partners must have a less positive outlook on the relationship and its future, a view that was not necessarily shared by their partners. The social interaction phase of the research revealed that, when discussing a serious relationship conflict, more anxious individuals appeared more distressed (as rated by observers). They also reported feeling more distressed, regardless of how positively their partners actually behaved toward them (as rated by observers).

We also examined a rather novel feature of Fraley and Shaver's (2000) model—that supportive events, which may signal that security goals are being met, might be perceived more positively by highly anxious than by less anxious people. Indeed, on days during the diary period when more support from partners was perceived, highly anxious individuals believed that they had a brighter relationship future. Highly anxious individuals also felt somewhat more satisfied and closer to their partners on days when they (highly anxious individuals) perceived greater support. It is important to note, however, that the positive impact of supportive events on highly anxious individuals was not evident when support occurred in the midst of relationship conflicts. Furthermore, even when their partners reported behaving more positively toward them (during the diary phase) and were rated by observers as behaving more positively toward them (during the conflict resolution task), highly anxious individuals continued to feel more distressed than less anxious individuals. Less anxious individuals, by comparison, felt less distressed following conflicts if their partners reported (in the diary) or were rated (in the conflict discussion) as behaving more positively toward them. Thus, for highly anxious individuals, the benefits of supportive experiences are noticeably diminished if they occur in connection with events that could portend eventual loss or rejection.

Collectively, these findings suggest that highly anxious people rely more heavily on daily perceptions of relationship events to assess the current and future quality of their relationships. This pattern of results is consistent with Holmes and Rempel's (1989) model of dyadic trust, which proposes that when individuals are unsure about their partners' love and affection, they should try to discern whether or not their partner truly cares for them. As a result, greater meaning should be granted to daily events that might signal rejection or abandonment. Moreover, if individuals remain uncertain of their partners' affection, positive behaviors should also be interpreted very positively, especially if they reduce uncertainty. This tendency could be aggravated by the fact that highly anxious individuals tend to have a more tenuous and contingent sense of self-worth (Bartholomew & Horowitz, 1991; Crocker & Wolfe, 2001), one that is heavily based on how positively their romantic partners currently view them and how well their relationships are currently functioning. This rather myopic here-and-now focus on daily relationship events could partially explain why highly anxious individuals and their romantic partners commonly report very low levels of relationship satisfaction (Simpson, 1990), sharp emotional swings over short time periods (Tidwell et al., 1996), and ardent beliefs that their relationships are always in flux (Hazan & Shaver, 1987). According to Kelley (1983), when individuals evaluate their relationships in response to the vicissitudes of daily relationship events and experiences rather than with reference to their longer term relationship goals and objectives, their relationships should feel and perhaps be more tumultuous.

In some ways, adopting a short-term focus toward daily relationship events may be an adaptive response to a history of receiving unpredictable or insufficient support (Bowlby, 1973), an interpersonal history that should motivate highly anxious people to pay more attention to, place greater weight on, and make stronger inferences about the implications of everyday relationship events. Over time, however, such a focus is likely to be maladaptive, especially when it is enacted by highly anxious people, whose working models may bias their perceptions of their partners and relationships toward overestimating the prevalence and negative impact of relationship-threatening events. Indeed, the new evidence we have presented suggests that these perceptual biases may extend even to the inferences that highly anxious individuals make about how their partners perceive the same potentially threatening events.

A Synthesis of the Findings

Most of the central findings revolve around the tendency for highly anxious individuals and their dating partners to perceive more frequent, severe, and expanded relationship conflict and for highly anxious persons to evaluate both the current and the future state of their relationships less positively on days when they perceive relationship conflict as stronger. Interpersonal conflicts serve as one principal trigger of the attachment system (Kobak & Duemmler, 1994), particularly for highly anxious people (Simpson & Rholes, 1994). Not only do relationship conflicts ignite worries about possible loss or abandonment in highly anxious individuals, but they also evoke hypervigilance (Cassidy & Berlin, 1994), amplify emotion-focused coping (Mikulincer & Florian, 1998), and increase dysfunctional interaction behaviors (Simpson et al., 1996), all of which deepen and exacerbate relationship conflicts.

The findings from the diary phase of our study also revealed that more anxious individuals perceive greater daily relationship conflict than less anxious people do, perceive more frequent daily conflicts, and acknowledge that daily conflicts are more likely to escalate and worsen. These findings are consistent with self-report studies showing that, when highly anxious individuals encounter negative relationship events, they feel more distressed and behave in ways that may instigate or aggravate relationship conflicts and may perpetuate them (Collins, 1996). These results fit with behavioral observation studies, which have demonstrated that highly anxious people display more destructive and relationship-damaging behaviors when they are trying to resolve serious relationship conflicts (Simpson et al., 1996).[1]

Indirect evidence for the biasing effects of anxious working models comes from the fact that highly anxious people typically perceived *more* daily conflict than their romantic partners did. Two perceptual processes might explain this outcome. First, highly anxious individuals might be better at detecting negativity in relationships given their stronger motivation to identify and avert loss and rejection. Second, their threshold for detecting negativity could be so low that they overdetect possible signs of negativity, generating a negative perceptual bias. Although our research was not designed to distinguish these different processes, some of the results in the diary phase of the study hint that the "negative bias" interpretation might be more correct. In the diary phase, highly anxious individuals reported greater relationship conflict, even when their partners' reports of daily conflict were statistically controlled. Furthermore, attachment scores within couples were not highly correlated, meaning that highly anxious people were *not* on average dating other highly insecure people (who might also have biased working models). Other research has confirmed that highly anxious individuals are inclined to infer more relationship conflict than is warranted (Collins, 1996) and to appraise normal life events in more threatening terms (Mikulincer, Birnbaum, Woodis, & Nachmais, 2000). Viewed together, this body of evidence suggests that highly anxious persons may occasionally "detect" daily relationship conflicts that do not exist.

Several of the most novel results in our diary and social interaction study involved statistical interactions between attachment anxiety and perceptions of conflict. In the diary data, for example, highly anxious individuals reported lower satisfaction and closeness and more negative views about the future of their relationships compared with less anxious individuals on days when they perceived greater relationship conflict. This myopic focus on daily relationship events is likely to have destabilizing effects on relationships over time. Kelley (1983) has conjectured that the stability of relationships should hinge on two variables: (1) the degree to which the benefits in a relationship typically exceed the costs and (2) the variance of this difference. For most relationships to be emotionally stable, therefore, the degree to which benefits outweigh costs must be great relative to the variability of the difference. In the case of highly anxious individuals, not only is the benefit-to-cost ratio likely to be lower, but it also should be more variable if highly anxious people continually evaluate their relationships in terms of daily relationship events. To complicate matters, highly anxious persons also presume that their partners are less satisfied or close and less optimistic on high-conflict days. On high-conflict days, highly anxious individuals might project their own pessimistic outlooks onto their partners. In support of this interpretation, when highly anxious people are upset, they overestimate their similarity with others (Mikulincer, Orbach, & Iavnieli, 1998).

Highly anxious individuals also believed that relationship conflicts during the diary period would have more negative long-term effects on their relationships, even when their partners reported behaving in a more positive and conciliatory fashion toward them during conflicts. Paralleling this result, highly anxious individuals in the social interaction phase of the study reported greater distress when they discussed the most important unresolved conflict from the diary period, even when their partners were rated by observers as behaving relatively more positively toward them. Thus, unlike less anxious individuals, who tend to be more securely attached, highly anxious persons are less likely to adjust their relationship evaluations in response to their partners' actions. There could be several reasons for these "noncontingent" partner behavior effects. Given the dubious and self-protective nature of their working models, highly anxious individuals might simply deny, dismiss, or discount their partners' positive overtures, particularly during conflict episodes in which positive gestures such as apologizing, showing remorse, or adopting a forgiving attitude could be interpreted as less than genuine. Highly anxious individuals might also become overwhelmed during relationship conflicts, limiting their capacity to monitor, notice, or give credit to their partners' positive overtures (Main, 1991). In line with this view, Mikulincer (1998) found that anger often overwhelms the cognitive system of highly anxious people, interfering with their ability to recruit resources to contain their negative feelings. Highly anxious individuals might also believe that, by giving their partners too much "credit" for their benevolent actions, they could be setting themselves up for major letdowns in the near future.

Less anxious (more secure) people, in contrast, responded to their partners' behavior in a more situationally contingent manner. Among others, Main (1991) has speculated that securely attached people perceive and evaluate relationship-relevant events in a more open and flexible manner than insecure persons do, chiefly because their working models do not distort attachment-relevant information. Similar situationally contingent effects of adult security have been found in other settings. Simpson, Rholes, Oriña, and Grich (2002), for instance, found that more securely attached women (assessed by the Adult Attachment Interview) are more likely to give their distressed male dating partners more comfort and support (as rated by observers) than are less secure women if their partners request or appear to need it, but they actually provide less support if their partners do not need it.

In the diary phase of our study, however, highly anxious individuals also felt better about the future of their relationships on days when they perceived greater support from their partners. This finding provides preliminary support for a central tenet of Fraley and Shaver's (2000) model of attachment anxiety—that perceptions of either greater relationship-based conflict or support ought to be more strongly linked to how highly anxious persons view and evaluate their relationships on a daily basis. Nevertheless, fewer effects emerged for perceptions of support than for perceptions of conflict. This is understandable when one considers that negative relationship events often have more important consequences for the well-being and stability of relationships than do positive events (see Fraley & Shaver, 2000; Gaelick et al., 1985).

Links with Other Theoretical Models

Although the current results fit well with Fraley and Shaver's (2000) ideas about activation of the appraisal/monitoring system, they can also be meaningfully understood and interpreted in terms of other theoretical models. Given the severe costs of social rejection, for example, Leary and Baumeister (2000) contend that humans may possess an evolved internal regulatory system—a self-esteem sociometer—that is responsive to cues of rejection, that warns people about possible rejection threats, and that motivates them to take action to avert or minimize possible threats. The current findings fit well with several aspects of this model. In fact, we suspect that highly anxious individuals have sociometers that are hypersensitive and overreactive to potential signs or cues of rejection and its complement (acceptance), given that so much of their self-worth hinges on the adequate functioning of their relationships.

Our results also fit well with findings from studies of dependency regulation and rejection sensitivity in relationships. Individuals with low self-esteem, many of whom are likely to be anxiously attached (Griffin & Bartholomew, 1994), tend to overinterpret relationship problems, often assuming that their partners' affection might be waning (Murray, Rose, Bellavia, Holmes, & Kusche, 2002). In addition, individuals who feel less positively regarded by their romantic partners—many of whom should be highly anxious—frequently read too much into relationship-threatening interactions, feel more hurt and worse about themselves on days after relationship-threatening interactions, and then behave more negatively toward their partners in turn (Murray, Bellavia, Rose, & Griffin, 2003). Similarly, highly rejection-sensitive individuals, many of whom are likely to be anxiously attached, expect, perceive, and overreact to ambiguous cues of possible interpersonal rejection (Downey & Feldman, 1996), and they tend to use conflict resolution tactics that exacerbate relationship difficulties and undermine their relationships (Downey, Freitas, Michaelis, & Khouri, 1998). It is important to note, however, that nearly all of the effects for attachment anxiety reported in this chapter remained significant when individuals' levels of chronic self-esteem *and* neuroticism were statistically controlled. Thus the unique variance that underlies attachment anxiety appears to play a distinct role in accounting for the findings discussed here.

The current findings might also have some interesting implications for interdependence theory. To the extent that highly anxious people are more attuned to and dependent on their partners' decisions and actions (either actual or perceived), their outcomes in relationships might be more strongly affected by their partners' decisions or actions—actual or incorrectly perceived—in certain types of interpersonal situations (see Kelley et al., 2003). This heightened "partner sensitivity" may be especially apparent when highly anxious individuals find themselves in situations that increase their dependence on their partners for good outcomes or in situations that make them feel uncertain or vulnerable about the stability and future well-being of their relationships. Future research should explore these issues.

CONCLUSIONS

In conclusion, the studies discussed here contribute to our understanding of why highly anxious people tend to have such tumultuous relationships. Not only does this research confirm that highly anxious individuals tend to perceive greater and more extensive daily conflict in their romantic relationships, but it also reveals that their working models may negatively bias their daily relationship perceptions and the inferences they make about the current and future well-being of their relationships. By basing their judgments of relationship quality on amplified perceptions of daily relationship conflict and strife, highly anxious individuals may unwittingly create what they fear the most—the destabilization of their romantic relationships.

NOTE

1. In a week-long daily diary study, Pietromonaco and Feldman Barrett (1997) found that highly anxious individuals did not report experiencing more extreme emotions when interacting with different types of partners (e.g., strangers, friends, romantic partners). They contend that conflict may provide these individ-

uals with an opportunity to achieve two deep-seated goals—to gain their partners' attention and to build greater intimacy and more felt security. On the surface, these findings seem to be at odds with those reported by Simpson et al. (1996), who found that more anxious individuals were rated by trained observers as displaying more dysfunctional conflict resolution tactics and more intense negative emotions when trying to solve major (but not minor) relationship-centered problems. In reality, the results of these studies are not inconsistent. When assigned to discuss a minor problem, more anxious individuals in the Simpson et al. (1996) study did not display either more negative emotions or more dysfunctional conflict resolution tactics than other individuals. Moreover, the major problem task and instructions used in Simpson et al.'s observational study were probably more threatening than the daily interactions investigated by Pietromonaco and Feldman Barrett (1997), many of which did not involve attachment figures (see also Pietromonaco, Greenwood, & Feldman Barrett, 2004).

REFERENCES

Bartholomew, K., Cobb, R. J., & Poole, J. A. (1997). Adult attachment patterns and social support processes. In G. R. Pierce, B. Lakey, I. G. Sarason, & B. R. Sarason (Eds.), *Sourcebook of social support and personality* (pp. 359–378). New York: Plenum.

Bartholomew, K., & Horowitz, L. M. (1991). Attachment styles among young adults: A test of a four-category model. *Journal of Personality and Social Psychology, 61*, 226–244.

Bowlby, J. (1969). *Attachment and loss: Vol. 1. Attachment*. New York: Basic Books.

Bowlby, J. (1973). *Attachment and loss: Vol. 2. Separation*. New York: Basic Books.

Bowlby, J. (1980). *Attachment and loss: Vol. 3. Loss: Sadness and depression*. New York: Basic Books.

Bradford, S. A., Feeney, J. A., & Campbell, L. (2002). Links between attachment orientations and dispositional and diary-based measures of disclosure in dating couples: A study of actor and partner effects. *Personal Relationships, 9*, 491–506.

Brennan, K. A., Clark, C. L., & Shaver, P. R. (1998). Self-report measurement of adult attachment: An integrative overview. In J. A. Simpson & W. S. Rholes (Eds.), *Attachment theory and close relationships* (pp. 46–76). New York: Guilford Press.

Campbell, L., Simpson, J. A., Boldry, J., & Kashy, D. A. (2005). Perceptions of conflict and support in romantic relationships: The role of attachment anxiety. *Journal of Personality and Social Psychology, 88*, 510–531.

Cassidy, J., & Berlin, L. J. (1994). The insecure/ambivalent pattern of attachment: Theory and research. *Child Development, 65*, 971–981.

Collins, N. L. (1996). Working models of attachment: Implications for explanation, emotion, and behavior. *Journal of Personality and Social Psychology, 71*, 810–832.

Collins, N. L., & Allard, L. M. (2001). Cognitive representations of attachment: The content and function of working models. In G. J. O. Fletcher & M. S. Clark (Eds.), *Blackwell handbook of social psychology: Interpersonal processes* (pp. 60–85). Malden, MA: Blackwell.

Collins, N. L., & Feeney, B. C. (2000). A safe haven: An attachment theory perspective on support seeking and caregiving in intimate relationships. *Journal of Personality and Social Psychology, 78*, 1053–1073.

Collins, N. L., & Feeney, B. C. (2004). Working models of attachment shape perceptions of social support: Evidence from experimental and observational studies. *Journal of Personality and Social Psychology, 87*, 363–383.

Collins, N. L., & Read, S. (1990). Adult attachment, working models, and relationship quality in dating couples. *Journal of Personality and Social Psychology, 58*, 644–663.

Crocker, J., & Wolfe, C. T. (2001). Contingencies of self-worth. *Psychological Review, 108*, 593–623.

Downey, G., & Feldman, S. I. (1996). Implications of rejection sensitivity for intimate relationships. *Journal of Personality and Social Psychology, 70*, 1327–1343.

Downey, G., Freitas, A. L., Michaelis, B., & Khouri, H. (1998). The self-fulfilling prophecy in close relationships: Rejection sensitivity and rejection by romantic partners. *Journal of Personality and Social Psychology, 75*, 545–560.

Feeney, J. A. (1999). Adult romantic attachment and couple relationships. In J. Cassidy & P. R. Shaver (Eds.), *Handbook of attachment: Theory, research, and clinical applications* (pp. 355–377). New York: Guilford Press.

Feeney, J. A., Noller, P., & Callan, V. J. (1994). Attachment style, communication and satisfaction in the early years of marriage. In K. Bartholomew & D. Perlman (Eds.), *Advances in personal relationships: Vol. 5. Attachment processes in adulthood* (pp. 269–308). London: Kingsley.

Fishstein, J., Pietromonaco, P. R., & Feldman Barrett, L. (1999). The contribution of attachment style and relationship conflict to the complexity of relationship knowledge. *Social Cognition, 17*, 228–244.

Fletcher, G. J. O., Simpson, J. A., & Thomas, G. (2000). The measurement of perceived relationship quality components: A confirmatory factor analytic approach. *Personality and Social Psychology Bulletin, 26*, 340–354.

Fraley, R. C., & Shaver, P. R. (2000). Adult romantic attachment: Theoretical developments, emerging controversies, and unanswered questions. *Review of General Psychology, 4*, 132–154.

Gaelick, K., Bodenhausen, G. V., & Wyer, R. S. (1985). Emotional communication in close relationships. *Journal of Personality and Social Psychology, 49*, 1246–1265.

Griffin, D. W., & Bartholomew, K. (1994). Models of the self and other: Fundamental dimensions underlying measures of adult attachment. *Journal of Personality and Social Psychology, 67*, 430–445.

Hazan, C., & Shaver, P. R. (1987). Romantic love conceptualized as an attachment process. *Journal of Personality and Social Psychology, 52*, 511–524.

Hazan, C., & Shaver, P. R. (1994). Attachment as an organizational framework for research on close relationships. *Psychological Inquiry, 5*, 1–22.

Holmes, J. G., & Rempel, J. K. (1989). Trust in close relationships. In C. Hendrick (Ed.), *Review of personality and social psychology* (Vol. 10, pp. 187–220). Newbury Park, CA: Sage.

John, O. P., & Srivastava, S. (1999). The big five trait taxonomy: History, measurement, and theoretical perspectives. In L. A. Pervin & O. P. John (Eds.), *Handbook of personality: Theory and research* (2nd ed., pp. 102–138). New York: Guilford Press.

Kashy, D. A., & Kenny, D. A. (2000). The analysis of data from dyads and groups. In H. T. Reis & C. M. Judd (Eds.), *Handbook of research methods in social psychology* (pp. 451–477). New York: Cambridge University Press.

Kelley, H. H. (1983). Love and commitment. In H. H. Kelley, E. Berscheid, A. Christensen, J. H. Harvey, T. L. Huston, G. Levinger, E. McClintock, L. A. Peplau, & D. R. Peterson (Eds.), *Close relationships* (pp. 265–314). San Francisco: Freeman.

Kelley, H. H., Holmes, J. G., Kerr, N. L., Reis, H. T., Rusbult, C. E., & Van Lange, P. A. M. (2003). *An atlas of interpersonal situations.* New York: Cambridge University Press.

Kirkpatrick, L. A., & Davis, K. E. (1994). Attachment style, gender, and relationship stability: A longitudinal analysis. *Journal of Personality and Social Psychology, 66*, 502–512.

Kobak, R. R., & Duemmler, S. (1994). Attachment and conversation: Toward a discourse analysis of adolescent and adult security. In K. Bartholomew & D. Perlman (Eds.), *Attachment processes in adulthood* (pp. 121–149). London: Kingsley.

Leary, M. R., & Baumeister, R. F. (2000). The nature and function of self-esteem: Sociometer theory. In M. P. Zanna (Ed.), *Advances in experimental social psychology* (Vol. 32, pp. 1–2). San Diego, CA: Academic Press.

Levy, M. B., & Davis, K. E. (1988). Lovestyles and attachment styles compared: Their relations to each other and to various relationship characteristics. *Journal of Social and Personal Relationships, 5*, 439–471.

Main, M. (1991). Metacognitive knowledge, metacognitive monitoring and singular (coherent) versus multiple (incoherent) models of attachment. In J. S. Stevenson-Hinde, C. M. Parkes, & P. Marris (Eds.), *Attachment across the lifecycle* (pp. 127–159). London: Routledge.

Mikulincer, M. (1998). Adult attachment style and individual differences in functional versus dysfunctional experiences of anger. *Journal of Personality and Social Psychology, 74*, 513–524.

Mikulincer, M., Birnbaum, G., Woddis, D., & Nachmias, O. (2000). Stress and accessibility of proximity-related thoughts: Exploring the normative and intraindividual components of attachment theory. *Journal of Personality and Social Psychology, 78*, 509–523.

Mikulincer, M., & Florian, V. (1995). Appraisal and coping with a real-life stressful situation: The contribution of attachment styles. *Personality and Social Psychology Bulletin, 21*, 408–416.

Mikulincer, M., & Florian, V. (1998). The relationship between adult attachment styles and emotional and cognitive reactions to stressful events. In J. A. Simpson & W. S. Rholes (Eds.), *Attachment theory and close relationships* (pp. 143–165). New York: Guilford Press.

Mikulincer, M., Gillath, O., & Shaver, P. R. (2002). Activation of the attachment system in adulthood: Threat-related primes increase the accessibility of mental representations of attachment figures. *Journal of Personality and Social Psychology, 83*, 881–895.

Mikulincer, M., & Horesh, N. (1999). Adult attachment style and the perception of others: The role of projective mechanisms. *Journal of Personality and Social Psychology, 76*, 1022–1034.

Mikulincer, M., Orbach, I., & Iavnieli, D. (1998). Adult attachment style and affect regulation: Strategic variations in subjective self–other similarity. *Journal of Personality and Social Psychology, 75*, 436–448.

Murray, S. L., Bellavia, G. M., Rose, P., & Griffin, D. W. (2003). Once hurt, twice hurtful: How perceived regard regulates daily marital interactions. *Journal of Personality and Social Psychology, 84*, 126–147.

Murray, S. L., Rose, P., Bellavia, G. M., Holmes, J. G., & Kusche, A. G. (2002). When rejection stings: How self-esteem constrains relationship-enhancement processes. *Journal of Personality and Social Psychology, 83*, 556–573.

Pietromonaco, P. R., & Feldman Barrett, L. (1997). Working models of attachment and daily social interactions. *Journal of Personality and Social Psychology, 73*, 1409–1423.

Pietromonaco, P. R., Greenwood, D., & Feldman Barrett, L. (2004). Conflict in adult close relationships: An attachment perspective. In W. S. Rholes & J. A. Simpson (Eds.), *Adult attachment: Theory, research, and clinical implications* (pp. 267–299). New York: Guilford Press.

Pistole, M. C. (1989). Attachment in adult romantic relationships: Style of conflict resolution and relationship satisfaction. *Journal of Social and Personal Relationships, 6*, 505–512.

Rholes, W. S., Simpson, J. A., Campbell, L., & Grich, J. (2001). Adult attachment and the transition to parenthood. *Journal of Personality and Social Psychology, 81*, 421–435.

Rosenberg, M. (1965). *Society and the adolescent self-image*. Princeton, NJ: Princeton University Press.

Shaver, P. R., & Brennan, K. A. (1992). Attachment styles and the "big five" personality traits: Their connections with each other and with romantic relationship outcomes. *Personality and Social Psychology Bulletin, 18*, 536–545.

Shaver, P. R., & Mikulincer, M. (2002). Attachment-related psychodynamics. *Attachment and Human Development, 4*, 133–161.

Simpson, J. A. (1990). The influence of attachment styles on romantic relationships. *Journal of Personality and Social Psychology, 59*, 971–980.

Simpson, J. A., & Rholes, W. S. (1994). Stress and secure base relationships in adulthood. In K. Bartholomew & D. Perlman (Eds.), *Attachment processes in adulthood* (pp. 181–204). London: Kingsley.

Simpson, J. A., Rholes, W. S., Oriña, M. M., & Grich, J. (2002). Working models of attachment, support giving, and support seeking in a stressful situation. *Personality and Social Psychology Bulletin, 28*, 598–608.

Simpson, J. A., Rholes, W. S., & Phillips, D. (1996). Conflict in close relationships: An attachment perspective. *Journal of Personality and Social Psychology, 71*, 899–914.

Tidwell, M. C. O., Reis, H. T., & Shaver, P. R. (1996). Attachment, attractiveness, and social interaction: A diary study. *Journal of Personality and Social Psychology, 71*, 729–745.

Part IV

Attachment, Sex, and Love

10

Attachment Styles, Sex Motives, and Sexual Behavior

Evidence for Gender-Specific Expressions of Attachment Dynamics

M. LYNNE COOPER, MARK PIOLI, ASH LEVITT,
AMELIA E. TALLEY, LADA MICHEAS,
and NANCY L. COLLINS

Shaver and colleagues (e.g., Hazan & Shaver, 1994; Shaver, Hazan, & Bradshaw, 1988) have argued that romantic love can be understood as an attachment process in which a committed, intimate relationship meets basic needs for comfort, closeness, and security. Although the need for felt security is seen as universal, individuals with different attachment styles are thought to seek different optimal levels of closeness versus independence in their relationships and to use different strategies for regulating their internal feeling states and interpersonal relations.

Building on these ideas, we argue that sexual behavior, governed in part by a behavioral system distinct from the attachment system described originally by Bowlby (1969/1982), provides an important set of strategies that people use to regulate emotional experiences and interpersonal relationships; that individuals with different attachment styles adopt different intra- and interpersonal goals and differ in the characteristic ways in which they use sex to achieve these goals; and, finally, that reliable differences in the regulatory functions of sex at least partly explain observed attachment-style differences in the nature and quality of sexual experience.

We begin this chapter by providing a thumbnail sketch of the three attachment types originally identified in Hazan and Shaver's (1987) seminal work, draw out the implications of these psychological portraits for human sexual behavior, and briefly review the empirical evidence examining attachment style differences in sexual behavior (see also Davis, Chapter 12, and Gillath & Schachner, Chapter 13, this volume). We then review theory and research on sexual motives and sexual behavior and develop a series of hypotheses that integrates these two lines of work. Finally, we present longitudinal data from a community sample of couples that directly tests the idea that differences in underlying sexual motives explain (or mediate) the links between attachment styles and sexual behavior.

ATTACHMENT STYLE DIFFERENCES IN THE REGULATION OF INTERNAL FEELING STATES AND INTERPERSONAL RELATIONSHIPS

Attachment scholars (beginning with Ainsworth, Blehar, Waters, & Wall, 1978) have identified at least three distinct patterns or styles of attachment—secure, avoidant, and anxious—that are thought to derive from early formative experiences with caregivers and to become embodied in the form of internal working models (or schemas) of self and others. Once developed, working models become core features of personality, features that are carried forward in time and continue to guide cognitive, emotional, and behavioral response patterns in attachment-relevant contexts (Bowlby, 1973; Collins & Read, 1994). A large number of studies have now been conducted on adult attachment styles (see Feeney, 1999; Mikulincer & Shaver, 2003; Shaver & Clark, 1994, for reviews), and a reliable portrait has emerged of the three kinds of individuals identified by this research.

Through a history of successful interactions with important others, *secure* individuals are thought to develop a sense of self-worth (i.e., a positive model of self), as well as a sense that other people are trustworthy and dependable (i.e., a positive model of others). As a result, they have generally positive expectations about relationship partners and are comfortable depending on others for support and seeking intimacy and closeness in relationships. At the same time, securely attached individuals are able to maintain a healthy balance between intimacy and autonomy needs because their own sense of self-worth does not hinge on the constant approval of others. Finally, securely attached adults, through a history of successful childhood experiences in regulating their distress (at first with attachment figures' support and guidance), have confidence in their ability to cope with negative emotions, tend to acknowledge feelings of anxiety and distress, and deal with them in constructive ways. A large body of research (reviewed by Mikulincer & Shaver, 2003) provides support for these contentions, showing that securely attached adults are better adjusted across a wide variety of both behavioral measures (e.g., secure individuals use more effective coping strategies) and emotional indices (e.g., they are generally less depressed, anxious, and neurotic). Not surprisingly, securely attached individuals also have relationships characterized by higher levels of trust, satisfaction, and commitment and lower levels of conflict, jealousy, and emotional ambivalence.

Through a history of inconsistent and sometimes intrusive caregiving, *anxiously attached* individuals are thought to have developed deep-seated doubts about their own worthiness (i.e., a negative self-model) and, consequently, to depend on other people's acceptance for a sense of personal worth and well-being. This leads to an exaggerated desire for closeness, coupled with a heightened concern about being rejected and unloved. As a consequence, anxiously attached adults are hypervigilant in relationships, seek constant reassurance of their worth, and are prone to bouts of jealousy and conflict. Further, anxiously attached adults tend to experience emotional extremes and have difficulty regulating their emotions. Ample empirical support exists for these contentions, indicating that anxious individuals are excessively reliant on others for approval, experience volatile relationships, and are poorly adjusted overall, although some evidence suggests that these effects are stronger for women than for men (e.g., Collins & Read, 1990; Feeney, 1999).

Presumably as a result of early attachment experiences with caregivers who were unresponsive and emotionally distant, *avoidant* individuals perceive attachment figures as unreliable and uncaring (i.e., have a negative model of others), and they prefer not to depend on others for support. Avoidant individuals value self-reliance and are uncomfortable with intimacy and interdependence. They attempt to maintain a positive self-image in the face of potential rejection by denying attachment needs, distancing themselves from others, and restricting expressions of emotionality. Consequently, such individuals tend to report low levels of satisfaction, intimacy, and commitment in relationships, though there is some evidence to suggest that these effects are stronger for men than for women (Collins & Read, 1994; Feeney, 1999). Finally, avoidant individuals are less socially skilled and experience higher levels of negative affect (relative to their secure counterparts), although they restrict both the acknowledgement and expression of these emotions.

ATTACHMENT STYLE DIFFERENCES IN SEXUAL BEHAVIOR

Shaver and colleagues (1988) have argued that adult love is an integration of the attachment, caregiving, and sexual systems and that the attachment system—because it deals with fundamental self-protection and comes into being first during development—shapes the functioning of the other two. Despite the theoretical importance of the attachment system to human sexuality, few studies have examined links between attachment and sexual experience, and most of these have been conducted among college students. Thus the extant database is limited and must be interpreted against the backdrop of normative developmental tasks during this life stage.

Developmental Considerations

Recently dubbed "emerging adulthood," the years that span the transition from adolescence into young adulthood (from roughly 18 to 24 years of age) are a period of profound change and importance (see Arnett, 2000, for a more complete discussion). Typically, emerging adults have moved beyond the dependency of adolescence but have not yet fully assumed the roles and responsibilities of adulthood. Thus, exploring a variety of possible life directions and identities, including love and sex, is a central developmental task undertaken in preparation for making the more enduring and life-constraining commitments of young adulthood. According to Arnett (2000), romantic relationships during this period last longer than in adolescence, involve a deeper level of intimacy, and are focused on answering questions about the kind of person one wants as a life partner. Not surprisingly, they also are more likely to involve sexual intercourse, often in the context of cohabitation. Romantic explorations during this period can also be ends in themselves—part of having a broad range of life experiences before taking on enduring adult responsibilities.

That sexual activity is a normal part of development during this period is supported by data from a recently published national study (Laumann, Gagnon, Michael, & Michaels, 1994) showing that 92% of 18- to 24-year-olds have had intercourse at least once. Moreover, nearly two-thirds of sexually experienced individuals in this age range have had two or more sex partners, and more than one-fourth of them have had five or more partners. Thus both having sex and having sex with multiple partners are (statistically) normative features of emerging adulthood and, presumably, serve important developmental needs.

Secure Attachment and Patterns of Sexual Behavior

In light of the normative developmental tasks thought to characterize this life stage, most securely attached individuals would be expected to have had sex by this time, possibly even with multiple partners. Presumably, securely attached youths would enter into sexual relationships as a way to express intimacy and caring for their partners, to explore the partners' suitability as a long-term mate, and to work out other aspects of their identities that are not yet fully formed.

Existing research supports these expectations. Securely attached individuals appear to be comfortable with their sexuality and to enjoy a variety of sexual activities, including physical touch (Hazan, Zeifman, & Middleton, 1994). Similarly, Tracy, Shaver, Albino, and Cooper (2003) found that securely attached adolescents reported the lowest levels of erotophobia (characterized by negative emotional reactions to sex, including guilt; Fisher, Byrne, & White, 1983) of the three attachment types. Consistent with the idea that securely attached youths like sex, they do not appear to delay the onset of intercourse or to have fewer sex partners (Chisholm, 1999; Cooper, Shaver, & Collins, 1998; Feeney, Peterson, Gallois, & Terry, 2000). They do, however, differ in the kinds of partners with whom, and the circumstances in which, they choose to have sex. They are more likely to have sex within the confines of a committed relationship and to have mutually initiated intercourse (Brennan & Shaver, 1995; Feeney, Noller, & Patty, 1993; Hazan et al., 1994). They also are less accepting of casual sex (Brennan & Shaver, 1995; Feeney et al., 1993; Stephan & Bachman, 1999) and, not surprisingly, less likely to have casual or promiscuous sex partners, one-night stands, or extrapair sex (Hazan et al., 1994; Paul, McManus, & Hayes, 2000). Similarly, in a representative community sample of adolescents, we found that securely attached adolescents were less likely to have had sex with a stranger or to have been the perpetrator or the victim of sexual aggression (Cooper, Shaver, & Collins, 1998; Tracy et al., 2003).

Anxious Attachment and Patterns of Sexual Behavior

Because anxiously attached youths lack a positive sense of self, are dependent on others for approval, and are intensely concerned about abandonment and rejection, we would expect them to have difficulty negotiating sexual relationships in healthy ways and to confuse sex with love. Due to these insecurities, we would expect anxiously attached individuals to be especially vulnerable to pressures to have sex, even when ill-advised. Thus they might initiate sex at a younger-than-optimal age; have more, and especially more risky, sexual partners; and be more likely to succumb to unwanted sexual advances and less likely to adopt safe sex practices, because doing so often requires asserting oneself even at the risk of offending one's partner (Impett & Peplau, 2002; Morokoff et al., 1997).

Empirical support for this profile has been surprisingly mixed, in part owing to the presence of important gender differences in how attachment anxiety is expressed in the sexual domain. For example, anxiety among males has been related to older age at first intercourse (Gentzler & Kerns, 2004), less frequent intercourse (Feeney et al., 1993), and fewer sex partners (Gentzler & Kerns, 2004). In contrast, anxiety among female adolescents has been linked to a higher likelihood of having ever had sex (Cooper, Shaver, & Collins, 1998) and, among female college students, to a younger age at first intercourse (Bogaert & Sadava, 2002; Gentzler & Kerns, 2004).

Anxiously attached females are also less likely to be in a sexually exclusive relationship (Feeney et al., 2000) and more likely to report having had extrapair sex (Bogaert & Sadava, 2002; Gangestad & Thornhill, 1997). Although both anxious males and females report feeling that their sexuality is controlled by others and have difficulty resisting pressures to have sex (Feeney et al., 2000), these experiences apparently translate into higher rates of unwanted (though reportedly consensual) sexual experience primarily among females (Gentzler & Kerns, 2004; Impett & Peplau, 2002).

Interestingly, anxiously attached individuals of both sexes prefer the intimate aspects of sexuality (i.e., touching, cuddling, kissing) to the sexual aspects per se (Hazan et al., 1994). This dislike or discomfort with the explicitly sexual aspects of sex is reflected in a more recent study showing that anxiously attached adolescents are significantly more erotophobic than their securely attached counterparts (Tracy et al., 2003). Finally, attachment anxiety appears to interfere with safe sex practices for anxious youths of both genders. Individuals high in anxiety avoid safe sex discussions, hold negative attitudes toward condoms (e.g., believe that they interrupt foreplay, reduce intimacy, destroy spontaneity) and, not surprisingly, report lower rates of consistent condom use (Feeney et al., 2000). Given this aversion to safe sex practices, it is also not surprising that attachment anxiety has been related to higher rates of unplanned pregnancy, especially among females (Cooper, Shaver, & Collins, 1998).

Avoidant Attachment and Patterns of Sexual Behavior

Sex—perhaps the most intimate human activity of all—presents a difficult dilemma for avoidant individuals, who typically eschew intimacy and closeness in relationships. In theory, however, this dilemma could be solved in one of several ways. Avoidants could avoid or delay the onset of sexual activity or have sex in contexts that make true intimacy unlikely. These are, of course, not mutually exclusive possibilities, and the evidence suggests that avoidant individuals use both strategies. In our earlier study, for example, we found that avoidant adolescents were less likely ever to have had sex, owing in part to their poor social skills (Cooper, Shaver, & Collins, 1998). This aversion to, or discomfort with, sex extended to the virgins in our sample as well, who reported fewer noncoital sexual behaviors (e.g., less making out, petting, etc.) than their nonavoidant virgin counterparts (Tracy et al., 2003). Evidence for delay comes from several other studies as well, in which sexually experienced avoidant youths reported an older age at first intercourse (Bogaert & Sadava, 2002; Gentzler & Kerns, 2004).

However, once avoidant individuals become sexually active, there is strong evidence that they, more than their nonavoidant counterparts, engage in a pattern of promiscuous and casual sex. Avoidant individuals endorse less restrictive attitudes toward sex (Gentzler & Kerns, 2004; Feeney et al., 1993), and they are both less likely to have sex with a steady or committed relationship partner (Gentzler & Kerns, 2004) and more likely to have one-night stands and sex with strangers (Cooper, Shaver, & Collins, 1998; Paul et al., 2000). Avoidants are also more likely to engage in solitary sexual activities such as masturbation (Bogaert & Sadava, 2002). Patterns such as these should allow avoidants to divorce intimate and affectionate behaviors (e.g., cuddling and kissing), which they dislike (Fraley, Davis, & Shaver, 1998; Hazan et al., 1994), from purely sexual behaviors. Avoidant individuals' discomfort with the intimate aspects of sexuality also appears to translate into an overall negative emotional response to sex, as indexed by higher scores on the erotophobia scale (Tracy et al., 2003).

Interestingly, avoidant men and women report feeling that their sexual experiences are controlled by others (Feeney et al., 2000) and are more likely to report having unwanted but consensual sex (Gentzler & Kerns, 2004), apparently out of a sense of obligation or responsibility (Impett & Peplau, 2002). Finally, avoidants report more positive attitudes toward condoms, and avoidant males in particular report that they are more likely to discuss HIV/AIDS risk and to use condoms every time they have sex (Feeney et al., 2000). Though decidedly beneficial from a health-risk perspective, these cautionary behaviors may be yet another mechanism to ensure that casual relationships do not evolve into more committed ones.

Summary of Attachment Style Differences in Sexual Behavior

In short, the distinctive psychological features of the different attachment types appear to translate into unique and theoretically meaningful patterns of sexual behavior. Securely attached individuals select partners and circumstances that foster mutuality, caring, and commitment in their sexual relationships. These experiences can be seen to provide important contexts for working on normative developmental tasks, including exploring alternative relationships and identities and meeting intimacy goals. In contrast, although anxiously attached individuals seek and value intimacy in their sexual relationships, the neediness and insecurities they bring to these relationships appear to undermine opportunities for the development of true intimacy. This is seen most clearly among anxiously attached females, who, despite their strong desire for intimate relationships, are actually less likely to be involved in sexually exclusive relationships and more likely to report extrapair sex. Finally, avoidant attachment is linked to two strategies for limiting intimacy in sexual relationships. Individuals with avoidant attachment styles both avoid sexual encounters and engage in sex with casual partners. As noted by Schachner and Shaver (2004; see also Fraley & Shaver, 2000), such findings are consistent with the notion that the sexual system is shaped by attachment-related motives and needs. To evaluate this possibility more carefully, we now turn to research and theory on sexual motivations.

MOTIVES FOR SEX AND SEXUAL BEHAVIOR

The notion that people use sex strategically to achieve different goals and that this in turn shapes the experience and expression of their sexuality is rooted in a functional perspective on behavior (Snyder & Cantor, 1998). According to this view, the key to understanding behavior lies in the goals and purposes served by the behavior. No matter how similar in outward appearance, behaviors undertaken in service of different needs or goals are psychologically distinct and should exhibit unique patterns of antecedents, correlates, and consequences. This perspective suggests that sexual behaviors that are motivated by different goals or needs (e.g., having sex to express love vs. to avoid rejection) should be triggered by unique antecedents, characterized by qualitatively different styles of behavior and emotions, and ultimately result in distinct consequences. In line with this view, the following sections identify the most important goals thought to be served by sexual behavior and review research linking these motives to unique patterns of sexual behavior and outcomes.

What Goals or Motives Underlie Sexual Behavior?

In our earlier work, Cooper and colleagues (Cooper, Shapiro, & Powers, 1998) hypothesized that two primary motivational dimensions underlie human sexual behavior and that these dimensions combine in unique ways to give rise to a relatively small number of discrete sexual motives (described subsequently). The first of these two dimensions distinguishes behaviors that involve the pursuit of positive or pleasurable experiences (appetitive or approach behaviors) from those that involve the avoidance of, or escape from, negative or painful ones (so-called aversive or avoidance behaviors). According to Gray (1987), aversive and appetitive behaviors are regulated by neurologically distinct motivational systems. The behavioral inhibition system (BIS) regulates aversive motivation and controls the experience of negative emotions, whereas the behavioral activation system (BAS) regulates appetitive motivation, causes movement toward goals (approach behavior), and controls the experience of positive emotions. Gray (1987) further hypothesized that individuals differ in a stable, traitlike manner in the relative sensitivity of the two systems. Consistent with this hypothesis, people who are high in behavioral inhibition are especially responsive to threat and punishment cues and are thus predisposed to experience negative affect and respond in an avoidant or fearful manner. Conversely, individuals who are high in behavioral activation are especially responsive to reward cues and are therefore predisposed to experience positive affect and engage in reward-seeking behaviors (see Carver & White, 1994; Larsen & Ketelaar, 1991, for supporting evidence). Indeed, high levels of the stable personality traits neuroticism and extroversion are thought to derive from overactive BIS and BAS, respectively (Larsen & Ketelaar, 1991). When applied to sexual behaviors, this distinction suggests that people can have sex to pursue positive outcomes, such as physical pleasure or excitement, or to avoid negative ones, such as rejection by socially significant others.

The second motivational dimension hypothesized to underlie human sexual behavior concerns the extent to which the behavior is motivated by an intraindividual or self-focused concern versus an interpersonal or other-focused concern. This distinction is closely related to the distinctions between agentic versus communal goals (Bakan, 1966), autonomy/competence versus relatedness goals (Skinner & Wellborn, 1994), and exploratory versus attachment goals (Bowlby, 1970). Thus sexual behaviors motivated by self-focused goals could serve agentic, identity, or autonomy/competence needs, such as having sex to affirm one's sense of identity or attractiveness or to manage one's internal emotional experience. The latter can be thought of as an agentic striving to the extent that it involves mastery and control of one's emotional experience (McAdams, 1984). In contrast, other-focused goals are motivated by attachment or communal needs, such as having sex to achieve intimacy and communion in a relationship or to gain another's approval. Thus, although intrapersonal motives may be pursued in an interpersonal context (as when one uses sex to self-affirm) and both intrapersonal and interpersonal motives can be seen as ultimately originating from a desire to manage one's emotions (either by direct manipulation of feeling states or indirectly by obtaining a valued outcome from a socially significant other), these motives nevertheless can be differentiated by the degree to which the outcomes sought are primarily self-focused and internal to the individual versus other-focused and external to the individual.

A factorial combination of these two dimensions yields four broad classes of motives: (1) appetitive self-focused motives, such as having sex to enhance physical or emotional pleasure (i.e., enhancement motives); (2) aversive self-focused motives, such as having sex to cope with threats to self-esteem or to minimize negative emotions (i.e., coping motives); (3) appetitive social motives, such as having sex to bond with socially significant others (i.e., intimacy motives); and (4) aversive social motives, such as having sex to avoid social censure or gain another's approval (i.e., approval motives).

As a first step toward validating the usefulness of this framework, Cooper, Shapiro, and Powers (1998, Study 1) asked undergraduates to list the most important reasons for their having had sex on a recent occasion of intercourse. Forty-nine percent of the resulting responses were categorized as enhancement reasons (e.g., "for pleasure and enjoyment"), 43% as intimacy reasons (e.g., "to strengthen the emotional bond with my partner"), and 8% as avoidant reasons, including both having sex to escape or cope with negative internal states (e.g., "So I could relieve stress") and to avoid rejection by one's peers or partner (e.g., "I felt that I had to because he was my boyfriend"). Subsequent factor analytic work in three independent samples revealed six discrete motives that could be nested in a hierarchical fashion under the four hypothesized motive classes. Specifically, higher-order factor models showed that the correlations among the six factors were equally well explained by a four-factor structure in which intimacy and enhancement were treated as indicators of discrete factors (i.e., appetitive other- and self-focused factors, respectively); affirmation and coping motives were treated as indicators of a single, higher order, aversive, self-focused factor; and peer and partner approval motives were treated as indicators of a single, higher order, aversive social factor (see Cooper, Shapiro, & Powers, 1998, Study 3). These data suggest that although multiple, specific manifestations of avoidance motives may exist, the four-motive typology is nevertheless a useful heuristic device for understanding the structure of sex motives. Finally, rates of endorsement in both college and community samples mirrored rates observed in the initial open-ended elicitation study; enhancement and intimacy were by far the most commonly endorsed reasons for having sex, followed (in descending order) by affirming ones' self-worth, coping with negative emotions, and gaining partner or peer approval (see Cooper, Shapiro, & Powers, 1998, Studies 2 and 3, for details).

In sum, findings from our research clearly indicate that people use sex to pursue a relatively small number of different goals and that these goals may be parsimoniously characterized in terms of underlying differences in approach–avoidance motivation and internal/self versus external/social focus.

Does Having Sex to Achieve Different Goals Matter?

As previously discussed, the functional perspective argues that sexual behaviors motivated by different goals should be driven by distinct causal processes, characterized by distinct patterns of sexual behavior and experience, and ultimately associated with distinct consequences. A growing body of evidence, reviewed here, lends strong support to these contentions.

Intimacy motives for sex index the extent to which one has sex to feel close or connected to one's partner, to express love, or to strengthen an emotional bond. In our earlier work (Cooper, Shapiro, & Powers, 1998, Studies 3 and 4), we found that intimacy motives were associated with positive feelings about sex (i.e., high erotophilia, low erotophobia)—a pattern consistent with the idea that intimacy motives are driven by appetitive or approach processes. Individuals who have sex for intimacy reasons were also found to have fewer, less risky, better known sexual partners (for similar results, see Browning, Hatfield, Kessler, & Levine, 2000; Hill & Preston,

1996; Levinson, Jaccard, & Beamer, 1995) and lower rates of unplanned pregnancies. Although intimacy motives also predicted more frequent intercourse and less condom use, these behaviors were more likely to occur within the context of an exclusive relationship. These findings suggest that people who are high in intimacy motives have more committed sexual partners, presumably because intimacy needs can be better satisfied in the context of such relationships. Consistent with this interpretation, Cooper, Shapiro, and Powers (1998, Study 4) found that individuals who were high in sex-for-intimacy motives were more likely to stay in committed relationships over time, or to move into such a relationship if they were not in one at baseline, and that this difference mediated the effects of having sex for intimacy reasons on changes in sexual behavior, including decreased risky sexual practices.

Enhancement motives for sex index the extent to which one has sex because it feels good (physically or emotionally), is exciting, or fulfills a need for adventure. Not surprisingly, individuals who are high in enhancement motives exhibit an entirely different pattern of behavior and outcomes compared with their high-intimacy-motive counterparts. Cooper, Shapiro, and Powers (1998, Studies 3 and 4) found that individuals who were high in enhancement motives reported strong positive feelings about sex (i.e., high erotophilia, low erotophobia), in addition to a strong desire for sex—again a pattern that connotes strong approach motivation. Approach motivations unfettered by concerns with intimacy, however, appear to translate into a pattern of promiscuous sex. Consistent with this idea, individuals who had sex for enhancement were more accepting of casual, uncommitted sex (cf. Browning et al., 2000; Hill & Preston, 1996; Levinson et al., 1995) and reported more frequent sex, more sexual partners (especially casual ones), more risky sexual practices, and higher rates of STDs. Not surprisingly, Cooper, Shapiro, and Powers (1998, Study 4) found in longitudinal analyses that individuals high in enhancement motives were less likely to enter or stay in committed relationships and that this difference mediated the effects of baseline enhancement motives on later sexual behavior.

Coping and affirmation motives are thought to share important common ground, psychologically speaking, in that both motives reflect an effort to use sex to escape, avoid, or minimize negative emotional states. According to Cooper, Shapiro, and Powers (1998), however, the origin of those negative feelings differs. Whereas coping motives tap a general tendency to use sex to minimize or avoid feelings of sadness, stress, or loneliness regardless of their source, affirmation motives specifically focus on the use of sex to alleviate unpleasant feelings stemming from a sense of personal inadequacy. This latter motive may manifest itself in different forms, including having sex to prove one's physical attractiveness or sexual desirability, to reassure oneself of one's lovability, or, more broadly, to enhance self-esteem or a sense of self-worth.

Consistent with the idea that these are related but distinct motives, coping and affirmation have been shown to exhibit partially overlapping patterns of associations with behavior and outcomes. Both motives have been positively related to need for sex, sexual desire, and erotophilia (Cooper, Shapiro, & Powers, 1998; Hill & Preston, 1996)—findings that, contrary to our view of these motives as aversive motivation processes, suggest an approach orientation to sex. However, both motives have also been positively related to erotophobia (Cooper, Shapiro, & Powers, 1998), thus suggesting an approach–avoidant or ambivalent orientation toward sex among those who use sex to cope or affirm. Thus the association of sex with ambivalent feelings (which are widely experienced as aversive; Priester & Petty, 1996), together with the strong positive correlations observed between both motives and neuroticism (Cooper, Shapiro, & Powers, 1998), can be seen as consistent with the contention that both motives are BIS-driven, aversive motivational processes.

Despite these commonalities, the two motives appear to relate to sexual behaviors in distinct manners. In our earlier research, for example, we found that having sex to affirm was negatively related to lifetime and 6-month frequency of sex in cross-sectional analyses and to smaller increases in frequency across time (though this last effect occurred primarily among individuals in committed relationships at baseline; Cooper, Shapiro, & Powers, 1998, Studies 3 and 4). Affirmation motives also prospectively predicted increases in the number of unplanned pregnancies, though no discernible effect on birth control use was found (Study 4). In contrast, individuals high in coping motives reported more frequent masturbation (Hill & Preston, 1996), more sex partners overall, and more casual and risky sex partners (Cooper, Shapiro, & Powers, 1998; Hill & Preston, 1996). In longitudinal analyses, those who were higher in coping motives also experienced steeper increases in the number of casual and risky sex partners, an effect that was mediated by their tendency to leave (or avoid) committed relationships at a higher rate than individuals who did not use sex to cope (Cooper, Shapiro, & Powers, 1998, Study 4). Finally, individuals scoring high on coping motives were also less likely to have unplanned pregnancies, which was partially explained by superior contraceptive practice among the subset of high-coping-motive individuals who were unattached.

Partner and peer approval motives are also thought to share important common ground in that both index the tendency to have sex to avoid censure or rejection by socially significant others, although who the "other" is differs. Theoretically, people who have sex in response to external social pressures (either real or perceived) lack strong positive, internal incentives for sex and are rendered vulnerable to external pressures by their own sense of personal inadequacy. Consistent with this psychological portrait, Cooper, Shapiro, and Powers (1998, Study 3) found that individuals high in partner- and peer-approval motives were also high in neuroticism, thus indicating a poor self-concept. Such individuals were also high in erotophobia, though they did not differ in erotophilia—findings that together suggest an absence of positive internal reasons for having sex. We also found that both motives were rare, with peer motives being the rarer of the two, especially among females. Finally, endorsement of both motives (but especially peer motives) declined with age, suggesting a more developmentally limited role for these motives.

Beyond these similarities, however, peer- and partner-approval motives were associated with distinct patterns of sexual behavior. For example, Cooper, Shapiro, and Powers (1998; Studies 3 and 4) found that having sex to impress one's peers—a phenomenon observed primarily among young adolescent males—was associated with a relative lack of sexual experience: such individuals reported fewer lifetime intercourse experiences, fewer lifetime sex partners, less frequent sex in the previous 6 months, and older age at first intercourse. Peer motives also prospectively predicted increased sexual risk taking, which may have been at least in part a "catch-up" phenomenon. In contrast, partner-approval motives were related to greater involvement in risky sexual practices, less birth control use, and higher rates of unplanned pregnancies, presumably reflecting reluctance to assert oneself and risk partner disapproval in sexual situations.

Summary

In sum, the foregoing review provides strong support for the idea that why people have sex matters. Indeed, sexual behaviors motivated by different goals were shown, in cross-sectional and longitudinal analyses and across samples, to be characterized by distinct patterns of behaving and by distinct consequences. In general, individuals who have sex for intimacy reasons have relatively frequent sex with fewer, less risky, and better known partners. Thus, although they like sex, their enjoyment of it is primarily restricted to partners with whom they have a close, committed relationship. In contrast, individuals who have sex for enhancement also like sex, but they appear to seek physical gratification for its own sake. Thus they hold permissive attitudes toward casual sex and engage in patterns of frequent and promiscuous sexual behavior. Although the four aversive motives were generally associated with negative feelings about sexuality—presumably owing to their roots in the BIS—and with dysfunctional patterns of sexual behavior, the specific patterns differed. Individuals who have sex to cope hold ambivalent feelings about sex, which in turn appear to be expressed in a pattern of promiscuous but "safe" (i.e., protected) sex. This pattern suggests a certain calculated quality to the sexual behavior of individuals who use sex to cope (cf. Gold & Skinner, 1993). In contrast, having sex to please one's partner is associated with failures to take precautions (e.g., use birth control) and the negative consequences of this failure (i.e., unplanned pregnancies), suggesting that those who are highly motivated to appease their partners sexually may find it difficult to assert themselves in sexual situations. Finally, having sex for affirmation or peer approval is associated with lack of experience (viz., being older at first intercourse, having less frequent sex and fewer partners).

ATTACHMENT, SEX MOTIVES, AND SEXUAL BEHAVIOR: AN EMPIRICAL EXAMINATION

As Gentzler and Kerns (2004) have pointed out, attachment researchers typically interpret attachment-style differences in sexual behavior as reflections of underlying differences in cognitions, emotions, and motivations. Ironically, however, few efforts to identify and test plausible mediators of attachment effects on sexual behavior have been reported in the literature, and none of these have examined specific sexual motivations as mediators. Drawing on the literature cited, we therefore test three broad sets of hypotheses about the motivational mediators of attachment-style differences in sexual behavior, using longitudinal data from a community sample of 224 couples. We focus on five of the six previously discussed motives (all but peer motives, which are extremely rare, especially among females) and on three primary behaviors: number of extrapair partners, number of extrapair partners who are casual or risky (e.g., IV drug users), and cheating (i.e., having sex outside the relationship in violation of the partner's understanding that the relationship is monogamous). We elected to focus on these particular indices because having sex outside one's primary relationship has been shown to be strongly linked to intimacy and commitment within the primary relationship (Drigotas, Safstrom, & Gentilia, 1999; Shackelford & Buss, 2000; see Drigotas & Barta, 2001, for a review). Thus we expected these behaviors to be particularly useful barometers of attachment-related dynamics within relationships.

Our hypotheses are schematically summarized in Figure 10.1. The hypothesized links between specific motives and behaviors follow directly from the previously summarized literature and hence are not discussed further here. However, the specific rationale underpinning each of our hypotheses regarding attachment effects on motives is summarized briefly.

Secure Attachment and Motives for Sex

Because securely attached individuals seek and value intimacy in close relationships and are more likely to have sex in contexts conducive to intimacy, they should be more likely to have sex for this reason. Because their sexual relationships are thought to be characterized by a healthy balance between intimacy and autonomy needs, securely attached individuals should be less

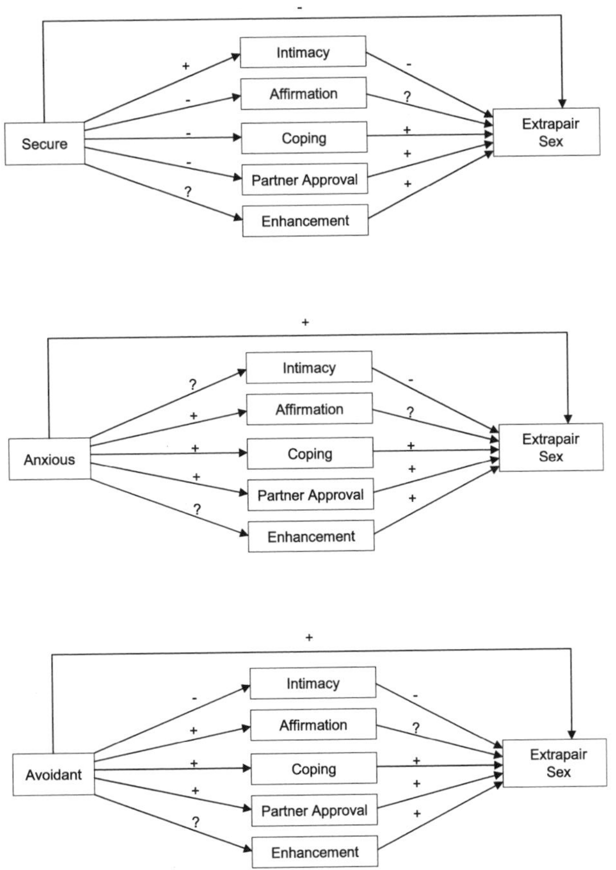

FIGURE 10.1. Hypothesized models linking attachment styles to extrapair sex via sex motives.

likely to have sex to please or appease their sex partners; and because they are generally confident and well-adjusted, they should also be less likely to have sex to affirm their self-worth or to cope with negative emotions. Predictions regarding enhancement motives are, however, less clear. Because securely attached people are generally comfortable with their sexuality and enjoy its physical aspects, they may report higher levels of enhancement motives than their insecure counterparts. However, enhancement goals are not thought to be central to the attachment system (Davis, Shaver, & Vernon, 2004); thus no clear theoretical rationale exists for expecting a relationship between attachment and enhancement motives.

Results from three cross-sectional studies lend preliminary support to these expectations. For example, an earlier study conducted by Tracy et al.

(2003) using data from a large community sample of adolescents (from which the couples participating in the present study were recruited) showed that securely attached adolescents were more likely to have sex to express love for their partners, and less likely to have sex out of fear that their partners would leave them. Although neither of the remaining two studies directly assessed attachment security (Davis et al., 2004; Schachner & Shaver, 2004), their findings were nevertheless consistent with the expectation that securely attached individuals are more likely to have sex for intimacy reasons and less likely to have sex for a range of more maladaptive reasons.

Anxious Attachment and Motives for Sex

Because anxiously attached individuals are intensely concerned about rejection and abandonment, they should be especially likely to have sex to please or appease their partners. Their poor self-concept and low self-esteem should also lead them to have to sex to reassure themselves of their worth. Anxiously attached individuals, who experience more frequent, intense negative affect and have difficulty regulating their affect, should also be prone to use sex to cope. Because anxious individuals desire intimacy in their relationships, they might also report stronger intimacy motives for sex. Finally, expectations regarding anxious attachment and enhancement motives are unclear. Although we might expect anxious individuals, who are uncomfortable with the explicitly sexual aspects of sex, to report low enhancement motives, enhancement goals, as previously discussed, are not central to the attachment system and thus may be unrelated to attachment anxiety.

Preliminary evidence from the aforementioned studies lends partial support to these predictions as well. All three studies found that anxiously attached individuals were more likely to have sex to avoid partner disapproval. In addition, both Schachner and Shaver (2004) and Davis and colleagues (2004) found that anxiously attached individuals were more likely to have sex to reassure themselves of their worth and to cope with negative emotions. (Tracy and colleagues, 2003, did not examine these specific motives.) However, none of the three studies found a relationship between attachment anxiety and increased intimacy motives.

Avoidant Attachment and Motives for Sex

Avoidant individuals, who are uncomfortable with intimacy and closeness, should be significantly less likely to have sex for intimacy reasons. However, avoidant individuals, who experience heightened levels of negative affect, should be more likely to use sex to avoid or suppress these troubling feelings (i.e., to cope). This expectation is reinforced by the fact that both attachment avoidance and coping motives have been associated with similar patterns of promiscuous but safe sexual behavior. Expectations regarding avoidant differences in the remaining motives are less straightforward, particularly in the present study, in which we have only a single measure of avoidance that is thought to confound two avoidant subtypes (Bartholomew & Horowitz, 1991): dismissing avoidants, who have a positive model of self but a negative model of others, and fearful avoidants, who have negative models of both self and others. Nevertheless, given evidence that avoidants, as assessed by the measure used in the present study, are high in neuroticism (Shaver & Brennan, 1992) and therefore presumably high in BIS sensitivity, we expect them to more strongly endorse each of the three aversive motives (coping, affirmation, and partner approval). Finally, predictions regarding avoidant differences in enhancement motives are unclear. On the one hand, because avoidants are high in erotophobia and dislike intimate touching, we might expect them to report low levels of enhancement motives for sex. On the other hand, however, avoidants like the purely sexual aspects of sex and have been shown to engage in a pattern of promiscuous sex—a preference and a behavior that are characteristic of individuals high in enhancement motives. Alternatively, as previously discussed, enhancement goals are not central to the attachment system, thus suggesting the possibility of no association between attachment avoidance and enhancement reasons.

Preliminary evidence from the previously described studies lends clear support to these hypotheses. Avoidant individuals are more likely to have sex to affirm their desirability, to cope with negative emotions, and to avoid partner disapproval, whereas they are less likely to have sex for intimacy reasons.

Gender Differences in Attachment Effects

As several researchers have pointed out (e.g., Schachner & Shaver, 2004), the notion that attachment effects should vary across gender groups is not intrinsic to the attachment-theoretic perspective. Nevertheless, sexual behavior is strongly gender specific, both biologically and culturally. For this reason, we expect to find gender differences in how attachment dynamics are expressed in the sexual arena. In particular, we expect to find stronger effects among women for attachment anxiety and stronger effects among men for attachment avoidance.

The expectation regarding gender differences in the expression of attachment anxiety rests partly on empirical evidence (reviewed previously) that shows stronger and more pernicious effects on sexual behavior among anxious women than men but also on the assumption that the effects of attachment anxiety on women are exacerbated in this culture by traditional stereotypes that place women in subordinate roles to men. Conversely, male sex-role norms—with their emphasis on independence and emotional control—may mitigate the adverse effects of attachment anxiety among men. Although the empirical evidence for sex differences in the effects of avoidant attachment on sexual behavior appears less strong, we nevertheless expect that attachment avoidance will exert stronger and more debilitating effects on sexual experience among men than women. Similar to the preceding logic, we assume that avoidant effects on men will be exacerbated by traditional stereotypes that stress independence and emotional control and that interpret emotional displays and vulnerability as signs of weakness. Conversely, the effects of avoidance among women may be at least partly neutralized by the countervailing feminine stereotype that stresses emotional expressivity, nurturance, and warmth as desirable traits.

AN EMPIRICAL TEST OF THE MEDIATION HYPOTHESES

In the following sections, we provide an empirical test of the models portrayed in Figure 10.1 using data from a longitudinal study of 224 black and white adolescents who were interviewed twice over a 5½-year period (see Collins, Cooper, Albino, & Allard, 2002, for details). This sample is a subset of the previously described community sample, on which we have published three papers concerning attachment (Cooper, Shaver, Collins, 1998; Cooper, Albino, Orcutt, & Williams, 2004; Tracy et al., 2003). Respondents were 16.8 years old on average at time 1 and 22.3 years at follow-up, when both they and their opposite-sex romantic partners were interviewed. Eighty-three of the primary respondents were male (37%), and 141 were female (63%); 100 respondents (45%) were black, and 124 (55%) were white.

Interviews were conducted face-to-face and in private at both times by trained same-sex interviewers, with more sensitive portions of the interview (e.g., all questions on sexual motivations and behavior) being self-administered. At follow-up, respondents' partners were 24 years old on average, and in all but 16 cases, both couple members were of the same race. Most couples (62%) said they were "dating seriously," whereas smaller and approximately equal percentages said they were married (13%) or engaged (17%); a small percentage (7%) described themselves as "casually dating." Couples had been together 2.9 years on average. Moreover, nearly all of the relationships (93%) began after our initial interview, thus making this a truly prospective study of attachment effects on dyadic sexual behavior.

Attachment style was measured at baseline using a modified version of Hazan and Shaver's (1987) questionnaire. Although this measure is limited in important ways (see Crowell, Fraley, & Shaver, 1999), it was the only measure available at the time of the initial interview. Respondents read descriptions of the three attachment styles, rated how self-characteristic each was on a 7-point scale, and chose which of the three styles was most self-descriptive. Following procedures used by Mikulincer and colleagues (Mikulincer, Florian, & Tolmacz, 1990), respondents who gave inconsistent answers to the continuous and categorical attachment measures (21% of the 282 respondents who completed the attachment measure) were excluded from analyses, thus yielding the final sample of 224. Although we use the continuous ratings in the present study, the distribution across the three attachment types was 19% avoidant, 27% anxious, and 54% secure, which is typical of the distributions in most large studies of American adults.

Both respondent and partner sexual behaviors were assessed using three measures. Extrapair partners were assessed by a single-item measure of the number of sexual partners outside the primary relationship in the previous 6 months; 25% of respondents and 24% of partners reported having one or more extrapair sex partners during the previous 6 months. Cheating was assessed by a dichotomy in which a "1" indicated that the respondent had had at least one extrapair partner in the previous 6 months even though his or her partner believed that the relationship was strictly monogamous. Fourteen percent of respondents and 12% of partners cheated on their partners, according to this definition. Finally, risky sex was assessed by a count of the number of different risky sex practices the respondent had engaged in during the previous 6 months, including having one-night stands, sex with strangers, and sex with intravenous drug users. The scale ranged from 0 (no risk behaviors) to 4 (four or more risk behaviors). Because most of the endorsed items involved sex with casual or risky partners, this measure is best considered a measure of promiscuous or risky-partner choice.

Motives for sex were assessed at follow-up with five of the six subscales developed by Cooper, Shapiro, and Powers (1998). These included intimacy, enhancement (for pleasure), coping, affirmation, and partner approval. Items were rated on a 5-point scale ranging from "almost never/never" to "almost always/always." Motives were assessed for both couple members. Coefficient alphas ranged from .83 (enhancement) to .89 (coping) among primary respondents and from .83 (enhancement) to .87 (intimacy) among partners.

Analyses were conducted in two stages. First, a series of regression analyses (OLS for continuous outcomes; logistic for dichotomous ones) were conducted to identify significant variables for inclusion in a final set of path models. Path models, testing mediation of attachment effects by motives, were then estimated in AMOS (Arbuckle, 2003). Race and age were controlled in all analyses in which they significantly predicted the outcome.

Do Attachment Styles during Adolescence Shape Sexual Experience in Young Adulthood?

A series of six regression models (three dependent variables × respondent/partner report) were estimated in which the sexual behavior measures were regressed on respondent gender, the three attachment style ratings, and the three gender × attachment style interaction terms. (See Table 10.1 for a summary of the results.) Results revealed only one main effect for attachment style: Attachment avoidance assessed during adolescence predicted more casual or risky extrapair sex partners 6 years later (beta = .12, $p < .10$). However, consistent with the expectation of important gender differences, there were six significant or marginally significant gender × attachment style interactions.

Plotting the interactions revealed, as expected, that avoidance was associated with more maladaptive sexual behaviors among men than women, whereas the reverse was true for anxiety. Specifically, men ($b = .18$, beta = .26, $p < .05$) but not women ($b = .002$) who were avoidant during adolescence reported more extrapair partners as young adults. Similarly, avoidance in adolescence was more strongly related among men than among women to one's own tendency to cheat ($b = .03$, beta = .14, $p < .20$), as well as to one's partner's tendency to cheat ($b = .03$, beta = .17, $p < .11$; both b's = .00 among women). Despite the significance of the interaction terms, however, neither of the simple slopes relating avoidance to cheating was significant among men, owing at least in part to the relatively small number of men in our sample ($n = 83$).

In contrast to the pattern observed for avoidance, but in line with the expected direction of gender differences for attachment anxiety, women who were anxiously attached during adolescence were more likely to cheat on their partners in young adulthood ($b = .022$, beta = .16, $p < .10$), whereas men who were anxiously attached during adolescence were actually *less* likely to cheat on their partners ($b = –.040$, beta = –.22, $p < .05$). Similarly, female partners of anxiously attached males reported fewer casual or risky extrapair sex partners ($b = –.11$, beta = –.29, $p < .05$), whereas the effect was not significant ($b = .04$) among the male partners of anxiously attached female respondents. Thus these data indicate that attachment anxiety is associated with adverse sexual consequences among women, as expected, but somewhat surprisingly, they may actually be protective among men.

Finally, gender interacted with attachment security in the prediction of casual and risky extrapair partners. Plotting the interaction revealed that the female partners of securely attached males had fewer casual or risky extrapair partners ($b = –.10$, beta = –.23, $p < .05$), whereas there was no association among the male partners of securely attached female respondents.

Do Attachment Styles during Adolescence Shape Sexual Motivations during Young Adulthood?

A series of 10 regression models (5 motives × respondent/partner report) were estimated in which motives (assessed at follow-up) were regressed on

TABLE 10.1. Summary of Regression Analyses: Attachment Style Differences in Sexual Behavior

	Extrapair partners		Cheating[a]		Risky behaviors	
Variable	R	P	R	P	R	P
Gender	0.195**	–0.150*	0.745/2.106†	–0.631/0.532	–0.009	–0.072
Avoidant	0.075	0.018	0.027/1.027	0.047/1.048	0.122†	0.038
Anxious	0.059	0.058	–0.057/0.944	–0.066/0.936	0.076	–0.041
Secure	–0.018	0.022	–0.148/0.863	0.062/1.064	0.018	0.022
G× Avoidant	0.223**	0.108	0.435/1.545†	0.565/1.759†	0.038	–0.013
G× Anxious	–0.128	–0.122	–0.566/0.568*	–0.353/0.703	–0.099	–0.181*
G× Secure	–0.026	0.049	0.307/1.360	0.579/1.784	–0.138	–0.197*

Note. R, respondent standardized beta weight; P, partner standardized beta weight; G, gender.
[a] Results from logistic regression reported as unstandardized b/odds ratio.
†$p < .10$; *$p < .05$; **$p < .01$.

gender, the three attachment style ratings, and the three gender × attachment interactions (see Table 10.2 for a summary of these regressions). Results revealed four attachment-style main effects, one of which was qualified by gender, as well as four additional gender × attachment interactions that were not associated with a significant attachment main effect. Given evidence that four of the eight attachment-motive relationships differed across gender groups, we estimated each of the attachment-motive relationships separately within gender groups. Results revealed that of the eight relationships, only one (avoidance → affirmation motives) was significant in both gender groups, and even this effect was significantly stronger among males than females (interaction $b = .14$, $p < .10$). Thus sex appears to serve different attachment-related goals for men and for women.

Specifically, men who were avoidant as adolescents were more likely than their less avoidant counterparts to use sex to cope ($b = .12$, beta = .23, $p < .05$), to bolster their egos ($b = .19$, beta = .32, $p < .01$), and to avoid partner disapproval ($b = .015$, beta = .23, $p < .05$). Women who were avoidant as adolescents were also more likely to use sex for ego enhancement (i.e., affirmation) reasons ($b = .06$, beta = .16, $p < .10$), but they did not differ from their less avoidant counterparts on the other motive dimensions. In contrast, men who were anxiously attached as adolescents actually exhibited a healthier profile of motives: Relative to their less anxious counterparts, they were less likely to use sex to cope ($b = –.11$, beta = –.26, $p < .05$) and less likely to have sex to bolster their egos ($b = –.09$, beta = –.20, $p < .10$), and their female partners were less likely to have sex to please or appease them ($b = –.01$, beta = –.25, $p < .05$). On the other hand, women who were anxiously attached as adolescents were significantly *more* likely than their less anxious counterparts to have sex to secure or maintain their partner's approval ($b = .01$, beta = .23, $p < .01$).

TABLE 10.2. Summary of Regression Analyses: Attachment Style Differences in Sexual Motivations

	Intimacy		Enhancement		Coping		Affirmation		Partner approval	
Variable	R	P	R	P	R	P	R	P	R	P
Gender	−0.007	0.103	0.098	−0.085	0.116†	−0.152*	0.117†	−0.139*	0.032	0.032
Avoidant	−0.043	0.059	−0.043	−0.024	0.110	0.106	0.223**	0.148*	0.094	0.111
Anxious	−0.028	−0.062	−0.078	−0.112	−0.032	−0.060	−0.005	−0.060	0.154*	−0.154*
Secure	0.050	0.063	−0.023	−0.005	0.005	0.036	0.062	−0.016	0.002	−0.005
G× Avoidant	−0.053	0.009	−0.078	0.023	0.158†	0.052	0.142†	0.046	0.138†	0.060
G× Anxious	−0.073	0.060	0.096	−0.021	−0.257**	−0.008	−0.203*	−0.040	−0.121	−0.108
G× Secure	0.005	0.058	0.071	0.042	0.025	0.023	−0.027	−0.013	−0.034	0.074

Note. R, respondent standardized beta weight; P, partner standardized beta weight; G, gender.
†$p < .10$; *$p < .05$; **$p < .01$.

Finally, and contrary to expectation, attachment security did not predict any of the sexual motivations. Moreover, the two insecure-attachment dimensions predicted only aversive sex motives; no differences were found in either of the appetitive sex motives. Although this was unsurprising for enhancement motives, the lack of effects for intimacy motives runs counter to expectation.

Do Sex Motives Mediate Attachment Style Differences in Sexual Behavior?

To provide a direct test of mediation by motives, we estimated a series of five path models, one for each of the previously described significant or nearly significant (at $p < .10$) attachment effects on sexual behavior. These included: attachment avoidance → casual or risky extrapair sex, estimated separately among men and women; and among men, attachment avoidance → extrapair partners; attachment anxiety → cheating; and attachment anxiety → partner casual or risky extrapair partners. Although attachment security among men also predicted their female partner's tendency to have fewer casual or risky extrapair partners, this path model was not estimated because security did not significantly predict any of the sex motives. Thus motives could not mediate this effect (see Baron & Kenny, 1986). For each of the estimated models, only those motives that were related in earlier analyses (described previously) to the relevant attachment measure (see Table 10.2), as well as to the relevant outcome measure (data not reported), were included as potential mediators. In addition, two of the path models were simplified by treating affirmation, coping, and partner-approval motives as indicators of a single latent aversive motivation factor rather than as correlated but distinct motives. This decision was justified by the fact that the three motives were moderately to highly correlated with one another ($.50 \leq r \leq .70$)

and were related in similar ways to avoidance, as well as to the two outcome measures in question. The results of these five models are summarized in Figure 10.2.

The top panel presents results of the attachment avoidance → casual extrapair partner analyses among women (on the left) and men (on the right). Separate models were estimated across gender groups because the potential mediators were found to differ. As the model on the left shows, women who were avoidant during adolescence were more likely in young

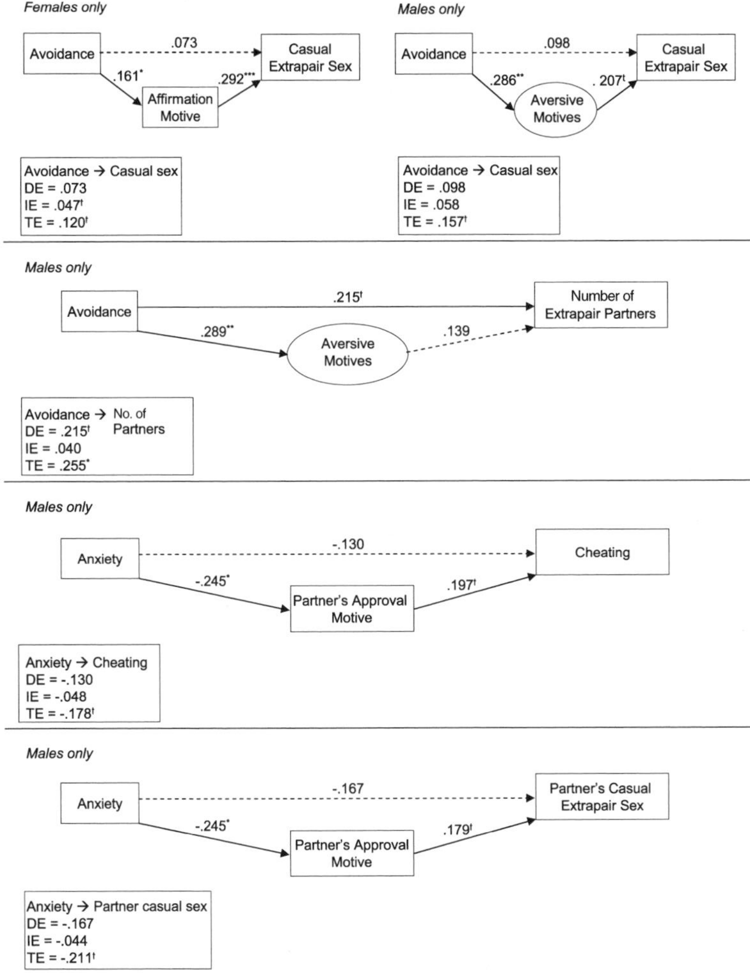

FIGURE 10.2. Estimated models linking attachment styles to extrapair sex via sex motives. DE, direct effect; IE, indirect effect; TE, total effect.
† $p < .10$; * $p < .05$; ** $p < .01$; *** $p < .001$.

adulthood to use sex to bolster their egos, which, in turn, was positively associated with having more casual or risky extrapair sex partners. As shown in the model on the right, men who were avoidant as adolescents were more likely to have sex for a variety of aversive reasons (i.e., affirmation, coping, partner approval), which in turn appears to have predisposed them to have casual or risky extrapair sex partners as young adults.

Results of the third model (second panel) indicate that motives do not mediate the effects of avoidance on the overall number of extrapair partners among men. Although the magnitude of the total effect was reduced, aversive motives did not directly predict number of partners in the multivariate context, which is a necessary condition for establishing mediation (Baron & Kenny, 1986). Moreover, the direct effect of avoidance on partners, though reduced, remained significant.

Interestingly, the last two models both reveal partial mediation of anxiety effects on sexual outcomes via the female partner's low likelihood of having sex to please or appease her anxiously attached male partner. As shown in the third panel, female partners of men who were anxiously attached as adolescents were less likely to have sex to gain their partner's approval, which in turn was associated with a lower likelihood of the male partner cheating. Similarly, as shown in the bottom panel, female partners of anxiously attached males were less likely to have sex to please their partners, which in turn was associated with a decreased likelihood of the female partner having risky or casual extrapair sex partners.

In sum, four of the five models provide support for partial mediation of attachment effects on sexual behavior by sex motives. In all four cases, however, the reduction in the total attachment effect due to motives was modest, ranging from 16% (avoidance → number of extrapair partners among men) to 39% (avoidance → casual extrapair partners among women), and in only one case (avoidance → casual extrapair partners among women) was the indirect effect statistically significant. However, given that there were more women than men (141 vs. 83) in our sample and that two of the nonsignificant indirect effects among men were actually larger than the significant indirect effect among women, it seems clear that the lack of statistical significance at least partly reflects the small sample size and hence low power among men.

SUMMARY AND DISCUSSION

In this chapter we have examined the notion that attachment styles, rooted in early childhood experiences with caregivers, shape the experience and expression of sexuality in adolescence and adulthood. Given the absence of prior longitudinal data on this topic, our study provides the most convincing evidence to date that the attachment system plays a formative role in shaping the sexual system, as well as the first explicit support for the assumption that this shaping occurs at least in part because individuals with different attachment styles use sex strategically to serve different attachment-related goals. Importantly, however, results of the present study also indicate that the expression of attachment dynamics in the sexual arena is channeled by gender-specific norms for sexual behavior. This finding represents an important extension or qualification of attachment theory, which does not specifically predict gender differences in the expression of attachment-related needs.

Gender differences were particularly striking for attachment anxiety, where anxiety in adolescence was associated with detrimental effects on sexual experience in young adulthood among women but positive effects among men. Indeed, males who were anxiously attached as adolescents were significantly less likely to use sex to cope with negative emotions or to bolster their self-esteem, and their female partners were less likely to have sex as a way to please or appease their partners. Interestingly, it was the influence on partner motivations for sex that best explained why males who were anxiously attached as adolescents were less likely to cheat on their partners, as well as why their female partners had fewer casual or risky extrapair sex partners. In contrast, women who were anxiously attached as adolescents were more likely to have sex to bolster their self-esteem, as well as to please or appease their partners. And ironically, given their intense need for safety and security in their romantic relationships, they were also significantly more likely to cheat on their partners. The particular ways in which anxious women used sex did not, however, account for the increased likelihood that they would cheat on their partners, given that neither affirmation nor partner approval motives predicted cheating among women.

In contrast, attachment avoidance was associated with similar patterns of sexual motives and behaviors among men and women, but the effects were stronger and more pervasive for men. Specifically, although both men and women who were avoidant as adolescents were more likely as young adults to use sex to reassure themselves of their worth, this effect was significantly stronger among men. In addition, men but not women who were avoidant as adolescents were also more likely to use sex to cope with negative emotions and to appease their partners. Thus avoidant men in particular appeared to use sex to meet largely intrapersonal rather than interpersonal goals. Finally, both men and women who were avoidant as adolescents reported having more casual or risky extrapair sex partners—a preference that was partly explained by the tendency to use sex to meet intrapersonal goals, which may be more easily met with impersonal partners. In addition, avoidant men also had more extrapair sex partners overall.

Considered as a whole, these data are consistent with the idea that prevailing gender norms may exacerbate (or buffer) the adverse effects of attachment insecurity on sexual experience. Thus the tendency of avoidant individuals to limit intimacy and closeness in relationships may be exacerbated among men by sex-role norms that restrict the expression of tenderness and vulnerability. Conversely, sex-role norms that encourage women to be warm, nurturant, and expressive may mitigate the destructive elements of attachment avoidance on sexual behavior. Similarly, the intense neediness and desire for approval that characterizes anxious attachment may be exacerbated among women by negative aspects of the female sex role that encourage dependency and excessive emotionality. In contrast, these same features of attachment anxiety may be mitigated among men by sex-role norms that encourage independence and self-reliance. Of course, sex-linked biological differences may also play an important role. Future research incorporating measures of adherence to sex-role norms would be one important step toward more carefully exploring these possibilities.

Although clear and theoretically meaningful portraits of attachment-style differences in sexual behavior emerged for anxiety and avoidance, the effects for attachment security were surprisingly weak. Indeed, we found only one significant effect: The female partners of men who were securely attached had fewer casual extrapair sex partners. Otherwise, security did not predict any of the remaining behaviors or any of the motives among either men or women. This may in part reflect limitations of our measure, given that past research has shown that Hazan and Shaver's (1987) secure prototype is endorsed by both avoidant and anxious individuals who agree with different elements of the prototype (Brennan, Shaver, & Tobey, 1991). Nevertheless, it seems unlikely that measurement issues alone can fully account for our null results given that this measure of security predicted meaningful profiles of differences in sexual behavior both cross-sectionally (Cooper, Shaver, & Collins, 1998) and longitudinally (Cooper et al., 2004) in prior research using a larger sample of which the present 224 individuals were part. Thus it is plausible that the lack of findings for security in the present sample reflects some peculiarity of this particular subset of respondents, or alternatively that security influences some aspects of sexuality, but not extrapair sex. Accordingly, future research both using better measures of attachment style and assessing a broad range of sexual behaviors will be needed to choose among these alternative explanations.

Contrary to expectation, the present study failed to find attachment-style differences in intimacy motives. Instead, insecurely attached males and their female partners differed in the extent to which they used sex for the more dysfunctional aversive reasons but not in the more normative appetitive reasons for having sex. It seems unlikely that the failure to obtain the expected effect for intimacy motives is due solely to measurement issues in that other studies using this measure of intimacy motives for sex have obtained the expected negative relationship between attachment avoidance and intimacy motives (Albino, 2004; Schachner & Shaver, 2004). One potential explanation lies in characteristics of our sample, which included only individuals who were in relationships at the time. As our past research has shown, such individuals should be higher on average in sex-for-intimacy motives, given that individuals who are high in intimacy motives are more likely to seek out close relationships, presumably because such contexts facilitate need satisfaction (Cooper, Shapiro, & Powers, 1998). Higher than average levels of intimacy motives, in turn, could lead to a restriction in range that would adversely affect our ability to detect significant effects in this measure. Consistent with this possibility, comparing the 224 individuals who participated in the couples' substudy with the 1,349 who did not revealed significantly higher levels of sex-for-intimacy reasons among the former than the latter group. The racial composition of this sample is another distinguishing feature that may contribute to our somewhat anomalous findings with intimacy motives. Consistent with this possibility, intimacy motives for sex were found to differ by race–gender subgroups in the full sample (Cooper, Shapiro, & Powers, 1998). Unfortunately, however, we did not have adequate power to explore both race and gender differences in the present sample. Whatever the explanation, this remains an important area for future research.

Caveats and Conclusions

Before concluding, several limitations of our data should be acknowledged. First, most of the significant effects involved two self-report measures and thus are vulnerable to inflation by monomethod bias. Offsetting this concern, however, these measures were obtained on discrete occasions, separated on average by 6 years. Thus momentary factors such as mood—typically a large component of monomethod bias—could not contribute to our findings. We also found corroborating evidence that attachment-style effects extend to the individual's partner, thus enhancing our confidence that the observed patterns reflect, at least to some extent, a shared social reality.

Although our findings were independent of important demographic influences, we cannot rule out the possibility that other factors that correlate with attachment, motives for sex, and extrapair sexual behavior are responsible for the observed effects. For example, it is well established that attachment styles are strongly correlated with relationship functioning. Thus it seems plausible that aspects of relationship quality, as opposed to either attachment or sex motives, might be responsible for the observed effects on sexual behavior. However, because attachment styles were assessed years prior to the beginning of these relationships in nearly all cases, temporal (and hence causal) precedence can be assigned to attachment styles over relationship factors. Thus, to the extent that relationship factors contribute directly to the explanation of extrapair sexual behaviors, they might plausibly serve as mediators of the link between attachment and extrapair sex, but they cannot serve as confounders on this relationship.

The argument is less clear, however, in the case of sex motives that were not assessed in the present study prior to relationship formation or, for that matter, prior to assessment of the sexual behaviors. Thus the causal status of sex motives in our model is less certain. Future research that imposes a clear temporal order on attachment, motives, and behavior will be necessary to enable more confident causal inference about the unique role of motivational factors in accounting for attachment effects on sexual behavior. In addition, future research will need to integrate important intrapersonal and interpersonal variables into a single model, as well as examine a broader range of outcomes, if we are to develop a more realistic understanding of the complex, multivariate processes that shape sexual behavior in relationships.

Finally, it is important to acknowledge that the observed attachment effects were modest in magnitude (ranging from 0.15 to 0.30 *SD*). However, for a variety of reasons, we believe it would be a mistake to dismiss them as trivial. First, these effects were obtained, despite the limitations of a single-item attachment measure, over a 6-year period and were evidenced in both self- and partner reports in relationships that did not exist at baseline. Furthermore, this particular 6-year period brackets the transition from adolescence into young adulthood—a period that, as previously discussed, is marked by dramatic changes in people's behavior, self-concept, and lifestyle. Finally, these effects were apparent despite the fact that many of our respondents changed their predominant attachment orientation during the intervening years. Together, we believe that these considerations make a strong argument for the importance of these effects, suggesting that processes and patterns of regulating internal processes and of relating to others that were set into motion during adolescence (or before) continue to influence behavior and experience in romantic relationships into young adulthood. Taken as a whole, these data add substantially to a growing body of evidence for the usefulness of attachment theory as a framework for understanding human functioning across the lifespan.

REFERENCES

Ainsworth, M. D. S., Blehar, M., Waters., E., & Wall, S. (1978). *Patterns of attachment: A psychological study of the Strange Situation.* Hillsdale, NJ: Erlbaum.

Albino, A. W. (2004). *Adult attachment and sexuality in heterosexual relationships.* Unpublished doctoral dissertation, University of Missouri, Columbia.

Arbuckle, J. L. (2003). *Amos 5.0 user's guide.* Chicago: SmallWaters.

Arnett, J. J. (2000). Emerging adulthood: A theory of development from the late teens through the twenties. *American Psychologist, 55,* 469–480.

Bakan, D. (1966). *The duality of human existence.* Chicago: Rand McNally.

Baron, R. M., & Kenny, D. A. (1986). The moderator-mediator variable distinction in social psychological research: Conceptual, strategic, and statistical considerations. *Journal of Personality and Social Psychology, 51*, 1173–1182.

Bartholomew, K., & Horowitz, L. M. (1991). Attachment styles among young adults: A test of a four-category model. *Journal of Personality and Social Psychology, 61*, 226–244.

Bogaert, A. F., & Sadava, S. (2002). Adult attachment and sexual behavior. *Personal Relationships, 9*, 191–204.

Bowlby, J. (1970). Disruption of affectional bonds and its effects on behavior. *Journal of Contemporary Psychology, 2*, 75–86.

Bowlby, J. (1973). *Attachment and loss: Vol. 2. Separation: Anxiety and anger.* New York: Basic Books.

Bowlby, J. (1982). *Attachment and loss. Vol. 1. Attachment.* New York: Basic Books. (Original work published 1969)

Brennan, K. A., Clark, C. L., & Shaver, P. R. (1998). Self-report measurement of adult attachment: An integrative overview. In J. A. Simpson & W. S. Rholes (Eds.), *Attachment theory and close relationships* (pp. 46–76). New York: Guilford Press.

Brennan, K. A., & Shaver, P. R. (1995). Dimensions of adult attachment, affect regulation, and romantic relationship functioning. *Personality and Social Psychology Bulletin, 21*, 267–283.

Brennan, K. A., Shaver, P. R., & Tobey, A. E. (1991). Attachment styles, gender, and parental problem drinking. *Journal of Social and Personal Relationships, 8*, 451–466.

Browning, J. R., Hatfield, E., Kessler, D., & Levine, T. (2000). Sexual motives, gender, and sexual behavior. *Archives of Sexual Behavior, 29*, 136–153.

Carver, C. S., & White, T. L. (1994). Behavioral inhibition, behavioral activation, and affective responses to impending reward and punishment: The BIS/BAS scales. *Journal of Personality and Social Psychology, 67*, 319–333.

Chisholm, J. S. (1999). Attachment and time preference: Relations between early stress and sexual behavior in a sample of American university women. *Human Nature, 10*, 51–83.

Collins, N. L., Cooper, M. L., Albino, A., & Allard, L. (2002). Psychosocial vulnerability from adolescence to adulthood: A prospective study of attachment style differences in relationship functioning and partner choice. *Journal of Personality, 70*, 965–1008.

Collins, N. L., & Read, S. J. (1990). Adult attachment, working models, and relationship quality in dating couples. *Journal of Personality and Social Psychology, 58*, 644–663.

Collins, N. L., & Read, S. J. (1994). Cognitive representations of attachment: The structure and function of working models. In K. Bartholomew & D. Perlman (Eds.), *Advances in personal relationships: Vol. 5. Attachment processes in adulthood* (pp. 53–90). London: Kingsley.

Cooper, M. L., Albino, A. W., Orcutt, H. K., & Williams, N. (2004). Attachment styles and intrapersonal adjustment: A longitudinal study from adolescence into young adulthood. In W. S. Rholes & J. A. Simpson (Eds.), *Adult attachment: Theory, research, and clinical applications* (pp. 438–466). New York: Guilford Press.

Cooper, M. L., Shapiro, C. M., & Powers, A. M. (1998). Motivations for sex and risky sexual behavior among adolescents and young adults: A functional perspective. *Journal of Personality and Social Psychology, 75*, 1528–1558.

Cooper, M. L., Shaver, P. R., & Collins, N. L. (1998). Attachment styles, emotion regulation, and adjustment in adolescence. *Journal of Personality and Social Psychology, 74*, 1380–1397.

Cooper, M. L., Wood, P. K., Orcutt, H. K., & Albino, A. (2003). Personality and the predisposition to engage in risky or problem behaviors during adolescence. *Journal of Personality and Social Psychology, 84*, 390–410.

Crowell, J., Fraley, R. C., & Shaver, P. R. (1999). Measures of individual differences in adolescent and adult attachment. In J. Cassidy & P. R. Shaver (Eds.), *Handbook of attachment: Theory, research, and clinical applications* (pp. 434–465). New York: Guilford Press.

Davis, D., Shaver, P. R., & Vernon, M. L. (2004). Attachment style and subjective motivations for sex. *Personality and Social Psychology Bulletin, 30*, 1076–1090.

Drigotas, S. M., & Barta, W. (2001). The cheating heart: Scientific explorations of infidelity. *Current Directions in Psychological Science, 10*, 177–180.

Feeney, J. A. (1999). Adult romantic attachment and couple relationships. In J. Cassidy & P. R. Shaver (Eds.), *Handbook of attachment: Theory, research, and clinical applications* (pp. 355–377). New York: Guilford Press.

Feeney, J. A., Noller, P., & Patty, J. (1993). Adolescents' interactions with the opposite sex: Influence of attachment style and gender. *Journal of Adolescence, 16*, 169–186.

Feeney, J. A., Peterson, C., Gallois, C., & Terry, D. J. (2000). Attachment style as a predictor of sexual attitudes and behavior in late adolescence. *Psychology and Health, 14*, 1105–1122.

Fisher, W. A., Byrne, D., & White, L. A. (1983). Emotional barriers to contraception. In D. Byrne & W. A. Fisher (Eds.), *Adolescents, sex, and contraception* (pp. 207–242). Hillsdale, NJ: Erlbaum.

Fraley, R. C., Davis, K. E., & Shaver, P. R. (1998). Dismissing-avoidance and the defensive organization of emotion, cognition, and behavior. In J. A. Simpson & W. S. Rholes (Eds.), *Attachment theory and close relationships* (pp. 249–279). New York: Guilford Press.

Fraley, R. C., & Shaver, P. R. (2000). Adult romantic attachment: Theoretical developments, emerging controversies, and unanswered questions. *Review of General Psychology, 4*, 132–154.

Gangestad, S. W., & Thornhill, R. (1997). The evolutionary psychology of extrapair sex: The role of fluctuating asymmetry. *Evolution and Human Behavior, 18*, 69–88.

Gentzler, A. L., & Kerns, K. A. (2004). Associations between insecure attachment and sexual experiences. *Personal Relationships, 11*, 249–265.

Gold, R. S., & Skinner, M. J. (1993). Desire for unprotected intercourse preceding its occurrence: The case of young gay men with anonymous partners. *International Journal of STD and AIDS, 4*, 326–329.

Gray, J. A. (1987). *The psychology of fear and stress.* Cambridge, England: Cambridge University Press.

Hazan, C., & Shaver, P. R. (1987). Romantic love conceptualized as an attachment process. *Journal of Personality and Social Psychology, 52*, 511–524.

Hazan, C., & Shaver, P. R. (1994). Attachment as an organizational framework for research on close relationships. *Psychological Inquiry, 5*, 1–22.

Hazan, C., Zeifman, D., & Middleton, K. (1994, July). *Adult romantic attachment, affection, and sex.* Paper presented at the International Conference on Personal Relationships, Groningen, Netherlands.

Hill, C. A., & Preston, L. K. (1996). Individual differences in the experience of sexual motivation: Theory and measurement of dispositional sexual motives. *The Journal of Sex Research, 33*, 27–45.

Impett, E. A., & Peplau, L. A. (2002). Why some women consent to unwanted sex with a dating partner: Insights from attachment theory. *Psychology of Women Quarterly, 26*, 360–370.

Larsen, R. J., & Ketelaar, T. (1991). Personality and susceptibility to positive and negative emotional states. *Journal of Personality and Social Psychology, 61*, 132–140.

Laumann, E. O., Gagnon, J. H., Michael, R. T., & Michaels, S. (1994). *The social organization of sexuality.* Chicago: University of Chicago Press.

Levinson, R. A., Jaccard, J., & Beamer, L. (1995). Older adolescents' engagement in casual sex: Impact of risk perception and psychosocial motivations. *Journal of Youth and Adolescence, 24*, 349–364.

McAdams, D. P. (1984). Human motives and personal relationships. In V. Derlega (Ed.), *Communication, intimacy, and close relationships* (pp. 41–70). New York: Academic Press.

Mikulincer, M., Florian, V., & Tolmacz, R. (1990). Attachment styles and fear of personal death: A case study of affect regulation. *Journal of Personality and Social Psychology, 58*, 273–280.

Mikulincer, M., & Shaver, P. R. (2003). The attachment behavioral system in adulthood: Activation, psychodynamics, and interpersonal processes. In M. P. Zanna (Ed.), *Advances in experimental social psychology* (Vol. 35, pp. 53–152). New York: Academic Press.

Morokoff, P. J., Quina, K., Harlow, L. L., Whitmire, L. E., Grimley, D. M., Gibson, P. L., et al. (1997). Sexual assertiveness scale (SAS) for women: Development and validation. *Journal of Personality and Social Psychology, 73*, 790–804.

Paul, E. L., McManus, B., & Hayes, A. (2000). "Hookups": Characteristics and correlates of college students' spontaneous and anonymous sexual experiences. *Journal of Sex Research, 37*, 76–88.

Priester, J. R., & Petty, R. E. (1996). The gradual threshold model of ambivalence: Relating the positive and negative bases of attitudes to subjective ambivalence. *Journal of Personality and Social Psychology, 71*, 431–449.

Schachner, D. A., & Shaver, P. R. (2004). Attachment dimensions and sexual motives. *Personal Relationships, 11*, 179–195.

Shackelford, T., & Buss, D. M. (2000). Marital dissatisfaction and spousal cost-infliction. *Personality and Individual Differences, 28*, 917–928.

Shaver, P. R., & Brennan, K. A. (1992). Attachment styles and the "big five" personality traits: Their connections with each other and with romantic relationship outcomes. *Personality and Social Psychology Bulletin, 18*, 536–545.

Shaver, P. R., & Clark, C. L. (1994). The psychodynamics of adult romantic attachment. In J. M. Masling & R. F. Bornstein (Eds.), *Empirical perspectives on object relations theories* (pp. 105–156). Washington, DC: American Psychological Association.

Shaver, P. R., Hazan, C., & Bradshaw, D. (1988). Love as attachment: The integration of three behavioral systems. In R. J. Sternberg & M. Barnes (Eds.), *The anatomy of love* (pp. 68–98). New Haven, CT: Yale University Press.

Skinner, E. A., & Wellborn, J. G. (1994). Coping during childhood and adolescence: A motivational perspective. In D. L. Featherman, P. B. Baltes, R. M. Lerner, & M. Perlmutter (Eds.), *Lifespan development and behavior* (Vol. 12, pp. 91–133). Hillsdale, NJ: Erlbaum.

Snyder, M., & Cantor, N. (1998). Understanding personality and social behavior: A functionalist strategy. In D. T. Gilbert, S. T. Fiske, & G. Lindzey (Eds.), *The handbook of social psychology* (Vol. 1, 4th ed., pp. 635–679). Boston: McGraw-Hill.

Stephan, C. W., & Bachman, G. F. (1999). What's sex got to do with it? Attachment, love schemas, and sexuality. *Personal Relationships*, 6, 111–123.

Tracy, J. L., Shaver, P. R., Albino, A. W., & Cooper, M. L. (2003). Attachment styles and adolescent sexuality. In P. Florsheim (Ed.), *Adolescent romantic relations and sexual behavior: Theory, research, and practical implications* (pp. 137–159). Hillsdale NJ: Erlbaum.

11

How **Do** *I Love Thee?*

Implications of Attachment Theory for Understanding Same-Sex Love and Desire

LISA M. DIAMOND

Hazan and Shaver's (1987) seminal notion that romantic love is an adult "version" of infant–caregiver attachment radically transformed our understanding of the nature and dynamics of adult intimate pair bonds, and the reverberations of this conceptual turning point continue to shape psychological research on adult romantic relationships. A key component of their theoretical model was the distinction between the evolved social-behavioral systems of *attachment*, *caregiving*, and *sexuality* (Shaver, Hazan, & Bradshaw, 1988). As they maintained, although experiences of adult romantic attachment typically integrate the feelings and behaviors of these systems, the systems themselves have distinct origins, functions, and underpinnings. Recent research on the brain substrates of both human and animal sexuality and pair bonding have confirmed this view (Bartels & Zeki, 2000; Fisher, Aron, Mashek, Li, & Brown, 2002; Williams, Catania, & Carter, 1992; Williams, Insel, Harbaugh, & Carter, 1994).

This conceptualization of romantic love and sexual desire as fundamentally distinct has profound implications for our understanding of the nature and development of same-sex sexuality, and yet these implications have gone largely unappreciated. Specifically, if love and desire are based in independent social-behavioral systems, then one's *sexual orientation* toward same-sex or other-sex partners need not correspond with experiences of *romantic attachment* to same-sex or other-sex partners. This, of course, runs directly counter to the implicit presumption among both scientists and laypeople that heterosexual individuals fall in love only with other-sex partners and lesbian and gay individuals fall in love only with same-sex partners.

Despite these presumptions, the last 30 years of social scientific research on same-sex sexuality have converged to indicate that inconsistencies between sexual and affectional feelings for same-sex versus other-sex partners constitute one of the primary forms of both interindividual and intraindividual variability in same-sex sexuality, both in contemporary Western culture and in other cultures and historical periods (Bell & Weinberg, 1978; Blackwood, 1985; Blumstein & Schwartz, 1977; Brown, 1995; Diamond, 2000a, 2004; Faderman, 1981; Gay, 1985; Golden, 1987; Nardi, 1992; Nichols, 1990; Rothblum, 1993; Savin-Williams, 1998; Shuster, 1987). Most notably, some individuals report falling in love with a same-sex friend in the absence of a generalized predisposition for same-sex *sexual* desire; in some cases, these emotional attachments engender situationally specific same-sex desires that remain restricted to the partner in question (reviewed in Diamond, 2003b).

Historically, such cases have been classed as instances of "spurious homosexuality" (Bergler, 1954) that have little to tell us about the basic nature and development of same-sex sexuality (DeCecco & Elia, 1993). Reflecting this view, studies investigating the potential genetic basis of sexual orientation have sometimes specifically excluded such individuals (Burr, 1996). It is certainly reasonable to posit that individuals whose same-sex desires are specifically limited to instances of same-sex emotional attachment represent different "types" of people than those with more generalized same-sex sexual predispositions. Yet it is difficult to evaluate this possibility given how many questions remain unanswered regarding the specific phenomenon of same-sex emotional attachment and its relationship to same-sex sexual desire (Brown, 1995; DeCecco, 1990).

In this chapter I briefly review a biobehavioral model of sexuality and attachment that I have advanced elsewhere (Diamond, 2003b) to address these unanswered questions, and I use longitudinal data on a sample of young sexual-minority (i.e., nonheterosexual) women to investigate the possibility that there are stable individual differences in the linkage between sexuality and attachment that shape women's experiences of same-sex and other-sex sexuality over time. Although these analyses must be considered preliminary, they raise fundamental questions about intra-individual variability in the links between love and desire that have important implications for understanding *both* attachment and sexual orientation.

A BRIEF REVIEW OF THE "UNORIENTATION" OF ATTACHMENT

It is commonly assumed that an individual's sexual orientation shapes not only his or her sexual desires but also experiences of romantic love. Tendencies to become romantically attached to same-sex versus other-sex partners are typically assessed as part of the standard measurements of sexual orientation (Kinsey, Pomeroy, & Martin, 1948; Pattatucci & Hamer, 1995; Russell & Consolacion, 2003; Sell & Petrulio, 1996), and, in fact, the majority of openly identified lesbian, gay, and bisexual individuals report desiring and participating in long-term romantic attachments with same-sex partners (reviewed in Diamond, in press), whereas heterosexuals typically form romantic attachments exclusively with other-sex partners.

Yet this is not always the case. As noted earlier, disjunctions between sexual and affectional feelings for same-sex and other-sex partners have been widely documented. Such disjunctions do not seem so peculiar, however, when one considers the biobehavioral architecture of romantic love. As Hazan and Shaver argued (1987), the dynamics of adult pair bonding are based in the *attachment* system, which originally evolved to keep infants in close proximity to caregivers (thereby maximizing their chances for survival) by establishing an intense affectional bond between them (Bowlby, 1982). In other words, adult pair bonding is an *exaptation*—a system that originally evolved for one reason (bonding infants to their caregivers) but came to serve another (bonding reproductive partners together) over the course of human evolution (see Hazan & Zeifman, 1999).

The fundamental correspondence between infant–caregiver attachment and adult pair bonding is supported by extensive research that documents that these phenomena share the same core emotional and behavioral dynamics: heightened proximity maintenance, resistance to separation, and utilization of the partner as a preferred target for comfort and security seeking (reviewed in Hazan & Zeifman, 1999). Even more powerful evidence is provided by voluminous animal research that documents that these two types of affectional bonding are mediated by the same opioid- and oxytocin-based neural circuitry (Carter, 1998).

Yet if the basic affective, behavioral, and neurobiological dynamics of pair bonding are based in the infant–caregiver attachment system—and, importantly, *not* in the sexual mating system—then consider the implications for sexual orientation. Quite simply, there is no reason to expect the orientation of an individual's *sexual* desires to fundamentally circumscribe his or her propensity for romantic attachment. If individuals were endowed with intrinsic affectional "orientations" driving them to form pair bonds *only* with partners of a particular gender, such orientations would have to be coded into the biobehavioral architecture of infant–caregiver attachment. Of course, this is implausible: Infants do not become selectively attached to same-sex versus other-sex caregivers, and it would be maladaptive if they did.

Consequently, it should be possible for lesbian or gay individuals to fall in love with other-sex partners and for heterosexual individuals to fall in love with same-sex partners, even in the absence of sexual desire. As it happens, both the anthropological and historical literatures are replete with descriptions of platonic same-sex "infatuations" between otherwise heterosexual individuals (Blackwood, 1985; Faderman, 1981; Gay, 1985; Hansen, 1992; Nardi, 1992; Sahli, 1979; Smith-Rosenberg, 1975). Although contemporary Western scholars typically ponder whether the participants were "really" lesbian or gay, this does not appear to have been true in most cases and was not typically suspected of the participants in the cultures and historical periods during which such bonds have been most prevalent (Faderman, 1981; Nardi, 1992).

For example, in 19th-century America, passionate attachments between women were actually viewed as appropriate outlets for intense intimacy during the adolescent years *because* of their platonic nature (Faderman, 1981). The diaries of young girls of this period frequently contained exclamations of enduring love for other girls (Smith-Rosenberg, 1975), and writers such as Henry Wadsworth Longfellow and Oliver Wendell Holmes explicitly described these intense friendships as forms of "rehearsal" for adult marital intimacy (Faderman, 1993). Even now, such passionate and platonic attachments continue to be observed (Crumpacker & Vander Haegen, 1993; Diamond, 2000a), most commonly among young women and most often in sex-segregated environments (reviewed in Diamond, 2003b).

PATHWAYS FROM LOVE TO DESIRE

Although the aforementioned cases demonstrate that one need not experience same-sex sexual desire in order to develop a same-sex attachment, it is important to note that in some cases, same-sex attachments appear to *precipitate* novel same-sex sexual desires among individuals who may have never before experienced such feelings (Diamond, 2000a) and who often claim that these desires are experienced *only* for the attachment figure in question. Although such cases have long been anecdotally reported in the literature on sexual identity and orientation (Cass, 1990; Pillard, 1990), they are often greeted with skepticism or puzzlement, given that our conventional understanding of sexual orientation maintains that it is impossible to have "just one" same-sex attraction (Blumstein & Schwartz, 1990).

Yet research increasingly suggests that such attachment-based same-sex desires are, in fact, possible and that they may be engendered by a certain degree of intrinsic plasticity in the human sexual response system (Cass, 1990), particularly among women (Baumeister, 2000). One potential explanation for these feelings is that although attachment and sexuality are distinct social-behavioral systems, there are cultural, psychological, and neurobiological interconnections between them that are intrinsically bidirectional, making it possible to "get" from love to desire just as individuals often begin with desire and progress toward love (for a full explanation of this possibility and the evidence for it, see Diamond, 2003b).

Interestingly, this might help to explain the widely documented but little understood phenomenon in which individuals (typically women) claim that they are not necessarily sexually oriented to one sex or the other but are rather drawn to "the person rather than the gender" (Blumstein & Schwartz, 1977; Golden, 1987; Weinberg, Williams, & Pryor, 1994). Such reports are difficult to reconcile with conventional conceptualizations of sexual orientation, in which love and desire are *always* fundamentally "about" gender. Yet, currently, we have little empirical or theoretical basis on which to interpret and evaluate such claims and to explore their significance for contemporary models of sexual orientation. One intriguing possibility, for example, is that there are considerable *individual differences* in the degree of interconnectedness between the social-behavioral systems of sexuality and attachment (perhaps even manifested in the functioning of their shared neurobiological substrates, as in Turner, Altemus, Enos, Cooper, & McGuinness, 1999) that make such "nongendered" desires possible. In other words, just as some individuals appear to possess sexual predispositions for other-sex or same-sex partners, other individuals might possess an orthogonal predisposition to develop full-blown adult attachments in the absence of sexual desire, or perhaps to develop sexual desires on the basis of such attachments, regardless of the other person's sex.

On this point, it is notable that some women who have experienced passionate but platonic same-sex attachments report having developed multiple such relationships at different stages of life (Cole, 1993), sometimes with playmates or even sisters in early childhood (Rothblum, 1993). This observation led Rothblum (1993) to speculate whether such relationships might serve as an influential developmental model, priming women to develop such bonds later on. Yet without knowing more about *how* interconnections between the systems of sexuality and attachment develop during childhood, puberty, and early adulthood, it is difficult to evaluate this possibility. Clearly, a systematic integration of research on attachment with research on sexual development has the potential to fundamentally advance our understanding of the nature and development of different forms of same-sex love and desire over the life course. In particular, it might help to evaluate the long-held presumption (critiqued by DeCecco & Elia, 1993) that individuals whose same-sex attractions and relationships are strongly influenced by situational and emotional factors are less "authentically" gay and less likely to maintain a lesbian/gay/bisexual identity over time than are individuals whose same-sex sexuality is motivated by generalized, early-appearing, and fundamentally sexual urges.

Toward this end, the research presented here provides a preliminary inquiry into some of these issues by exploring two attachment-relevant phenomena that have remained unexplained in the extant literature on sexual orientation: (1) being attracted to "the person and not the gender," and (2) requiring a strong emotional bond in order to develop a physical attraction. Using a sample of young sexual-minority women whose trajectories of same-sex and other-sex love and desire have been documented over an 8-year period, the goal is to provide a rough snapshot of the prevalence of these phenomena, to assess whether they appear fundamentally related to one another, and to investigate whether women reporting either of these experiences appear to represent unique "types" of sexual minorities, with distinctive patterns of emotional and physical attractions, relationships, and developmental histories.

OVERVIEW OF STUDY METHODS

Participants were 79 nonheterosexual women between the ages of 18 and 23 years who were initially interviewed in person as part of a longitudinal study of sexual identity development among young women (Diamond, 1998, 2000a, 2000b, 2003a). Of the original sample of 89 women, 42% identified as lesbian, 30% identified as bisexual, and 28% declined to adopt a sexual identity label. Time 1 (T1) assessments were scripted, face-to-face interviews conducted with each woman by the primary investigator, approximately 90% of which lasted between 1 and 1.5 hours. When possible, interviews were conducted in a university office. When this was not feasible, interviews were conducted at a location of the participant's choosing, usually her home. Because of the sensitivity of the subject matter, interviews were not tape-recorded. Detailed notes were taken during the interview by the primary investigator and transcribed immediately afterward. The primary investigator reinterviewed participants over the phone 2 years later (T2), after an additional 3 years (T3), and after an additional 2 years (T4). The T2, T3, and T4 interviews followed a standard script reassessing the major variables assessed at T1 and lasted between 20 and 30 minutes. Verbatim typed transcriptions were taken of the T2 interviews while they were being conducted; T3 and T4 interviews were tape-recorded and transcribed. Eleven women could not be located for follow-up by time 4. At the first assessment, the mean and median age of the participants was 19; at the fourth assessment, the mean and median age of the participants was 28. There were no significant age differences across recruitment sites or sexual identity categories.

Initial sampling took place in two moderately sized cities and a number of smaller urban and rural communities in central New York state. The settings that were sampled included (1) lesbian, gay, and bisexual community events (i.e., picnics, parades, social events) and youth groups; (2) classes on gender and sexuality issues taught at a large university with a moderately ethnically diverse—but largely middle-class—student population; and (3) lesbian, gay, and bisexual student groups at a large public university with a predominantly white but more socioeconomically diverse population and at a small, private women's college with a predominantly white and middle-class student population. This recruitment strategy succeeded in sampling sizable numbers of bisexual women as well as nonheterosexual women who declined to label their sexual identity; both groups are underrepresented in most research on sexual minorities. However, the sample shares a chronic drawback with other samples of sexual minorities in that it comprises predominantly white, highly educated, middle- to upper-class individuals. Nearly all of the college-age participants had enrolled in college at one point, and 75% came from families in which at least one parent had completed college. Sixty-three percent of women came from families in which at least one parent had a professional or technical occupation, and 84% were white.

As reviewed in previously published reports on this sample (Diamond, 1998, 2000a, 2000b, 2003a), at the beginning of each interview, each woman was asked, "How do you currently label your sexual identity to yourself, even if it's different from what you might tell other people? If you don't apply a label to your sexual identity, please say so." Lesbian- and bisexual-identified women were categorized according to their chosen identity labels. Women who declined to attach a label to their sexuality were classified as *unlabeled*. Women were also asked to recall the process by which they first questioned their sexuality and to recount any changes they had recently undergone since the previous interview regarding their experience or conceptualization of their sexuality. At time 1, they also provided information on the age at which they first consciously questioned their sexual identity, first experienced a same-sex attraction, first engaged in same-sex contact, and first openly adopted a sexual-minority identity. To assess their same-sex attractions, at each interview women were asked to estimate the general percentage of their current attractions that were directed toward the same sex on a day-to-day basis; separate estimates were provided for sexual versus romantic/affectional attractions. This yields an estimate of the *relative frequency* of same-sex versus other-sex attractions, regardless of the intensity of these attractions or the total number of sexual attractions experienced on a day-to-day basis. Also, at T4 women were asked to rate, on a 5-point Likert scale, their agreement with the following statements describing different aspects of sexual orientation and its development: "I'm the kind of person who's attracted to the person rather than to their gender"; "I feel my sexuality is something I was born with"; "I feel my sexuality has been influenced by my environment"; "I would have a hard time becoming physically attracted to someone without having an emotional connection to them."

RESULTS

Overall, 60% of the sample agreed or strongly agreed with the statement that they were generally attracted to the person rather than their gender ($M = 3.64$, $SD = 1.23$), and 45% agreed or strongly agreed with the statement that they needed an emotional connection with someone to become physically attracted them ($M = 3.11$, $SD = 1.45$). Notably, responses on these items were not associated with one another (Table 11.1 presents correlations among these variables and the major variables under analysis). A one-way analysis of variance found that endorsement of "nongendered" attractions differed significantly among the sexual identity groups (using time 1 identity labels), $F(2, 76) = 4.56$, $p = .01$. Specifically, bisexually identified individuals more strongly endorsed nongendered attractions than both lesbians and unlabeled women, both Bonferroni-corrected p values $< .05$. Because the majority of respondents changed identity labels over the 8 years of the study (Diamond, 2005), this analysis was repeated using T2, T3, and T4 identity labels (note, for example, that 42% of the T4 bisexuals had a different identity label at T1). The results were unchanged.

In contrast, a two-group t test found that emotionally based attractions (i.e., needing an emotional connection to become physically attracted to someone) were more strongly endorsed among women who selected "unlabeled" as their sexual identity during at least one assessment over the 8 years of the study, $t = 2.45$, $p < .02$. Emotionally based attractions were also significantly associated with reidentification as heterosexual: Of the 11 women who reidentified as heterosexual over the 8-year study period (note that 5 of these women ended up going back to lesbian/gay/unlabeled identities by the last assessment, so that only 6 women identified as heterosexual at T4), all but one of these women either agreed or strongly agreed with the statement describing emotionally based attractions, $\chi^2 (1, n = 79) = 6.0$, $p = .01$. The only other consistent distinguishing characteristic of women with emotionally based attractions was that they tended to begin questioning their sexuality at later ages.

Endorsement of nongendered attractions showed a broader pattern of associations: As shown in Table 11.1, it was significantly associated with having less exclusive (i.e., more bisexual) attractions and with being more

TABLE 11.1. Correlations among Study Variables

	1	2	3	4	5	6	7	8
1. Attracted to person, not gender								
2. Need emotional bond to become attracted	–.10							
3. Percentage of day-to-day physical attractions to women, averaged across the 4 assessments	–.45***	–.10						
4. Percentage of day-to-day emotional attractions to women, averaged across the 4 assessments	–.27*	–.03	.82***					
5. Gap between emotional and physical attractions (emotional minus physical), computed for each assessment and averaged	.29*	.10	–.39***	.18				
6. Belief that the environment has influenced one's sexuality	.45***	–.05	–.22†	–.05	.27*			
7. Belief that one was "born" with her sexuality	–.14	–.12	.16	.15	–.01	–.35**		
8. Age of first conscious same-sex attraction	–.04	.08	–.20	–.01	.27*	.15	–.12	
9. Age of first conscious questioning of sexual identity	–.09	.25*	–.15	–.02	.15	.15	–.07	.53***

†$p < .10$; *$p < .05$; **$p < .01$; ***$p < .001$.

emotionally than physically drawn to women (assessed by subtracting each woman's percentage of physical attractions from her percentage of emotional attractions in order to yield a difference score, with positive values indicating same-sex attractions that were more emotional than physical and negative values indicating same-sex attractions that were more physical than emotional). These effects are represented in Figure 11.1, which contrasts the 8-year averages for percentages of same-sex physical and emotional attractions among women with gendered versus nongendered attractions and also displays the gaps between these attractions at each of the four assessments.

Nongendered attractions were also associated with believing that one's sexuality was, to some extent, environmentally influenced, although it was *not* associated with the age of women's first same-sex attractions, the age of their first sexual questioning, the degree to which they believed they were

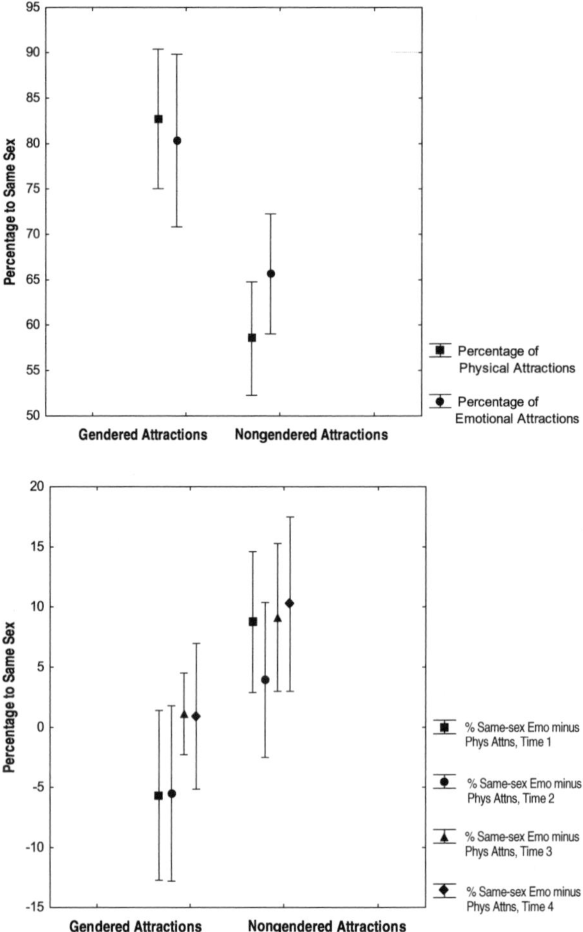

FIGURE 11.1. Percentages of same-sex physical and emotional attractions among women with gendered versus nongendered attractions, averaged across assessments, and differences between emotional and physical attractions at each assessment.

"born" with their sexuality, or the likelihood of reidentifying as heterosexual. This contrasts with the conventional wisdom, noted earlier, that individuals who are attracted to "the person, not the gender" are less "essentially" gay (and therefore, presumably, less likely to experience an early onset of their same-sex attractions).

The pattern of associations in Table 11.1 clearly demonstrates that nongendered attractions and emotionally based attractions are two distinct phenomena, representing different patterns of same-sex and other-sex sexuality. In order to explore their implications for the degree of linkage over time in women's physical and emotional attractions, hierarchical linear modeling was used to test whether these two individual difference dimensions moderated within-person covariation between physical and emotional attractions from T1 to T4.

Hierarchical linear modeling (Bryk & Raudenbush, 1992) is a technique designed for multilevel data structures in which observations at one level of analysis (in this case, self-reported percentages of physical and emotional same-sex attractions at times 1–4) are nested within higher levels of analysis (individuals). This technique estimates within-person and between-person effects simultaneously. At the within-person level (known as level 1), the model estimates a separate regression equation for each participant, modeling physical same-sex attractions at time *i* as a function of emotional attractions at time *i*. Then the coefficients for each of these *n* equations (one for each participant) become the dependent variables for the between-person (level 2) analysis, where they are modeled as a function of the following variables: overall percentage of physical same-sex attractions (averaged across all assessments), gap between emotional and physical attractions (averaged across all assessments), the degree to which one's attractions are emotionally based, and the degree to which they are gendered versus nongendered. Thus the model is essentially testing whether these individual-difference dimensions moderate the degree to which a specific woman's physical and emotional attractions have covaried over the 8 years of the study. Inclusion of the overall percentage of same-sex attractions and also the gap between emotional and physical attractions as potential moderators was designed to assess whether—independent of women's subjective experience of their attractions as emotionally based or nongendered—those with more exclusive same-sex attractions showed more correspondence over time between their physical and emotional attractions and whether there was less correspondence among women who had consistently reported large discrepancies between physical and emotional attractions. Including these attraction measures is also important given that both are correlated with women's self-reports of nongendered attractions. All level 2 variables were centered before entry into the equation.

The results indicated significant moderating effects. Specifically, women who described themselves as having nongendered attractions showed greater covariation between their physical and emotional attractions over time, $G = .016$, $t = 3.17$, $p = .002$. Covariation was not associated, however, with endorsement of emotionally based attractions. Notably, greater covariation was also found among women with larger overall percentages of same-sex physical attractions, $G = .008$, $t = 8.94$, $p < .001$, whereas there was *less* covariation among women whose attractions to women were more emotional than physical (i.e., larger difference scores when subtracting their percentage of physical attractions from their percentage of emotional attractions), $G = -.004$, $t = -5.70$, $p < .001$.

DISCUSSION

These findings confirm that the degree of correspondence between sexual-minority women's physical and emotional attractions for same-sex and other-sex partners is neither perfect nor uniform. Rather, the women in the sample showed notable interindividual variability in the nature and degree of linkage between these two different types of attractions, and hence potentially between their underlying mating and attachment systems. These findings underscore the importance of investigating attachment-related phenomena in the context of research on sexual identity and same-sex sexuality.

Attractions to "the Person and Not the Gender"

Importantly, these results suggest that the experience of being attracted to "the person and not the gender" is appreciably distinct from the experience of needing an emotional bond with another person in order to experience physical attraction to them. There was no significant association between these two types of experiences, and each was found to be associated with a distinct profile of sexual and emotional attractions to same-sex and other-sex partners over time. Nongendered attractions were strongly associated with bisexuality in terms of both the distribution of women's same-sex and other-sex attractions and their self-identifications. At each of the four assessments, women with nongendered attractions were disproportionately likely to identify as bisexual, despite the fact that the exact composition of the "bisexual" identity group changed from assessment to assessment. Clearly, many contemporary sexual-minority women consider a capacity for desire based on "the person and not the gender" to be consistent with their own definitions and conceptualizations of bisexuality. Notably, the same finding has been obtained in older cohorts of bisexuals. Weinberg et al. (1994) found that an "open gender schema" with regard to patterns of attractions characterized many of the adult bisexual men and women they surveyed in the 1980s.

Of course, not all individuals with this profile view "bisexual" as an appropriate identity label. Some of the women in the present study explicitly noted during their interviews that they had elected *not* to identify as bisexual specifically because they felt that the term placed too much emphasis on gender:

> "I don't even identify as a bisexual, just because my definition of bisexuality is one who maybe craves both, either at the same time or . . . or just can see themselves with both parties whereas with me I'm all about one person. I've gotten to the point now in my life where it's not even like a sexual or gender identification; it's just, like, I'm attracted to certain

things about a . . . about a whole person and if and when I find that *sexuality* doesn't really matter that much for me anymore. It's just about the person."

Nongendered attractions were also significantly associated with the experience of being more emotionally than physically drawn to women (based on gaps between women's self-reported percentages of day-to-day physical attractions to women and their percentages of day-to-day emotional attractions) and with greater covariation between physical and emotional attractions across the 8 years of the study. These findings hint at a potential difference between women with nongendered versus emotionally based attractions: Although women who were attracted to "the person and not the gender" generally experienced more emotional than physical attractions to women, changes in one domain over the 8 years of the study were associated with corresponding changes in the other. This might indicate a high propensity for the type of bidirectional plasticity between sexuality and attachment that makes the phenomenon of nongendered attractions possible, particularly given that some of these women experienced a generally low frequency of day-to-day physical attractions to women. In contrast, the experience of "needing" an emotional attachment in order to develop physical attractions seems to suggest a pattern of interconnections between sexuality and attachment that is more unidirectional, more commonly progressing from attachment to sexuality than vice versa.

Emotionally Based Attractions

Although some women with nongendered attractions preferred to reject sexual identity labels altogether, this tendency was much more pronounced among women who reported that they needed an emotional connection to another person in order to become attracted to them; furthermore, such women were also disproportionately likely to readopt *heterosexual* identities over time. Thus, despite the fact that women with "emotionally based" attractions were comparable to the rest of the sample with regard to their overall proportion of same-sex attractions and the degree to which they felt they were "born with" their sexuality, they nonetheless perceived that their particular pattern of attractions was inconsistent with contemporary conceptualizations of lesbian and bisexual orientations.

This was directly reflected in women's stated reasons for declining to adopt an identity label. For example, numerous unlabeled women remarked that they were unsure whether emotionally based attractions "counted" as a reliable index of their underlying sexual orientation, and they were therefore reluctant to consider themselves lesbian or bisexual even if they had done so in the past. As one woman noted:

> "I guess my attraction to women isn't really all that sexual. . . . My immediate gut-level physical response is to men, but I want to marry a woman because I find women more beautiful, and I have more enduring emotional bonds with a woman. I guess I find women magnetic. I'm not sure that's the same as a sexual attraction."

Certainly, her reservations might be shared by scientists and laypeople who believe that individuals with same-sex attractions that are primarily situationally or interpersonally based are fundamentally different "types" of sexual minorities than those whose same-sex attractions are experienced as broad, cross-situational predispositions.

Yet the present findings cannot be taken as straightforward confirmation for this view. Although nearly all of the women who ended up concluding that they were "really" heterosexual had emotionally based attractions, this was a fairly uncommon pattern. Overall, the majority of women with emotionally based attractions maintained sexual-minority identifications over time. Thus, to the extent that we can identify a phenomenon of "situational" same-sex sexuality that represents an emergent property of emotionally intimate same-sex bonds, this phenomenon may, in fact, be meaningfully linked to the phenomenon of emotionally based attractions. However, the converse is not necessarily true: Experiencing one's attractions as emotionally based does not necessarily mean that one's same-sex sexuality is exclusively situational. As with the phenomenon of nongendered attractions, we clearly require a greater understanding of the basic biobehavioral links between the systems of attachment and sexuality in order to understand the bases and developmental implications of these phenomena.

CONCLUSION

Although these findings raise more questions than they definitively answer, they certainly demonstrate the importance of investigating attachment phenomena in order to understand individuals' sexual self-concepts and behaviors over time. The standard practice of classifying individuals into discrete sexual categories solely on the basis of their physical attractions for same-sex versus other-sex partners provides an incomplete picture of the complex interconnections between emotional intimacy and physical eroticism that shape individuals' subjective experiences of their sexuality.

Interestingly, taking greater account of attachment phenomena might productively change not only the way we investigate the development of same-sex sexuality but also the way we study other-sex sexuality. As Brown (1995) noted, perhaps instead of asking why some individuals grow up to be gay, lesbian, or bisexual, we might ask why *heterosexual* individuals who may have experienced intense, emotionally intimate same-sex bonds in childhood or adolescence either lost such bonds or never sexualized them. Brown's point highlights how little we know about the constellation of intrapsychic, cultural, and perhaps even neurobiological mechanisms through which sexuality and attachment become interconnected over the course of social and sexual development. One intriguing possibility is that certain types of erotic *or* emotional experiences during the childhood or early adolescent years influence the nature and strength of these interconnections. On this note, it is interesting to consider that women with emotionally based attractions typically began questioning their sexuality at around age 16½ (notably, later than the rest of the sample), which corresponds to the age at which Hazan and Zeifman found that adolescents generally first begin developing full-blown attachment relationships with peers rather than parents (Hazan & Zeifman, 1994). Clearly, in order for future research to clarify the bases and developmental implications of nongendered or emotionally based attractions among sexual-minority women, we need more substantive basic research on links between sexuality and affectional bonding among *all* kinds of individuals over the life course.

Thus, whereas the first 50 years of systematic psychological research on same-sex sexuality largely ignored questions of romantic love, the next generation of scientific research on the topic cannot afford to. Understanding the ways in which desire, caregiving, and attachment are interbraided in our experiences of physical and emotional intimacy with same-sex and other-sex partners is clearly fundamental to understanding our basic sexual and affectional nature.

REFERENCES

Bartels, A., & Zeki, S. (2000). The neural basis of romantic love. *Neuroreport, 11*, 3829–3834.

Baumeister, R. F. (2000). Gender differences in erotic plasticity: The female sex drive as socially flexible and responsive. *Psychological Bulletin, 126*, 247–374.

Bell, A. P., & Weinberg, M. S. (1978). *Homosexualities: A study of diversity among men and women*. Bloomington: Indiana University Press.

Bergler, E. (1954). Spurious homosexuality. *Psychiatric Quarterly Supplement, 28*, 68–77.

Blackwood, E. (1985). Breaking the mirror: The construction of lesbianism and the anthropological discourse on homosexuality. *Journal of Homosexuality, 11*, 1–17.

Blumstein, P., & Schwartz, P. (1977). Bisexuality: Some social psychological issues. *Journal of Social Issues, 33*, 30–45.

Blumstein, P., & Schwartz, P. (1990). Intimate relationships and the creation of sexuality. In D. P. McWhirter, S. A. Sanders, & J. M. Reinisch (Eds.), *Homosexuality/heterosexuality: Concepts of sexual orientation* (pp. 307–320). New York: Oxford University Press.

Bowlby, J. (1982). *Attachment and loss: Vol. 1. Attachment* (2nd ed.). New York: Basic Books.

Brown, L. (1995). Lesbian identities: Concepts and issues. In A. R. D'Augelli & C. Patterson (Eds.), *Lesbian, gay, and bisexual identities over the lifespan* (pp. 3–23). New York: Oxford University Press.

Bryk, A. S., & Raudenbush, W. W. (1992). *Hierarchical linear models: Applications and data analysis methods*. Newbury Park, CA: Sage.

Burr, C. (1996). *A separate creation: The search for the biological origins of sexual orientation*. New York: Hyperion.

Carter, C. S. (1998). Neuroendocrine perspectives on social attachment and love. *Psychoneuroendocrinology, 23*, 779–818.

Cass, V. (1990). The implications of homosexual identity formation for the Kinsey model and scale of sexual preference. In D. P. McWhirter, S. A. Sanders, & J. M. Reinisch (Eds.), *Homosexuality/heterosexuality: Concepts of sexual orientation* (pp. 239–266). New York: Oxford University Press.

Cole, E. (1993). Is sex a natural function? Implications for sex therapy. In E. D. Rothblum & A. D. Brehony (Eds.), *Boston marriages* (pp. 187–193). Amherst: University of Massachusetts Press.

Crumpacker, L., & Vander Haegen, E. M. (1993). Pedagogy and prejudice: Strategies for confronting homophobia in the classroom. *Women's Studies Quarterly, 21*, 94–106.

DeCecco, J. P. (1990). Sex and more sex: A critique of the Kinsey conception of human sexuality. In D. P. McWhirter, S. A. Sanders, & J. M. Reinisch (Eds.), *Homosexuality/heterosexuality: Concepts of sexual orientation* (pp. 368–386). New York: Oxford University Press.

DeCecco, J. P., & Elia, J. P. (1993). A critique and synthesis of biological essentialism and social constructionist views of sexuality and gender. In J. P. DeCecco & J. P. Elia (Eds.), *If you seduce a straight person, can you make them gay? Issues in biological essentialism versus social constructionism in gay and lesbian identities* (pp. 1–26). New York: Harrington Park Press.

Diamond, L. M. (1998). Development of sexual orientation among adolescent and young adult women. *Developmental Psychology, 34*, 1085–1095.

Diamond, L. M. (2000a). Passionate friendships among adolescent sexual-minority women. *Journal of Research on Adolescence, 10*, 191–209.

Diamond, L. M. (2000b). Sexual identity, attractions, and behavior among young sexual-minority women over a two-year period. *Developmental Psychology, 36*, 241–250.

Diamond, L. M. (2003a). Was it a phase? Young women's relinquishment of lesbian/bisexual identities over a 5-year period. *Journal of Personality and Social Psychology, 84*, 352–364.

Diamond, L. M. (2003b). What does sexual orientation orient? A biobehavioral model distinguishing romantic love and sexual desire. *Psychological Review, 110*, 173–192.

Diamond, L. M. (2004). Emerging perspectives on distinctions between romantic love and sexual desire. *Current Directions in Psychological Science, 13*, 116–119.

Diamond, L. M. (in press). The intimate same-sex relationships of sexual minorities. In D. Perlman & A. L. Vangelisti (Eds.), *The Cambridge handbook of personal relationships*. New York: Cambridge University Press.

Diamond, L. M. (2005). A new view of lesbian subtypes: Stable vs. fluid identity trajectories over an 8-year period. *Psychology of Women Quarterly, 29*, 119–128.

Faderman, L. (1981). *Surpassing the love of men.* New York: Morrow.

Faderman, L. (1993). Nineteenth-century Boston marriage as a possible lesson for today. In E. D. Rothblum & K. A. Brehony (Eds.), *Boston marriages* (pp. 29–42). Amherst: University of Massachusetts Press.

Fisher, H. E., Aron, A., Mashek, D., Li, H., & Brown, L. L. (2002). Defining the brain systems of lust, romantic attraction, and attachment. *Archives of Sexual Behavior, 31*, 413–419.

Gay, J. (1985). "Mummies and babies" and friends and lovers in Lesotho. *Journal of Homosexuality, 11*, 97–116.

Golden, C. (1987). Diversity and variability in women's sexual identities. In Boston Lesbian Psychologies Collective (Ed.), *Lesbian psychologies: Explorations and challenges* (pp. 19–34). Urbana: University of Illinois Press.

Hansen, K. V. (1992). "Our eyes behold each other": Masculinity and intimate friendship in antebellum New England. In P. Nardi (Ed.), *Men's friendships* (pp. 35–58). Newbury Park, CA: Sage.

Hazan, C., & Shaver, P. R. (1987). Romantic love conceptualized as an attachment process. *Journal of Personality and Social Psychology, 52*, 511–524.

Hazan, C., & Zeifman, D. (1994). Sex and the psychological tether. In D. Perlman & K. Bartholomew (Eds.), *Advances in personal relationships: A research annual* (Vol. 5, pp. 151–177). London: Kingsley.

Hazan, C., & Zeifman, D. (1999). Pair-bonds as attachments: Evaluating the evidence. In J. Cassidy & P. R. Shaver (Eds.), *Handbook of attachment: Theory, research, and clinical applications* (pp. 336–354). New York: Guilford Press.

Kinsey, A. C., Pomeroy, W. B., & Martin, C. E. (1948). *Sexual behavior in the human male.* Philadelphia: Saunders.

Nardi, P. M. (1992). "Seamless souls": An introduction to men's friendships. In P. Nardi (Ed.), *Men's friendships* (pp. 1–14). Newbury Park, CA: Sage.

Nichols, M. (1990). Lesbian relationships: Implications for the study of sexuality and gender. In J. C. Gonsiorek & J. D. Weinrich (Eds.), *Homosexuality: Research implications for public policy* (pp. 350–364). Newbury Park, CA: Sage.

Pattatucci, A. M. L., & Hamer, D. H. (1995). Development and familiality of sexual orientation in females. *Behavior Genetics, 25*, 407–420.

Pillard, R. C. (1990). The Kinsey Scale: Is it familial? In D. P. McWhirter, S. A. Sanders, & J. M. Reinisch (Eds.), *Homosexuality/heterosexuality: Concepts of sexual orientation* (pp. 88–100). New York: Oxford University Press.

Rothblum, E. D. (1993). Early memories, current realities. In E. D. Rothblum & K. A. Brehony (Eds.), *Boston marriages* (pp. 14–18). Amherst, MA: University of Massachusetts Press.

Russell, S. T., & Consolacion, T. B. (2003). Adolescent romance and emotional health in the U.S.: Beyond binaries. *Journal of Clinical Child and Adolescent Psychology, 32*, 499–508.

Sahli, N. (1979). Smashing: Women's relationships before the fall. *Chrysalis, 8*, 17–27.

Savin-Williams, R. C. (1998). " . . . *And then I became gay": Young men's stories.* New York: Routledge.

Sell, R. L., & Petrulio, C. (1996). Sampling homosexuals, bisexuals, gays, and lesbians for public health research: A review of the literature from 1990 to 1992. *Journal of Homosexuality, 30*, 31–47.

Shaver, P. R., Hazan, C., & Bradshaw, D. (1988). Love as attachment: The integration of three behavioral systems. In J. Sternberg & M. L. Barnes (Eds.), *The psychology of love* (pp. 193–219). New Haven, CT: Yale University Press.

Shuster, R. (1987). Sexuality as a continuum: The bisexual identity. In Boston Lesbian Psychologies Collective (Ed.), *Lesbian psychologies: Explorations and challenges* (pp. 56–71). Urbana, IL: University of Illinois Press.

Smith-Rosenberg, C. (1975). The female world of love and ritual: Relations between women in nineteenth century America. *Signs, 1*, 1–29.

Turner, R. A., Altemus, M., Enos, T., Cooper, B., & McGuinness, T. (1999). Preliminary research on plasma oxytocin in normal cycling women: Investigating emotion and interpersonal distress. *Psychiatry, 62*, 97–113.

Weinberg, M. S., Williams, C. J., & Pryor, D. W. (1994). *Dual attraction: Understanding bisexuality.* New York: Oxford University Press.

Williams, J. R., Catania, K. C., & Carter, C. S. (1992). Development of partner preferences in female prairie voles (*Microtus ochrogaster*): The role of social and sexual experience. *Hormones and Behavior, 26*, 339–349.

Williams, J. R., Insel, T. R., Harbaugh, C. R., & Carter, C. S. (1994). Oxytocin administered centrally facilitates formation of a partner preference in female prairie voles (*Microtus ochrogaster*). *Journal of Neuroendocrinology, 6*, 247–250.

12

Attachment-Related Pathways to Sexual Coercion

DEBORAH DAVIS

Recent evidence has linked insecure attachment, especially avoidance or a combination of anxiety and avoidance (called "fearful avoidance"; Bartholomew & Horowitz, 1991), to both perpetration of sexual coercion, ranging from verbal pressure and arguments to violent criminal sexual offenses (e.g., Burk & Burkhart, 2002; Davis, 2004; Feiring, Deblinger, Hoch-Espada, & Haworth, 2002; Lyn & Burton, 2004; Smallbone & Dadds, 1998, 2001; Tracy, Shaver, Albino, & Cooper, 2003; Ward & Marshall, 1996; Ward, Hudson & McCormack, 1997; Ward, McCormack, & Hudson, 1997; Ward, Polaschek, & Beech, 2005) and sexual victimization (e.g., Davis, 2004; Davis, Follette, & Vernon, 2001; Flanagan & Furman, 2000; Tracy et al., 2003; Wekerle & Wolfe, 1998). Likewise, insecure attachment has been linked more generally with partner coercion involving violence and partner abuse (e.g., Dutton, 1999; Fonagy, 1999; Roberts & Noller, 1998; see also Bartholomew & Allison, Chapter 5, this volume).

In this chapter, I propose a model of attachment-related pathways to sexual coercion, a model that addresses (1) the overall relationship of attachment style to coercive sexual behavior, (2) the specific mechanisms through which attachment style affects coercion, and (3) the distinctive pathways through which anxious versus avoidant attachment can lead to coercion. I begin with an overview of my general model of sexual coercion. Following this, I discuss the individual components of the model, considering the association between attachment style and each component. Finally, I summarize proposed separate pathways through which attachment anxiety and avoidance are likely to affect the propensity toward sexual coercion.

OVERVIEW OF THE MODEL OF SEXUAL COERCION

Most experts agree that causes of sexual coercion vary, such that no single model of rape can account for all causes or all types of sexually coercive actions (e.g., Crowell & Burgess, 1996; Scully, 1990). Even within specific categories of coercion, such as rape, causes, as well as personal vulnerabilities and specific internal and external instigators, sexual actions, targets, and use of violence, may vary. Hence, I do not claim that my model fits all types and variations of sexual coercion. Instead, the model is intended to characterize common pathways to sexual coercion, with particular attention to those potentially affected by attachment style.

My general model of sexual coercion (see Figure 12.1) is based on the assumption that the potential for sexual coercion begins with internal or external triggers of sexual motivation (defined here as the desire to engage in sexual activity, regardless of the underlying reason for that desire—whether sexual pleasure, relationship management, impressing peers, exertion of control, or other motives). Given the arousal of sexual motivation, a person's expectations regarding the likely success of efforts to engage in sexual activity will affect the likelihood and nature of efforts to satisfy sexual urges. Overall, I expect that if a person believes that efforts to engage in consensual sexual activities will be successful, he or she is likely to attempt consensual sex. But if the person believes such attempts will not be successful, he or she may either choose to use coercion as a secondary strategy, choose other strategies such as prostitution or masturbation, or simply forgo sexual activity altogether. In some cases a person may prefer coercion as a primary strategy, as, for example, when he or she has other goals and desires, such as expression of hostility or a need to exert control over a partner or to assert status.

If the person chooses to initiate consensual sexual activity, his or her efforts may either succeed or fail. However, *accurate understanding* of a partner's willingness is also crucial. The initiator of sexual relations may perceive rejection where none exists and, therefore, either give up unnecessarily or resort to unnecessary coercive behaviors. Likewise, he or she may erroneously perceive consent and hence unknowingly coerce the partner. That is, a partner's refusal may go completely unrecognized or be misperceived as

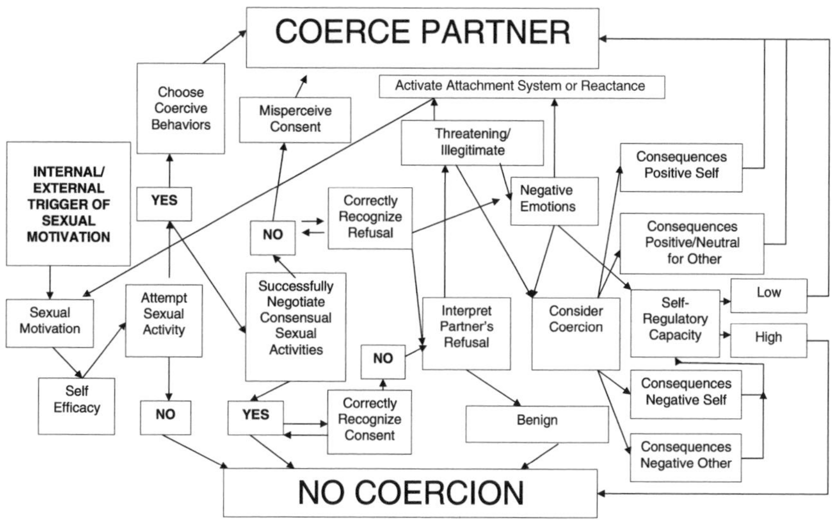

FIGURE 12.1. A general model of attachment-related pathways to sexual coercion.

simply token resistance or as insincere, resulting in sexual behaviors that are not recognized as coercive.

If the person succeeds in achieving truly consensual sex, coercion is unnecessary and unlikely. If the effort fails, however, and the person recognizes the failure, the resulting construal of the partner's refusal will affect the choice of a response, including the likelihood of attempts to coerce the partner into having sex. The refusal may be construed as either legitimate (e.g., the partner is someone else's spouse who has not led the pursuer on) or illegitimate (e.g., "He led me on" or "I paid for her dinner") and in either threatening or benign terms. The rebuffed person may feel threatened on several grounds, including concerns about the status of the relationship, his or her self-esteem or sense of control, social status or peer admiration, and confidence in sexual prowess, among other concerns. The specific construal of a partner's refusal is likely to be affected by the nature of the initial trigger of sexual motivation. For example, if sexual motivation was initially triggered by the need to be reassured of the partner's love, the partner's refusal is more likely to be interpreted as reflecting lack of love than it would be if the desire for sex was triggered by nonrelational motivations such as sexual arousal or stress reduction.

Threatening construals of a partner's refusal may then directly increase sexual motivation and may also trigger negative emotions such as anger, humiliation, frustration, or reactance. Hence, sexual frustration, the sense of threat triggered by a partner's refusal, and the enhanced sexual motivation and negative emotions they jointly trigger will motivate the person to somehow address them. The person may then consider various options, including coercing the partner to have sex.

Benign attributions for a partner's refusal do not necessarily prevent coercion, although they render it less likely. If the pursuer perceives that a partner is not in the mood as the result of a bad day at work, for example, he or she may still choose to pursue sexual activity, either overestimating the potential to overcome the bad mood, underestimating the aversive effects for the partner, or simply disregarding the partner's needs in favor of his or her own.

The person may or may not actively consider the consequences of coercion. However, even if such consequences are considered, they may not be accurately assessed for either oneself or one's partner. Perceptions may be colored by the original motive for pursuing sex with the target; by the degree of sexual arousal; or by the person's acute emotional state, acute incapacities such as intoxication, chronic or acute motivational states, or chronic deficits in perspective taking. And even if the undesirability of coercion is realized, the person may lack the self-regulatory capacity to suppress the urge to coerce the target. This capacity may be directly overcome by the negative emotions triggered by the partner's refusal or may be reduced by an acute state (such as intoxication) or chronic predispositions (such as insecure attachment). If the person believes that coerced sexual activity will satisfy immediate needs, either failure to recognize or to care about additional negative consequences of coercion or failure to inhibit coercive impulses despite recognition of such consequences will increase the likelihood of coercive behavior.

As I explain in subsequent sections of this chapter, attachment style influences each component of this model, ranging from the initial triggers of sexual motivation through the final assessment of potential responses to refusal and the ultimate decision to coerce and/or rape a partner. I now turn to consideration of the specific pathways through which avoidant or anxious attachment might lead to coercion and of the specific internal and external circumstances likely to trigger coercion for those with each form of attachment insecurity.

ATTACHMENT-RELATED PATHWAYS TO SEXUAL COERCION

Triggers of Sexual Motivation

The model suggests that the potential for sexual coercion begins when sexual motivation is triggered. Such triggers vary, as illustrated in Figures 12.2–12.4. Clearly, sexual motivation may be triggered by purely physical urges, which tend to be more frequent among men than women (see Baumeister & Tice, 2000). However, sex may serve a variety of additional social and nonsocial motives, prominently including attachment motivations (see Davis, Shaver & Vernon, 2004; Cooper et al., Chapter 10, and Gillath & Schachner, Chapter 13, this volume).

Marshall (1989, 1993; Hudson & Ward, 2000; Ward et al., 2005; Ward, Hudson, Marshall, & Siegert, 1995) suggested that because insecurely attached men suffer deficits in interpersonal skills, low self-confidence, and lack of empathy, they experience difficulties in achieving intimacy through appropriate courtship behaviors and establishing satisfying intimate relationships. They may therefore be more likely to satisfy intimacy needs through sexual behavior. Smallbone and Dadds (1998) suggested that sexual behavior may be activated differently in secure than in insecure adults. They suggested that for secure persons, sexual motivation tends to be activated within a contexts that include security, reliability, and mutuality (i.e., contexts similar to the parental environment that promotes security). Further, they suggested that attachment behaviors activated by other conditions, such as distress, are functionally separated in a secure person's mind from the sexual behavior system, such that even if the two kinds of behavior do coincide, proximity-seeking behavior will still be constrained by the set goal of mutuality.

In contrast, for insecure persons, sexual behavior may be activated with less regard for commitment or mutuality. Moreover, such behavior may be activated in response to "negative cognitive and affective states similar to those experienced during problematic early attachment experiences. Disorganized attachment-related behaviors in adults may result in less functional separation between the attachment and sexual behavior systems, and coercive or contradictory sexual behavior strategies may be employed" (Smallbone & Dadds, 1998, p. 558). Indeed, there is support for such an argument.

Davis et al. (2004) proposed that sexual behavior can sometimes function as a form of proximity seeking and therefore may be triggered by the same three classes of triggers known to activate the attachment system and trigger proximity seeking: threats of losing an attachment figure's love and availability, internal threats such as distress or illness, and external threats and dangers (Bowlby, 1969/1982). In contrast to Marshall (1989), however, my colleagues and I argued that the use of sexual behavior to serve attachment functions is likely to be particularly characteristic of anxious persons, rather than of all insecure persons. Consistent with this reasoning, we found that many of our survey respondents reported feeling more interested in sex when experiencing insecurity about the relationship and that this tendency was related to attachment anxiety. Respondents also generally reported having sex to reduce stress (i.e., in response to internal distress) and to protect themselves from unpleasant partner moods (in response to an external threat). They also reported having sex to accomplish attachment-related goals such as controlling the partner (presumably to achieve proximity and to receive caregiving or other comforts), to be reassured of a partner's love, and others. In this context, it is interesting to note that many rapists report having committed rape (including rape of a stranger) shortly after upsetting events, some involving wives or girlfriends (e.g., Scully, 1990).

As my colleagues and I expected, most motivations for sex were related to attachment anxiety. Figures 12.2 and 12.3 depict zero-order correlations from two studies between attachment anxiety, avoidance, and various self-reported motives for sex. Results from the Davis et al. (2004) study are presented in the top row of each box, and those of a replication and extension by Schachner and Shaver (2004) are presented in the bottom rows. For the peer influence–social identity motive, two measures from Schachner and Shaver's (2004) study are presented: peer influence and desire to fit in.

As depicted in Figure 12.2, attachment anxiety was most strongly related to having sex to obtain reassurance of a partner's continuing love and regard, but anxiety was also related to all of the other motives for sex except those of purely physical pleasure and desire to impress peers and to fit into a peer group. Notably, several of the motives associated with attachment anxiety have previously been identified as contributors to sexual coercion, including manipulation and control of one's partner (Baumeister, Catanese, & Wallace, 2002), self-regulation of emotion (Burk & Burkhart, 2003; Hudson, Ward, & McCormack, 1999), and enhancement of self-esteem (Baumeister et al., 2002). Attachment anxiety was also associated,

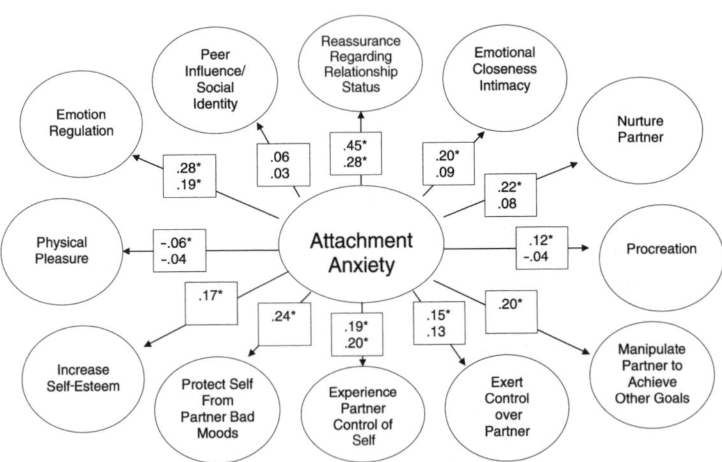

FIGURE 12.2. Relationships between attachment anxiety and subjective motivations for sex. Zero-order correlations between anxiety and each motive for sex are presented in the boxes. Correlations in the top row are from Davis et al. (2004); those in the bottom row are from Schachner and Shaver (2004). Correlations for the motive of peer influence/ social identity are both from Schachner and Shaver and indicate a desire to influence peers and to fit in. *Significant beyond .05.

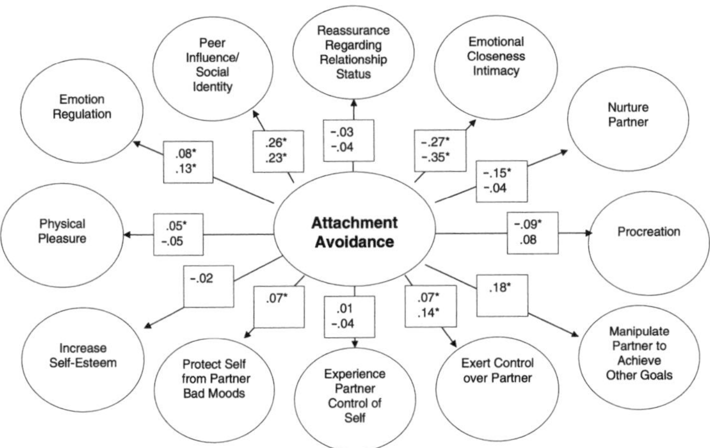

FIGURE 12.3. Relationships between attachment avoidance and subjective motivations for sex. Zero-order correlations between avoidance and each motive for sex are presented in the boxes. Correlations in the top row are from Davis et al. (2004); those in the bottom row are from Schachner and Shaver (2004). Correlations for the motive of peer influence/social identity are both from Schachner and Shaver and represent the desire to influence peers and to fit in. *Significant beyond .05.

however, with the additional motives of experiencing a partner's control over oneself, protecting oneself from a partner's bad moods, and using sex to please or nurture a partner.

Avoidant attachment, in contrast, was strongly and negatively associated with having sex to achieve emotional closeness or intimacy and somewhat negatively associated with having sex to nurture one's partner (see Figure 12.3). Instead, avoidance was most strongly associated with having sex to influence or impress peers and to fit in (see Schachner & Shaver, 2004). Like attachment anxiety, avoidance was also associated with having sex to manipulate or control a partner and, less strongly, with having sex to regulate one's emotions or to protect oneself from a partner's bad moods.

Bowlby (1969/1982) argued that the primary evolutionary function of attachment behavior is protection from harm through proximity to a caregiver. Sadly and ironically, even in the face of punishing interactions with such caregivers, distressed infants tend to seek proximity and cling to, rather than to avoid, the punishing figure (e.g., Harlow, 1961; Main & Hesse, 1990; see Smallbone & Dadds, 1998, for review). Apparently, insecure adults tend to use sexual interaction to satisfy attachment needs while simultaneously diffusing or deflecting potentially dangerous or unpleasant behaviors from their partners.

Burk and Burkhart (2003) have argued that disorganized attachment (involving both anxiety and avoidance) is associated with using sex to regulate emotions and that the tendency to use sex in this way is associated with coercion. It is also important to consider that attachment-related needs for control may lead to coercive behaviors for their own sake. Rapists report power and control as central to their motives for and gratification received from rape (e.g., Groth, 1979), and dominance as a motive for sex has predicted laboratory aggression against women (e.g., Malamuth, 1988). Avoidant attachment has been linked to need for control (see Mikulincer & Shaver, 2003), and this attachment-related need for control has been specifically described as promoting violence and coercion (e.g., Burk & Burkhart, 2003; Follingstad, Bradley, Helff, & Laughlin, 2002; Fonagy, 1999).

Given the somewhat different motives for sex associated with anxious and avoidant attachment, one might expect anxious persons to be most prone to sexual coercion when feeling threats to relationship status or closeness, to the ability to control a partner, to one's safety from a partner's negative affect, or to self-esteem or when in need of emotional comfort. In contrast, avoidant persons (particularly those who are dismissingly avoidant, hence least motivated by attachment-related concerns) might be most prone to sexual coercion of strangers, in new dating relationships, and under circumstances in which emotion regulation, peer influence, or desire to impress peers are served by sexual activity.

Models of sexual coercion have suggested that peer cultures may encourage coercion (see Lalumière, Harris, Quinsey, & Rice, 2005, for review), and that coercion may be facilitated by social identity needs and needs for partner admiration or social status concerns, particularly among narcissists (e.g., Baumeister et al., 2002). These sorts of motives may be triggered either internally (such as by chronic relationship insecurities or narcissism) or externally (such as by peer pressure or the appearance of romantic rivals).

The Relationship of Triggers of Sexual Motivation to Construals of Partner Refusals

As already noted, specific triggers of sexual motivation may predict reactions to partner refusals. As depicted in Figure 12.4, if sexual motivation is triggered by motives unrelated to self-esteem, to relationship reassurance or intimacy goals, or to social identity (such as physical urges or perceived partner needs), negative construals involving threats to crucial self-regulation goals and the negative emotions they tend to evoke may be less likely; whereas if sexual motivation is instead triggered by self-esteem, need for emotion regulation, or relationship-related or social identity goals, negative construals and negative emotions are more likely.

For example, because attachment anxiety is associated with stronger motivation to have sex when feeling insecure about one's relationship and

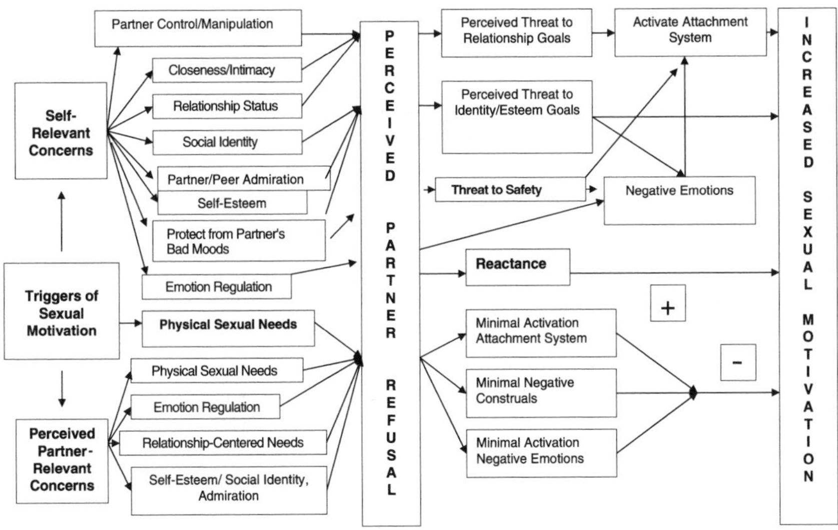

FIGURE 12.4. The relationship of triggers of sexual motivation to construals of partner unavailability.

with relationship-oriented goals such as achieving closeness and intimacy or gaining reassurance of a partner's love (and with the same chronic self-regulation goals), it may also be associated with the tendency to interpret partner refusals as threatening to these goals. Indeed, we (Davis et al., in press) obtained some evidence of this tendency in that anxiety was associated with the tendency to view sexual behavior as a "barometer of relationship status" (as measured by such items as "If we're not having sex pretty frequently, I feel like something is wrong with the relationship"; "When my partner doesn't want to have sex, it makes me worry about whether (s)he still loves me"). Davis (2004) also found that the "barometer" scale predicted self-reports of sexually coercive behaviors and mediated the significant zero-order relationships linking both avoidance and anxiety with sexual coercion.

Avoidant attachment is associated with different self-regulation goals, such as independence and feelings of mastery, competence, and control (see Mikulincer & Shaver, 2003, for a review). Further, avoidance is associated with having sex to promote peer admiration and peer acceptance (Schachner & Shaver, 2004). Hence partner refusals, particularly in circumstances in which such goals are salient, may be construed as threatening one's power and reputation, thereby encouraging coercion on the part of avoidant individuals.

Frequency and Strength of Sexual Motivation

My model assumes that the potential for sexual coercion is greater among those who experience stronger or more frequent sexual motivation. Indeed, rape researchers have shown that rapists appear to be higher in sexual motivation, in that they engage in more "mating effort" (defined as "energy expended in acquiring and keeping sexual partners"; Lalumière et al., 2005, p. 63) and have more sexual partners and higher rates of orgasm than other men (Kanin, 1985; Lalumière, Chalmers, Quinsey, & Seto, 1996; Mahoney, Shively, & Traw, 1986; see Lalumière et al., 2005, for a review).

In the general population, gender is perhaps the strongest determinant of the frequency and strength of sexual urges and mating effort (Baumeister & Tice, 2000), although some evidence suggests that anxious attachment is positively related to sexual motivation, whereas avoidant attachment is negatively related. For example, Davis et al. (2004) found that attachment anxiety was positively associated with average ratings of all motivations for sex and to reported maintenance of sexual passion for specific partners over time. In contrast, avoidance was unrelated to average motivations for sex but positively related to loss of passion over time. Further, Davis et al. (2001) found that avoidant attachment was related to reports of having more sex than desired (especially among avoidant women) and to having voluntary unwanted sex (Davis et al., 2001; Davis, 2004; Impett & Peplau, 2002). Hence attachment-related differences in overall sexual motivation may contribute to the propensity for coercion among anxious persons.

It should be noted that the strength of sexual motivation or arousal can directly affect important perceptual processes, such as the ability to recognize cues reflecting consent or to accurately assess potential consequences of coercion. Arousal-motivated failures to perceive a partner's emotional reactions and communications accurately or to accurately project consequences for oneself or a partner can contribute to the tendency toward coercive behavior.

Sexual Self-Efficacy

As is true for most behaviors, the tendency to attempt sexual activity with a partner, as well as the choice of *how* to attempt such activity, will be affected by assessments of likely success. Although not dealing specifically with *sexual* self-efficacy, substantial data suggest that insecure attachment is related to negative expectations regarding one's own ability to elicit love and care from others.

Both forms of insecurity are assumed to develop in response to a history of unresponsive, ineffective, and/or unreliable caregivers. Attachment anxiety generally results when caregivers are inconsistent and unreliable in responding and awkward, self-centered, or intrusive in providing care. This awkwardness and inconsistency causes a child to develop a "hyperactivating" style of affect regulation, involving *hypersensitivity* to threats (because threats have been ineffectively managed by caregivers) and *hypervigilance* regarding the availability and sensitivity of relationship partners (because caregivers have been inconsistently available and responsive). Attachment avoidance generally results when caregivers respond consistently but negatively to bids for proximity, support, or protection, reacting coolly, angrily, or disapprovingly, particularly in response to displays of need or distress. Parents of avoidant children actively discourage expressions of negative emotion and tend to withdraw from their children when they express negative (but not positive) emotion. As a result, avoidant children are less likely to communicate with their parents when upset. Instead, they learn to seek support without displays of distress or to become "compulsively self-reliant" (Bowlby, 1969/1982). Over time, such children learn to deactivate their attachment systems and habitually refrain from seeking closeness, comfort, and support from others, a pattern well documented in studies of adults (Main, 1990; Mikulincer & Shaver, 2003).

By definition, insecure attachment is associated with negative "working models" of self as worthy of love and caregiving from others (attachment anxiety) or of others as reliable providers of love and caregiving (attachment avoidance), which are developed in response to the parenting patterns just described (Bartholomew, 1990; Bartholomew et al., 1991; Collins, 1996; Mikulincer, 1998a, 1998b). Attachment anxiety is associated broadly with lower self-esteem (see recent review in Park, Crocker, & Mickelson, 2004), whereas dismissing avoidance (low anxiety but high avoidance) is associated with high self-esteem selectively based on self-assessments of personal competence rather than on personal lovability or supportive relationships (Brennan & Bosson, 1998; Brennan & Morris, 1997; Park et al., 2004).

Additional support for the notion that insecure people suffer from relatively negative expectations concerning the support and cooperation of others comes from research on caregiving (reviewed by Collins & Feeney, 2000; Feeney & Collins, 2001), which has established that insecure individuals (particularly those who are avoidant) are less likely to seek support or care from their partners in times of stress or need (see Simpson, 1990; Simpson et al., 1992, 2002). This reluctance to communicate and negotiate with a romantic partner about one's needs seems to be based partly on lack of trust (e.g., Mikulincer, 1998b; Pistole, 1993), lack of openness (Mikulincer & Arad, 1999), negative expectations regarding partner responsiveness and support sensitivity to rejection (Downey, Freitas, Michaelis, & Khouri, 1998), and perceived relative costs versus benefits of seeking support from others (Collins & Feeney, 2000; Ognibene & Collins, 1998). This is also reflected in greater use of extreme strategies, such as use of cosmetic surgeries, in an effort to attract and keep a partner's love (Davis & Vernon, 2002).

Hence, general expectations of the availability and cooperativeness of others are more negative among the insecurely attached.

Insecure attachment is also associated with less popularity with peers (Priel & Shamai, 1995) and with less confidence and assertiveness in social situations (Collins & Read, 1990). Arguably, a history of lesser popularity would undermine sexual self-efficacy, particularly with regard to new or potential partners. Although there is not yet clear-cut evidence of a negative association between sexual self-efficacy and insecure attachment, the preceding results are consistent with such an expectation. Indeed, Feeney, Peterson, Gallois, and Terry (2000; see also Tracy et al., 2003) found that both anxiety and avoidance were related to external sexual "locus of control" beliefs and that anxiety was related to poor self-efficacy regarding sexual negotiations. Further, my colleagues and I (Davis, Follette, Vernon, & Shaver, 2001; Davis et al., in press) have found that both forms of insecurity are associated with inhibited expression of sexual needs to partners, as well as with inhibited expression of needs more generally (Davis & Follette, 2000a).

Some theorists (e.g., Marshall & Barbaree, 1990) have suggested that lack of self-confidence and self-efficacy contribute to sexual coercion indirectly through their influence on the development of negative attitudes and beliefs toward others and the resultant failure to develop social skills and close relationships. Consistent with such a notion, Hudson and Ward (1997) examined the relationship of attachment to attitudes toward women in a sample of incarcerated sex offenders. Fearful and dismissing men scored higher on measures of fear of intimacy, anger expression, and anger suppression. Fearful men reported the greatest hostility toward women, whereas dismissing men reported the greatest acceptance of rape myths. The authors proposed that the emotional loneliness associated with insecurity leads to hostile attitudes toward women, as well as acceptance of interpersonal violence and actual physical violence (see Ward, Hudson, & McCormack, 1997, for a review). Further, they suggested that the fusion of need for emotional closeness with sexual behavior can lead to sexual preoccupation, promiscuity, and the possibility of sexual offending as efforts to gain intimacy through sexual contact escalate (see also Marshall, 1989, 1993).

A host of studies have documented the relationship between sexual coercion and hypermasculinity, hostility toward women, adversarial sex-role beliefs, acceptance of interpersonal violence, rape-supportive attitudes, and a variety of other cognitive distortions (Keenan & Ward, 2000; Lalumière et al., 2005; Ward, 1995; Ward, 2000; Ward, Hudson, Johnston, & Marshall, 1997; Ward, Keenan, & Hudson, 2000). These attitudes are associated with narcissism (e.g., Bushman, Bonacci, van Dijk, & Baumeister, 2003). Davis, Carlen & Gallio (2006) found that both anxiety and avoidance were likewise associated with these rape-supportive attitudes in male and female college students. These attitudes in turn may provide a pathway to rape. This path may begin when such attitudes promote lower self-efficacy beliefs with respect to obtaining consensual sex in the absence of coercion. Adversarial beliefs entailing distrust of women and beliefs that needs must be negotiated through competitive tactics of manipulation may be reflected in preference for coercion as a primary strategy, perhaps in most cases more likely to involve manipulative tactics for seduction rather than outright physical coercion. In the event of partner refusals, such beliefs are likely to promote negative construals of partner refusals, which may feed reactance and desire to assert control, thereby directly promoting coercive strategies.

Attempted Sexual Activity

If a person does opt for sexual activity, several pathways are available—such as masturbation, prostitution, having sex with consenting partners, or coercion. Presumably, attempts to achieve consensual sex with a partner will be most commonly chosen. However, in some circumstances, or for some persons, coercion may be preferred as a primary strategy in the absence of any prior attempt at consensual sex. Indeed, several prominent models of sexual offending (e.g., Hall & Hirschman, 1991; Malamuth, Heavey, & Linz, 1993) include sexual arousal to deviant sexual behaviors among their predictors of coercion, and studies of phallometric responses to coercive versus noncoercive pornographic materials have shown that rapists tend to respond more positively to physical coercion, graphic violence, and victim humiliation than normal controls do (see review by Lalumière et al., 2005), indicating that such strategies are attractive. These, as well as lower level coercive preferences, may result, as described earlier, in response to lack of trust or self-efficacy regarding consensual sex or in response to hostility and adversarial belief systems. However, they may also be the simple result of lack of self-efficacy due to low perceptions of one's own mate value.

Thornhill and Palmer (2000), for example, have argued that low ability to attract consenting partners is associated with a particular evolutionary adaptation toward coercion. That is, rape may be a biological adaptation whereby men lacking characteristics necessary to attract mates (such as status and resources) must target youthful, attractive, fertile victims vulnerable to coercion in order to successfully mate and reproduce. Similarly, attachment theorists have argued that low self-esteem and poor intimacy skills resulting from poor attachment histories prevent a person from developing successful adult relationships. Hence, emotional loneliness leaves the person vulnerable to seeking intimacy indirectly through sex, even if it must involve coercion (e.g., Marshall et al., 1993; Ward, Hudson, Marshall, & Siegert, 1995; see Ward, Hudson, & McCormack, 1997, for a review).

Generally, attachment theorists have argued that secure strategies of interaction are organized in terms of what Bowlby called a "goal-corrected partnership," whereby attempts to influence an attachment figure are based on open communication of needs and cooperative strategies based on mutual needs—which would include consensual sexual activities. In contrast, the strategies of insecure persons are more likely to be self-centered, noncompliant, and coercive. In cases involving abuse or violence, disorganized strategies may be strongly contradictory, including alternation between intense approach behaviors, angry displays, and avoidant strategies (see Crittenden, 1997; Lyons-Ruth, 1996; Smallbone & Dadds, 1998). In the context of adult sexuality, such strategies may involve intense sexual motivation combined with either coercive attempts to achieve sexual contact or avoidant strategies involving self-stimulation or nonintimate sex.

What might be called a low-level preferred coercive style (attempts to achieve sex through lying, partner manipulation, or persuasion) has been associated with the avoidant attachment style. For example, Hendrick and Hendrick's (1987) *ludic* "love style" involves a "game playing" style of relationship behaviors whereby a person engages in little intimate disclosure to a partner, exhibits high sensation seeking, and is prone to casual and sometimes manipulative sexuality. Rules govern behavior, and the love object is expected to understand and play by those rules (perhaps including such rules as "If you engage in foreplay, you must engage in intercourse" or "If I pay for your dinner, you must put out"; Hendrick & Hendrick, 1987). Subsequent research has associated avoidant attachment with this ludic style (Fricker & Moore, 2002; Feeney & Noller, 1990; Hendrick & Hendrick, 1989; Levy & Davis, 1988; Shaver & Hazan, 1988). In turn, the ludic style is associated with angry temperament (Worobey, 2001) and sexual coercion (Kalichman, Sarwer, & Johnson, 1993).

Negotiation of Consensual Sexual Activity

Although coercion may be in some cases be the preferred sexual choice, it is perhaps more frequently a backup strategy employed in response to unsuccessful attempts to achieve consensual sex. The reasons a person may fail to achieve consensual sex with desirable targets are many, beginning with selection of appropriate targets and appropriate circumstances. The person may be insufficiently attractive to the chosen targets for a variety of reasons ranging from physical attractiveness to social status or social skills, among others. It is beyond the scope of this chapter to consider all such potential pathways to rejection. Here, I focus on the contributions of relationship satisfaction and communication skills as attachment-related pathways to coercion.

Before turning to these issues, however, I should mention that the importance of any pathway to rejection will depend on the context of the sexual attempt. For example, factors that affect coercion within existing couple relationships are likely to differ from those that contribute to date rape among new partners or stranger rape. Insufficient physical attractiveness, social skills, or social status may trigger rejection of new suitors, for example, whereas they may rarely trigger rejection in established relationships. In contrast, couple distress or conflict may trigger rejection in ongoing relationships but play no role in rejection of new suitors. This being said, I now consider factors related to attachment style with potential to cause rejection in both contexts.

Relationship Satisfaction

Considerable research has documented associations between relationship satisfaction and sexual satisfaction (e.g., Baumeister & Tice, 2000; see Karney & Bradbury, 1995, for a review). Though causality may flow in both directions, one is less likely to achieve sex at all (or satisfactory sex) with a disaffected partner. Insecure attachment is associated with relationship dissatisfaction (Davis & Follette, 2000b; Davila, Karney, & Bradbury, 1999; Davis, Kirkpatrick, & Levy, 1994; Feeney, 2002; Frei & Shaver, 2002; Davis, 1999; Kirkpatrick & Davis, 1994) and specifically with sexual dissatisfaction (e.g., Davis et al., in press). Further, rapists and other violent offenders report less satisfaction and less supportive relationships with romantic partners (Ward, McCormick, & Hudson, 1997). Hence, although not yet documented, it is likely that insecure and sexually coercive individuals suffer a higher rate of rejection of sexual advances due to the association of these characteristics with overall relationship dissatisfaction.

Sexual Communication

Rejection of sexual advances may also result from poor communication and negotiation of sexual needs. There is extensive evidence of attachment-related deficits in communication skills. Intimate self-disclosure to romantic partners, for example, has been found to correlate negatively with attachment avoidance (e.g., Anders & Tucker, 2000; Bradford, Feeney, & Campbell, 2002; Pistole, 1993), whereas failure to disclose socially undesirable sexual preferences such as homosexuality (e.g., Elizur & Mintzer, 2001; Holtzen, Kenny, & Mahalik, 1995; Mohr & Fassinger, 2003; Ridge & Feeney, 1998) and generally being secretive have been associated with both avoidance and anxiety (e.g., Vrij, Paterson, Nunkoosing, Soukara, & Oosterwegel, 2003). Avoidant attachment is related to evasive approaches to problem solving in conflict situations (i.e., failure to discuss or resolve a problem; e.g., Black, Jaeger, McCartney, & Crittenden, 2000; Creasey, 2002; Creasey & Hesson-McInnis, 2001; Davis & Follette, 2000b; Feeney, Noller, & Callen, 1994). Hence, when there is conflict over preferences or needs, avoidant individuals tend to let the problem persist rather than negotiate a resolution compatible with their own and their partners' needs. Generally, both forms of insecurity are associated with dysfunctional communication and problem solving (e.g., Baron & Ortiz, 2002; Creasey, 2002; Creasey & Hesson-McInnis, 2001; Davis & Follette, 2000a, 2002b; Feeney, 1999; Pistole & Arricale, 2003; Shi, 2003; Simpson, Rholes, & Phillips, 1996; see Treboux, Crowell, & Waters, 2004, for a recent review), inhibited communication (Davis & Follette, 2000a), and with lower communication competence and assertiveness, which is in turn related to less satisfactory recruitment of social support (e.g., Anders & Tucker, 2000).

Research on couple communication has associated anxious attachment with coercion, high levels of relationship conflict (e.g., Feeney et al., 1994; Mikulincer & Nachshon, 1991; Pistole, 1989), angry and volatile styles of conflict management (e.g., Davis & Follette, 2000b; Creasey, 2002), and emotional "flooding" during conflict (Davis & Follette, 2000b). Insecure attachment more generally has been associated with impaired communication skills (e.g., Roberts & Noller, 1998), and impaired communication specifically regarding sex (Davis, Follette, Vernon, & Shaver, 2001; Davis et al., 2005; Feeney, Kelly, Gallois, Peterson, & Terry, 1999; see Feeney & Noller, 2004, for a review). Relationship researchers have also observed links between dysfunctional communication and general violence toward partners (e.g., Dutton, 1999; Roberts & Noller, 1998).

Indeed, Davis (2004) found that inhibited communication of sexual needs was correlated with self-reported coercive behaviors (such as lying to partners to achieve sex). I proposed that poor communication skills serve as an attachment-related pathway to coercion, because both attachment anxiety and avoidance were previously associated with inhibited expression of sexual needs (Davis et al., in press). In addition, however, the angry emotional states and coercive styles characteristic of anxious persons, as well as the overall poor quality of problem-solving communications among insecure persons, are likely to contribute directly to failure to achieve consensual sex and thereby to the potential for coercive sex.

Although research addressing the role of social skills has yielded inconsistent associations with sexual coercion (see Baumeister et al., 2002; Hudson & Ward, 2000, for reviews), little research has addressed the effects of intimate communication skills and propensities, problem-solving skills, and specifically sexual communication. These skills are arguably more related to successful negotiation of consensual sex (and to attachment style) than are social skills as typically operationalized. Relationship skills and intimacy deficits have been proposed by authors of studies of incarcerated sexual offenders as primary pathways to sexual deviance. These researchers argue that poor early attachment experiences render a person unable to form intimate relationships with other adults (e.g., Craissati, McClurg, & Browne, 2002; Marshall, 1989; McCormack, Hudson, & Ward, 2002; Ward et al., 1995). However, such skills have not been directly assessed in research with offenders, and given the use of offender populations without control-group comparisons, their relationship to propensity to rape cannot be adequately tested.

Accurate Perception of Consent

Regardless of a partner's actual willingness to engage in consensual sexual activity, the initiator may misperceive the partner's intentions. Indeed, this misperception may occur before or during the attempt to initiate sex, after the partner has communicated his or her reactions to the attempt, and even after completed coercion or rape. Poor choice of targets, for example, may reflect exaggerated perceptions of one's own attractiveness to a specific target or class of targets. Baumeister et al. (2002) suggested that this sort of general overestimation of one's own sexual attractiveness on the part of men and broad expectations of sexual willingness among desirable women contribute to narcissistic reactance in response to rejection. On the other hand, failure to attempt sexual contact with a target or target class may reflect underestimation of one's attractiveness to desired targets. Again, this general perception of the unavailability of desirable partners has been proposed to create resentment, reactance, and the potential for coercion (Baumeister et al., 2002).

Misperception of sexual consent has, of course, been central to theories of rape. Victim reports of rape and sexual coercion vastly outnumber male reports of perpetrating them, perhaps in part reflecting men's failure to accurately perceive cues of nonconsent (e.g., Laumann, Gagnon, Michael, & Michaels, 1994). Studies of rapists have also revealed a large subset who deny having committed any rape (e.g., Groth, 1979; Johnson & Ward, 1996; Lalumière et al., 2005; Scully, 1990; Ward, 2000; Ward, Hudson, Johnston, & Marshall, 1997). Finally, laboratory studies of communication and perception of sexual interest and intent have shown that men "overperceive" sexual interest or consent in women's behavior (see Abbey, Zawacki, & Buck, 2005; Henningsen, 2004, for recent reviews). Indeed, some research indicates that rapists are selectively impaired in decoding women's negative cues only but are no worse in reading women's positive cues or men's cues of either sort. Apparently, this reflects motivated information processing, particularly of cues inconsistent with sexual motivation (McDonel & McFall, 1991).

Clearly, most men are able to perceive rejection of their sexual advances more or less accurately. Hence it becomes of interest to ask what individual differences may be associated with failure to do so. The studies discussed previously indicate that rapists are generally less able to recognize real refusals and lack of interest. Baumeister et al. (2002) presented evidence that male narcissists tend to overperceive female confederates' attraction to them and that narcissists may be generally less able to recognize cues of disinterest or rejection (although particularly likely to respond with hostility and rejection when they are recognized).

Alcohol-induced sexual motivation is in part reflected in inability to perceive lack of interest in others. Marx and Gross (1995) developed an experimental procedure in which research participants were confronted with a hypothetical audiotaped vignette involving a woman in a scenario depicting progressively more attempted sexual contact by her male date. Participants were asked to determine when the man's behavior had become inappropriate. In that study, both men who had consumed alcohol and those who only believed they had consumed alcohol took longer to recognize situations in which a man should cease attempts for further sexual contact, and differences in discernment between sexually coercive and noncoercive men disappeared among those who had consumed alcohol (see Davis & Loftus, 2004, for review, and Abbey, Zawacki, & Buck, 2005, for a recent replication and extension). Because insecure attachment is associated with substance use for stress management (see Mikulincer & Shaver, 2003, for review) and in sexual situations (Tracy et al., 2003), intoxication is likely to provide an additional attachment-related pathway to sexual coercion, including through its effects on perception of consent-related cues.

Construal of Partner Refusals

Unsuccessful efforts to achieve consensual sex are likely to trigger attributions concerning the legitimacy, causes, and implications of the lack of success, some benign and some relatively threatening.

Particularly among people who take a "rules"-oriented approach to sexual interaction, a woman's right to refuse may be perceived as invalid under certain circumstances. Especially among those with "rape-supportive" attitudes of various kinds (Ward, 1995), the woman may be viewed as obligated to provide sex if, for example, she has engaged in foreplay, has gone out with a man for a certain amount of time, has dressed provocatively or engaged in other suggestive behaviors, has accepted financial or other favors, or is married to her pursuer (see Lalumière et al., 2005, for a review of the link between such attitudes and rape). These factors may contribute to men's tendency to view resistance under such circumstances as insincere "token resistance," a practice that almost half of college women have admitted to engaging in (Muehlenhard & Hollabaugh, 1988; Sprecher, Hatfield, Cortese, Potapova, & Levitskaya, 1994). Further, as argued by Baumeister et al. (2002), some men (particularly narcissists) may view it as their prerogative to bed desirable women of their choice and therefore view any refusals as illegitimate.

As depicted in Figure 12.4, three major categories of construals of causes and implications can be identified.

Benign Construals

My model assumes that benign, nonthreatening construals are most likely when the initial triggers of sexual motivation do not involve attachment-related or self-esteem–social identity concerns. That is, if a person initiates sex either for purely physical reasons or in response to perceptions that the partner may desire sex for some reason, the partner's refusal is less likely to be construed in negative terms. Granted, refusal may still activate negative attachment, esteem, or social identity construals even in these circumstances. However, I suggest that they are less likely when the initiator did not begin the encounter with such concerns already in mind.

Attachment-Related Construals

The first category of potentially threatening construals concerns the relationship implications of refusing to have sex. That is, when sexual advances are rejected, the initiator may make such inferences as (1) the target does not love or want the pursuer or does not perceive the pursuer as desirable, (2) the target does not want to be intimate with the pursuer, or (3) the pursuer cannot control the target or gain access to the target. Davis et al. (2004) also suggested that sexual behavior can be motivated by the need to protect oneself from a partner's negative affect and behavior (i.e., sex as an attempt to diminish threatening partner behavior—a motive we found to be associated strongly with attachment anxiety and more weakly but significantly associated with avoidance; see Figures 12.2 and 12.3). Negative construals in this category threaten the attachment-related goals of safety and partner availability and responsiveness and can be expected to activate the attachment system. Davis et al. (2004) argued that threats to attachment goals can enhance sexual motivation, in that sexual activities can reassure a person of a partner's love and availability and facilitate control of the partner and regulation of distress.

Anxious attachment is associated with hypervigilance and concern with attachment-related goals and cues regarding the availability and responsiveness of attachment figures. Not surprisingly, given this chronic activation of the attachment system and attachment-related goals, anxious individuals are more likely to see attachment-related implications in their partners' behavior and to react more strongly and negatively, and with stronger and more persistent proximity-seeking, to perceived relationship threats (see Feeney, 1999; Mikulincer & Shaver, 2003, 2005; Mikulincer, Shaver, & Pereg, 2003, for reviews). For anxious persons, sexual motivation is also more likely to be initially triggered by attachment-related concerns, as demonstrated by the previously reviewed data indicating that anxious persons are more likely to report feeling more interested in sex when feeling insecure about their relationships and for the purposes of maintaining a partner's love, gaining reassurance of love, achieving closeness and intimacy, controlling a partner, and achieving emotion regulation. Hence, in the face of a partner's refusal, anxious persons can be expected to make more negative attachment-related construals than those with other attachment styles. In turn, such perceived threats to attachment goals will further activate the attachment system and fuel sexual motivation, creating even greater frustration if the partner's refusal persists.

Anxious Attachment and the Coercive Style. Crittenden (1997; see also Lyons-Ruth, 1996) argued that a coercive strategy of need satisfaction is characteristic of children with inconsistent caregivers. The coercive strategy is used to elicit satisfaction of attachment-related needs from an attachment figure—including increased closeness, physical comfort, distress regulation, and protection. The coercive strategy involves, in effect, a "win stay, lose change" strategy of alternation between the two poles of aggressive/threatening behavior (crying, screaming, throwing tantrums) and "coy"/disarming behavior. "This strategy involves displaying angry threats and/or aggression at high intensity until the parents respond. If the parent's response is appeasing, the display of anger usually escalates until the need is satisfied. If, on the other hand, the parent's response is angry, the child switches to coy behavior. Coy, feigned helplessness is used to 'bribe' the parent until he or she becomes exasperated with that also; then the child switches back to threatening aggressiveness" (Crittenden, 1997, p. 56). Because coy and coercive behaviors can be used only in the physical presence of the attachment figure, anxious individuals should have a strong need to be in this figure's presence.

In adulthood, sexuality provides one of the main avenues to closeness. To the extent that sexual behaviors correspond to either the coy or the aggressive pole of the coercive strategy, they may be used to control a partner and simultaneously satisfy needs for physical closeness and reassurance of the partner's availability and love. In fact, Crittenden (1997) pointed out that coy behaviors are, in many instances, morphologically identical to flirtatious, sexually seductive behaviors. For example, feigning helplessness or incompetence is a common flirtation/seduction strategy used by both men and women—as are such strategies as acting cute, talking baby talk, and making flirtatious glances. To the extent that anxious people use coy strategies to elicit caregiving, they may also use sexual flirtation and sex itself for this purpose.

Sex to Disarm and Protect. According to Crittenden's (1997) analysis of the coercive strategy, anxious individuals sometimes use the coy strategy to defuse or deflect a caregiver's anger or aggression, as suggested in our previous discussion of motives for sex. Implicit in this analysis of the coercive strategy is the idea that sex may provide a means to control or exert power over one's partner and, further, that the coy strategy (and its analog, sex) is used for this purpose. This suggests that anxious adults may use sex to control both benevolent and dangerous behaviors of their partners. Because anxiety is associated with the tendency to use the coercive strategy, anxious individuals should both use sex as a coercive strategy and use the coercive strategy to obtain sex.

Generally, the coercive strategy includes the use of aggression as a relatively prominent strategy for achieving attachment-related goals, perhaps including sex with a reluctant partner. Coercive stalking of lost or unavailable partners is associated with anxious attachment (Davis, Ace, & Andra, 2002; Davis, Frieze, & Maiuro, 2002). Likewise, Davis, Shaver, and Vernon (2003) found that anxious individuals reported a strongly ambivalent pattern of acting out in response to relationship dissolution. That is, attachment anxiety was associated with both positive romantic behaviors and angry, aggressive acting out in response to a breakup initiated by a desired partner. Hence, like anxious/ambivalent children, anxious adults employed both poles of Crittenden's coercive strategy to attempt to achieve their attachment goals with the lost partner. Similar results have been obtained in studies of partner abuse. Dutton (1999) described the cycle of abuse as consisting of an episode of partner abuse followed by a phase of sweet, appeasing attempts to apologize and restore intimacy. He further found that abuse was associated with attachment anxiety (i.e., fearful and preoccupied attachment). Also, as noted earlier, both anxiety and avoidance are associated with reports of having sex in order to control partners.

Rape researchers have also observed that rape can be instigated by perceived threats to attachment goals. Sexual activity itself serves attachment goals (Davis et al., 2004), and when denied, these goals can inspire sexual aggression. However, rape often takes place when attachment goals are threatened by such factors as potential romantic rivals or feared or actual abandonment by one's partner (see Lalumière et al., 2005, for a review of such factors associated with spousal rape). Rape under such circumstances may well be most likely among the anxiously attached, who tend to experience more jealousy and are generally both more vulnerable to perceiving attachment-related threats (and hence more likely to make negative construals of partner refusals to have sex) and more likely to employ coercive strategies for achieving attachment-related needs. Rapists also tend to perceive attachment-related insults. Lisak and Roth (1988), for example, found that rapists report having been hurt, betrayed, used, exploited, or manipulated by women and hence assert their needs for control or revenge through rape (see also Keenan & Ward, 2000; Ward, 2000; Ward et al., 1997; Ward et al., 2000, for discussion of various cognitive distortions among rapists). Moreover, many rapists (80%) report upsetting or relationship-threatening experiences (often with their wives or girlfriends) prior to rapes (even of strangers; Scully, 1990; see also Kanin, 1965). Further, incarcerated rapists score significantly higher on sensitivity to rejection than other groups of offenders, except pedophiles (Ward, McCormack, & Hudson, 1997). Given such patterns, sexual coercion among the anxious should be most commonly directed toward relationship partners to whom the perpetrators feel attached, as opposed to strangers or casual partners.

Finally, it is interesting to note that rapists often suffer from the delusion that they have achieved attachment goals via coerced sex. Baumeister et al. (2002; see also Ward, 2000) reviewed substantial evidence that rapists (even those in jail for the crime) believe that their victims think fondly of them, perceive them as fabulous lovers, enjoyed the rape, and had participated voluntarily. The authors interpreted such misperceptions as examples of narcissistic self-aggrandizement, but wishful attachment-related thinking may also have contributed. In fact, there is evidence that narcissism is associated with uncertainty and jealousy (Neumann & Bierhoff, 2004). Hence attachment goals may affect the construals of narcissists as well.

Self-Regulation Goals and Insecure Attachment. As noted earlier, Burk and Burkhart (2003) argued that disorganized attachment (involving both anxiety and avoidance) is associated with using sex to regulate emotions. As shown in Figures 12.2 and 12.3, the previously described studies of subjective motivations for sex have indeed shown that both anxiety and avoidance are associated with having sex to regulate emotion. Burk and Burkhardt (2003) further argued that use of sex for emotion regulation is associated with coercion. Attachment theory suggests that internal distress activates the attachment system, leading a person to turn to attachment figures for distress regulation. When sex is sought for the purpose of emotion regulation, a partner's refusal both fails to reduce distress and further activates the attachment system through the threat to partner availability and responsiveness. This additional threat is likely to enhance negative emotions (particularly among anxious persons), thereby further activating the attachment system and further increasing sexual motivation.

Construals Related to Self-Esteem and Social Identity Concerns

As depicted in Figure 12.4, a second category of negative construals concerns threats to one's self-concept and social identity. Such threats can involve either one's internal feelings of self-esteem, competence, attractiveness, and so on or anticipated reactions of others who might know of one's sexual outcomes. Substantial evidence indicates that sexual coercion often occurs in the context of considerable peer pressure to engage in sexual conquests and, in part, as a result of needs to impress or fit in with one's peer group (e.g., Kanin, 1985; Lalumière et al., 2005). In fact, Kanin (1985) found that date rapists were more likely than nonrapist controls to report peer pressure to seek sexual conquests. Lalumière et al. (2005) propose that sexual conquests in response to peer pressure are particularly characteristic of the "young male syndrome" of adolescent antisocial behavior, which includes rape. They suggest that rape due to such influences is likely to be characteristic of rapists in the "adolescence limited" category. Males in this category tend to engage in sexual coercion only during this period of life and to do so in the context of competitive male social groups such as gangs, sports teams, the military, fraternities, or other campus groups.

However, there is also evidence that such self-concept and social identity concerns play a role in rape in other life contexts as well. It is primarily these sorts of concerns that are addressed in Baumeister, Catanese, and Wallace's (2002) "narcissistic reactance" theory of sexual coercion. According to this theory, when a man desires sex with a particular partner, he may simply perceive her as unavailable, or she may actively reject his advances. Some men may take her unavailability as a deprivation of freedom—that is, the freedom to have sex with the woman he desires. If the man has reason to expect that he should or would be able to have sex with the woman, this unavailability is particularly likely to elicit "psychological reactance" (Brehm, 1966; Brehm & Brehm, 1981). Further, the authors argue that a man's general sense that many or most women might be unavailable may create reactance, although it is more likely when specific women refuse him. On experiencing reactance, the man is likely to experience the three common responses: (1) to desire the woman more than ever, (2) to attempt to reassert his freedom to have sex with her, and (3) to aggress against her, as the source of the restriction of his freedom.

Notice that this theory shares features with an attachment analysis of sexual coercion. In attachment terms, the threat to the love or accessibility of an attachment figure activates the attachment system, which further increases desire and overt efforts to reestablish the figure's availability. Further, as Bowlby (1973) explained, frustration of attachment needs produces anger toward the attachment figure, which can result in overt aggression (see Dutton, 1999, for a detailed discussion of attachment-related anger and aggression). Finally, both theories suggest that the strongest reactions will occur under conditions in which the initiator has reason to expect sex with the target. In attachment terms, the more established and important the attachment relationship, the stronger would be expectations and desires for the love of and access to the attachment figure. In reactance terms, the more the person expects or values a particular freedom, the more reactance will be experienced when that freedom is threatened. Both theories also suggest that the goal of sexual coercion is to reestablish access to or control over the partner, rather than simply to achieve or enjoy sex (see Baumeister et al., 2002, for a review of evidence of lack of physical gratification among rapists). Hence the two theories produce similar predictions up to this point.

The "narcissistic reactance" theory, however, focuses largely on construals of partner availability and its effects on self-esteem and social identity rather than on attachment-related construals. In addition, narcissistic reactance theory relates these construals specifically to the nature of the narcissistic mind. Narcissism is expected to increase the likelihood (1) that a person will expect sexual access, (2) that the person will experience reactance upon being refused, and (3) that the person will resort to coercion to obtain sex. Baumeister et al. (2002) argue that the characteristic exaggerated sense of "entitlement" among narcissists leads them to believe that they deserve to have sex when and with whom they desire at a higher rate than other men, and therefore experience greater reactance to partner unavailability.

Although not stated in these terms, the authors essentially point to narcissistic construals of partner unavailability that would further increase reactance, anger, and other negative emotions. That is, they suggest that narcissists are more likely to view refusal as a personal affront and to construe it in more self-centered, as opposed to partner-centered or situational, terms. Such self-focused attributions include insults to narcissists' inflated sense of sexual prowess, attractiveness, and superiority, as well as perceived threats to social identity, such as damage to one's reputation with peers, and frustration of one's general need for admiration and social status. Finally, the authors point to evidence that narcissists are especially prone to anger, hostility, and aggression when criticized or shown disrespect (e.g., Bushman & Baumeister, 1998; Bushman, Bonacci, van Dijk, & Baumeister, 2003; Morf & Rhodewalt, 2001).

On the basis of such reasoning, Baumeister et al. (2002) suggested that narcissists would tend to rape under conditions that promote their inflated expectations of access, such as when they have achieved a recent elevation in social status, when romantically infatuated, or when the target has consented to other sexual activities such as petting (see Bushman et al., 2003, for evidence that narcissists respond more positively to depictions of rape preceded by consensual affectionate activity than to rape alone). They would also be more likely to rape when there have been previous instances of consensual sex with the target, when the target has granted access to other men and is therefore seen as easily available, or in circumstances in which failure to gain sexual access threatens their sense of self-esteem or competence, opens them to criticism from peers, or denies them an opportunity to brag about their sexual prowess or attractiveness. Narcissists should tend to rape attractive victims, because sexual access to attractive partners may impress others and inflate social status. Although Baumeister et al. (2002) present considerable evidence to support these propositions, narcissists may rape under conditions affecting attachment motivations as well, as suggested by Neumann and Bierhoff's (2004) findings that narcissists suffer from romantic insecurities and jealousies.

Avoidance. There is reason to expect that attachment avoidance will result in rape through pathways similar to the narcissistic pathways suggested by Baumeister et al. (2002). First, avoidance is associated with having sex in relatively uncommitted, unattached contexts, such as with multiple uncommitted sexual partners (e.g., Brennan & Shaver, 1995; Feeney, Noller, & Patty, 1993; Ridge & Feeney, 1998; Schachner & Shaver, 2002). Baumeister et al. (2002) suggested that this preference may necessitate coercion, because fewer women are interested in sex in casual or uncommitted contexts. Also, the more different women a man attempts to have sex with, the more opportunities for coercion (i.e., rejection) will arise.

Further, sexually coercive young men are more likely than other men to have had sex with a woman recommended as sexually available by other men, a strategy compatible with the preference for casual sex among avoidants. Baumeister et al. (2002) argue that having to report failure with promiscuous partners will be particularly threatening to social identity, in that failure with someone easily accessible to others is particularly humiliating. Hence, men in such a situation may be particularly likely to coerce the woman to avoid social embarrassment.

Negative Emotions

Negative construals of all kinds are likely to activate or exacerbate negative emotions. As shown in Figures 12.1 and 12.4, negative emotions can activate the attachment system (Bowlby, 1969/1982), which in turn can further activate sexual motivation. In addition to simple reactance and the consequent desire to reassert the prerogative to engage in the desired sexual activity, a partner's sexual unavailability can lead to feelings of frustration, shame, embarrassment, and anger. These emotions can further contribute to sexual coercion through several pathways.

Activation of the Attachment System

First, as depicted in Figures 12.1 and 12.4, negative emotions can trigger the attachment system and heighten desire for comfort from a partner, even when the partner has been the source of the negative emotions. Particularly when the target is a partner in an ongoing relationship, negative emotions may further trigger sexual desire as a mechanism of emotion regulation.

Anger, Controlling Behavior, and Partner Violence

Negative emotions such as anger may lead directly to attempts to control a partner, and thereby to violence. Follingstad and colleagues (2002) presented evidence that anxious attachment is associated with angry temperament, which is in turn associated with attempts to control relationship partners, which in turn directly predicts relationship violence. Other authors have proposed that a variety of attachment-related negative emotions directly contribute to coercive sexual behavior, including negative feelings toward partners, negative attributions regarding partners' behaviors, loneliness, distrust, and anger (e.g., Ward et al., 1995; Ward, Hudson, & Marshall, 1996). Finally, negative emotional responses to relational events and dysfunctional responses to anger tend to be stronger among insecure persons, although the specific negative emotions and behaviors among anxious and avoidant persons tend to differ (Mikulincer, & Florian, 1998; Mikulincer et al., 2003; Mikulincer & Shaver, 2005).

Negative Emotions and Judgment

Negative emotions can also distort judgments of the desirability of coercive behaviors. A number of studies have documented the direct effects of affect on judgment (e.g., see Forgas & East, 2003; the January 2002 issue of *Psychological Inquiry*, Vol. 13 [1], devoted to Forgas's affect infusion model and related data), as well as the effects of motivational processes on judgment (e.g., see Higgins & Spiegel, 2004; the January 1999 issue of *Psychological Inquiry*, Vol. 10 [1], on motivated cognition). Also, extreme emotion can narrow the focus of attention to only the most salient stimuli or issues (e.g., Safer, Christianson, & Autry, 1998), rendering the person susceptible to selective influence from the factors that have triggered the strong emotions. In situations that provoke coercion, this would involve focusing on the victim's provocative behaviors, and hence would accentuate cognitions justifying coercion or violence. For anxious persons in particular, negative emotions (even those not triggered by the partner) tend to distort judgments of a relationship partner's behaviors (Mikulincer et al., 2003).

Negative Emotions and Self-Regulation

Even if a person is able to perceive short- and long-term consequences of coercion accurately, he or she must still be able to act in accordance with these judgments (see upcoming section). Unfortunately, negative emotions tend to interfere with self-regulation (see Baumeister & Vohs, 2004, for reviews). Hence, when experiencing strong impulses toward sexual coercion, a potential rapist experiencing anger and other negative emotions may be unable to inhibit them.

Evaluating the Alternatives

When deciding whether to engage in sexually coercive behavior, one may consider consequences for the self, for the other, both, or neither. These perceptions are likely to influence the ultimate decision of whether to coerce a partner or not (e.g., Baumeister et al., 2002; Hamilton & Yee, 1990; O'Donohue, Yeater, & Fannetti, 2003). Acute and chronic characteristics of the person, as well as contextual factors, can influence the extent to which consequences are considered at all, as well as the weight they are given.

The Relationship of Triggers of Sexual Motivation to Perceived Consequences of Coercion

My model assumes that cognition at all points in the process leading to coercion will be colored by chronic and acute self-regulation goals and concerns. Hence, just as the goals that initially trigger sexual motivation, as well as the overall strength of sexual arousal, can affect the ability to perceive partner refusals correctly or one's construal of a partner's unavailability, so can they also affect evaluation of possible responses, including coercion. If the initiator is motivated to pursue a particular target because of social identity concerns, for example, evaluation of what to do in response to a partner's resistance to sexual overtures will focus on those same concerns. The person may choose coercion to avoid the embarrassment of failure. Likewise, if the primary need is attachment-related, alternative partners will not suffice; whereas if the need is purely for sexual gratification, a variety of options may suffice, including approaching alternative partners or engaging in masturbation. Finally, regardless of the initial trigger of sexual motivation, once arousal is sufficient, the person may be unwilling to forgo sex.

Impaired Processing

A person's ability to consider consequences may be impaired by chronic or acute characteristics or circumstances. Some characteristics, such as psychopathy (see Lalumière et al., 2005, for a review specifically focused on rape), seem to impair judgment with regard to consequences for both oneself and others. Other characteristics, such as narcissism (see Baumeister et al., 2002) or failures of empathy (e.g., Lisak & Ivan, 1995; Marshall, Hudson, Jones, & Fernandez, 1995; O'Donohue et al., 2003) seem to impair consideration of consequences for others. Baumeister et al. (2002) also reviewed evidence that rapists and narcissists may be *able* to empathize and read social cues from others but selectively choose not to when it would not serve their current motives.

Both forms of attachment insecurity are associated with less empathy and perspective taking (see Mikulincer & Shaver, 2003, for review) and with generally more self-centered rather than other-regarding motives for behavior (e.g., Feeney & Collins, 2003), which have been suggested as one pathway through which insecure attachment can lead to violence and sexual coercion (e.g., Burk & Burkhart, 2003; Fonagy, 1999; Fonagy & Target, 1997). Fonagy and Target (1997; Fonagy, 1999) suggested that disorganized attachment involves multiple segregated internal attachment representations that inhibit the development of reflective mental functions, such as the ability to recognize the role of mental states in the behaviors of oneself or others (see also Keenan & Ward, 2000; Ward, Keenan, & Hudson, 2000). Presumably, the absence of this function contributes to sexual coercion through impairment of empathy and the sense of personal responsibility and through perceiving other people as objects. Likewise, Marshall, Hudson, and Hodkinson (1993) argued that poor attachments "make the transition at puberty to peer relationships more difficult and make attractive those social messages that objectify others, portray people as instruments of sexual pleasure, emphasize power and control over others, and deny the need for social skills and compassion for others" (p. 109).

Insecure people may be less able to correctly anticipate interpersonal consequences of coercive behavior and less likely to care about those consequences even when they do foresee them. Even though anxious people are generally concerned about the relationship implications of all behaviors, including sexual ones, this enhanced concern tends to be reflected in stronger motivation to ensure that they engage in sexual activity in order to feel loved and reassured of their partners' interest. Combined with lack of perspective-taking skills and empathy, such extreme needs for sex may promote coercion.

Intoxication

Intoxication represents perhaps the most common source of acute impairment of processing resources involved in sexual coercion (see Davis & Loftus, 2004, for review). Specifically, alcohol appears to impair perception of the consequences of coercion. Norris, George, Davis, Martell, and Leonesio (1999) found that intoxicated men perceived less negative reactions in rape victims depicted in violent pornography. In part, the reduction in ability to know when sexual behavior should cease (reviewed earlier), or when it is causing pain and distress, may be the result of impaired perception. However, it is also arguably a matter of elevated personal sexual motivation coloring interpretation of that of others.

Failures of Self-Regulation

As noted earlier, regardless of the accuracy with which one perceives potential consequences of various responses to partner unavailability, one must still be able to act accordingly. Hence, even those who recognize (and care about) negative, and even catastrophic, potential results of sexual coercion for themselves and/or their partners may yet succumb to the urge (see Ward, Hudson, & Keenan, 1998; Wiederman, 2004, for discussions of the relationship of self-regulation to sexual behavior and offending; and Vohs &

Ciarocco, 2004, for discussion of the importance of self-regulation for general interpersonal functioning).

It is worth noting that failures of self-regulation may contribute to partner coercion in the absence of negative construals of any kind and in the absence of any negative emotions other than frustrated sexual desire. That is, delay of gratification is one form of self-regulation, and coercion may result when a person simply cannot tolerate delay in satisfaction of sexual urges and is insufficiently deterred by awareness of and concern for the impact of coercive behaviors on a partner. However, when other strong negative emotions are present, failures of self-regulation become more likely, as noted earlier.

Intoxication will tend to contribute to this tendency (see Hull & Slone, 2004, for a review of the effects of alcohol on self-regulation). Perhaps as a result of alcohol myopia (Steele & Josephs, 1990) and the tendency toward enhanced focus on sexual stimuli when intoxicated with a member of the opposite sex (see Davis & Loftus, 2004, for a review), alcohol appears to impair one's ability to *suppress* or *inhibit* arousal. Laboratory demonstrations of this phenomenon have taken two forms. First, some authors have exposed men to erotic stimuli while instructing them to suppress sexual arousal. Measures of penile tumescence have shown that as intoxication increases so does penile girth, despite instructions to avoid arousal. Other studies have examined penile tumescence following exposure to deviant sexual stimuli, such as pictures of rape or child molestation, among sex offenders and nonoffenders. For offenders, desire to suppress arousal to such stimuli is assumed. Among offenders, arousal in response to deviant stimuli increases while intoxicated, whereas arousal in response to nondeviant stimuli remains unchanged. The reverse is true for nonoffenders. Thus, deviants—who would be expected to try to suppress arousal to deviant stimuli—are less able to do so when intoxicated (see review by George & Stoner, 2000).

George and Stoner (2000) suggest that the widely reported association between alcohol use and sexual risk taking is in part the result of inability to suppress arousal while intoxicated. That is, they argue that alcohol-induced inability to suppress arousal renders a person insensitive and unresponsive to cues that might normally prevent sexual engagement (such as the risk of pregnancy, disease, or sexual assault; see also Abbey, Saenz, & Buck, 2005, for a recent demonstration). Particularly pertinent to sexual coercion, Steele and Josephs's (1990) alcohol myopia model specifies that intoxication causes disinhibition of behavior only in cases in which a person faces strong conflict between instigatory and inhibitory motives. It follows, then, that those who otherwise feel some desire both to coerce and to avoid coercive behavior will experience the greatest disinhibitory effects of alcohol.

Insecure attachment provides yet another source of vulnerability to self-regulation failure. Poor emotion regulation is associated with anxious attachment (see Calkins, 2004; Mikulincer & Shaver, 2003; for recent neurological evidence, see Gillath, Bunge, Shaver, Wendelken, & Mikulincer, in press). Moreover, insecure persons are more prone to use of drugs or alcohol for emotion regulation, which would further impair self-regulation. This can be relevant to rape in that coercion or rape does not always follow immediately upon refusal. The would-be rapist may become angry over either the *perceived* unavailability of a desired partner or actual rejection, later become intoxicated in response to that anger, and then proceed at that point to coerce or rape the victim. Indeed, both major forms of attachment insecurity, anxiety and avoidance, have been shown to relate to alcohol or drug use before or during sex (e.g., Feeney et al., 2000; Tracy et al., 2003).

SUMMARY AND CONCLUSIONS

The model of pathways to rape presented in this chapter provides the basis for understanding attachment-specific pathways to sexual coercion and rape. That is, attachment is assumed to affect the initial triggers of sexual motivation, the overall degree of sexual motivation, perceived sexual self-efficacy, the initial choice of coercive versus consensual strategies to achieve desired sexual activity, effective negotiation of consensual sex, accurate recognition of consent and nonconsent, construals of and emotional reactions to partner unavailability or refusal, understanding and valuing of the consequences of coercion for self and partner, and finally the ability to inhibit coercive urges when they are present. Through examination of the relationship of anxious versus ambivalent attachment to these various components of the model, I have shown that both anxious and avoidant persons are likely to exhibit greater rates of sexual coercion than secure persons. However, although the two different forms of insecurity share some vulnerabilities related to coercion, there are also attachment-related differences that have implications for the internal and external conditions likely to promote coercion.

Common Pathways of the Two Insecure Styles

The common vulnerabilities of anxious and avoidant individuals primarily concern the overall tendencies (1) to communicate ineffectively and negotiate unsuccessfully regarding consensual sex, (2) to misinterpret cues of consent and nonconsent, (3) to construe the meaning and implications of partner unavailability or refusal inaccurately and destructively, (4) to experience negative emotions, (5) to appraise the consequences of coercion inaccurately or to care too little about the likely negative consequences, and (6) to lack the ability to self-regulate and inhibit coercive impulses when they arise. Further, the greater tendency of both anxious and avoidant persons to become intoxicated in sexual situations will exacerbate some of these processes. In contrast, the pathways that differ between anxious and avoidant individuals concern (1) the relationship context in which coercion is likely to occur, (2) the initial triggers of sexual motivation, (3) the initial preference for coercive versus consensual attempts to have sex, and (4) the specific kinds of negative construals that shape responses to partner unavailability or refusal.

Anxiety-Specific Pathways to Coercion

Most rapes take place within established relationships. Indeed, among female respondents in the National Health and Social Life Study (NHSLS) national survey who reported having been forced to engage in sex against their will, 46% reported that this occurred with "someone with whom they were in love"—more than twice as many as the next most frequent category ("someone the respondent knew well"; Laumann et al., 1994). Further, some findings indicate that most victims have reported having sex with the attacker on previous occasions (e.g., 59%; O'Sullivan, Byers, & Finkelman, 1998) and that many victims go on to consent to having sex with the rapists on later occasions (e.g., 40%; Koss, 1998). Finally, some men also sexually assault their wives (9%; Laumann et al., 1994). Apparently, rape often takes place in response to relatively unusual refusals of women to consent to have sex with men they are otherwise intimate with, and this is particularly likely to occur under conditions that seem to threaten the attachment relationship, such as sexual competition from rivals, suspected or actual partner infidelity, impending separation, or even the arrival of competition in the form of a baby (see review by Lalumière et al., 2005).

The evidence reviewed here suggests that anxious persons may be most prone to coercion within established relationships. Because they report having sex to achieve relationship closeness, intimacy, and reassurance, sexual motivation is likely to be triggered by such motives among anxious persons. When a person is pursuing these goals, partner rejection is particularly likely to be perceived as goal relevant and to be experienced as a threat to the attachment relationship. Such a threat will further activate the attachment system, causing the person to desire the reassurance provided by sexual contact all the more. To the extent that coercion is triggered by attachment-related concerns in anxious persons, anxiety should also be related to the tendency to rape or coerce partners under conditions associated with insecurity about the relationship, such as those involving jealousy of rivals (including the arrival of new children), cues indicating that the partner may be about to leave the relationship, or after actual relationship dissolution.

Avoidance-Specific Pathways to Coercion

In apparent contradiction to the previously noted findings in the representative sample of the NSHLS that most women are coerced by someone they love, some studies with college students have shown that sexual aggression is most common in pickup, first-date, or occasional-date situations and that it occurs in more advanced dating relationships in which intercourse has not yet occurred consensually (e.g., Kanin, 1969, 1971). This pattern may fit the "young male syndrome" pattern of sexual coercion discussed by Lalumière et al. (2005) and is perhaps more representative of circumstances in which avoidant men are more likely to engage in sexual coercion—that is, coercion intended to gain initial access to a desired target rather than in response to threatened attachment needs within an established relationship.

In light of the uncommitted, game-playing, "ludic" style of sexual relating associated with avoidance, avoidant persons may also be particularly prone to rape in conditions that appear to violate "rules" such as that consensual petting should lead to intercourse or that if a man spends a lot of money on a woman, he can expect sex. In some ways, the patterns of sexual coercion among avoidant men can be expected to resemble those of narcissists, whereby the view of women as sex objects and the possession of generally adversarial sexual attitudes promotes negative construals of women generally and of sexual negotiations specifically.

These suggestions represent only a few of the many ways my model suggests that pathways to sexual coercion may differ for anxious and avoidant persons. Most of these remain untested, although there is some relevant evidence.

Existing Evidence Concerning Attachment and Sexual Coercion

Unfortunately, existing studies suffer from methodological difficulties that compromise our ability to assess attachment-specific pathways with certainty. Most rapes tend to occur between relationship partners, and these rapes tend to go unreported by the victims and may be unacknowledged by the perpetrators, who commonly distort their perceptions of these encounters (see Lalumière et al., 2005; Laumann et al., 1994; Ward, 2000). Of necessity, most research involves interview or questionnaire studies of those among general populations who *admit* rape and other coercive behavior or of convicted rapists. Convicted rapists may differ from controls in respects other than the propensity to rape and may differ from other rapists in intelligence or other characteristics that render them susceptible to detection. Finally, although some studies distinguish between categories of rapists (usually violent vs. nonviolent), neither these studies nor the self-report studies conducted with college and other general populations assess the many distinctions important to my analysis (such as the initial triggers of sexual motivation, construals of partner unavailability, the relationship context of the sexual encounter, the social context, and so on). These and other methodological issues pose problems for attempts to interpret available studies of attachment and sexual coercion.

Studies of Convicted Offenders

A number of studies have examined attachment among convicted sex offenders, typically in comparison with other violent and nonviolent non-sex offenders. Generally, offenders of all types tend to be insecure relative to the overall population. For example, McCormack and colleagues (2002) found that over 75% of the offender population (including sexual and non-sexual offenders) were classified as insecure, in contrast to normative samples, which tend to be 55% to 65% secure. The authors also found that all offenders tended to report very high levels of negative relationships with parents and dysfunctional family dynamics. Hence, findings of relative insecurity in populations of incarcerated rapists must be considered in light of this relationship between insecurity and all forms of antisocial behavior.

Nevertheless, some distinctive findings regarding rapists have emerged. For example, rapists generally share a number of characteristics with other violent offenders, including a dismissing attachment style (e.g., Ward et al., 1996), whereas child molesters tend to be more fearfully avoidant (see McCormack et al., 2002, for review). These relationships appear to reflect the preferences for lack of intimacy among avoidants who rape strangers, as well as the enhanced needs for intimacy among the child molesters, who court and seek love relationships with children perceived as less threatening, more available, and more accepting than age peers. Baker and Beach (2004), and Smallbone and Dadds (1998), present contrasting results indicating no adult attachment differences between sex offender types, although both studies were based on very small samples, 15–20 and 16 per group. Smallbone and Dadds (1998) nevertheless did find more insecure attachment among sex offenders than among nonoffenders or nonsex offenders and reported differences in parental behaviors consistent with anxious attachment among pedophiles and avoidant attachment among rapists.

Rapists and violent offenders tend to have had particularly negative relationships with their fathers, including higher rates of reported rejection, neglect, and physical abuse, and were more likely to experience disruptions of attachments through death, divorce, abandonment, or sexual abuse (see Alexander, 1992; Craissati et al., 2002; Hudson & Ward, 1997; McCormack et al., 2002; Ward, Hudson, & McCormack, 1997) than other offenders. Overall, the early attachment experiences of all offenders tend to be overwhelmingly negative, but for rapists and violent offenders, the most negative experiences appear to be with their fathers (whereas those of pedophiles tend to be with their mothers; see Craissati et al., 2002; McCormack et al., 2002; Smallbone & Dadds, 1998; Ward, Hudson, & McCormack, 1997). Unfortunately, much of this work involved nonrandom samples, even within incarcerated offenders (e.g., men who were mandated to undergo assessment or treatment, with measures collected under conditions of limited confidentiality) and very small *n*s. Hence, the reliability and validity of such data remain uncertain.

Studies of General Populations

Several studies have examined coercive sexual behavior among college students. Smallbone and Dadds (2000, 2001) examined the effects of attachment to parents and adult attachment style on coercive sexual behavior, antisociality, and aggression. Both studies indicated that insecure childhood attachment was associated with sexually coercive behavior, independently of its association with antisociality and aggression. Secure adult attachment was negatively correlated with sexually coercive behavior, antisociality, and aggression, whereas anxiety was correlated with sexual coercion in the second study and avoidance was associated with sexual coercion in both. Davis (2004) also found associations between both anxiety and avoidance and sexual coercion.

DIRECTIONS FOR FUTURE RESEARCH

I have presented considerable evidence suggesting that insecure attachment is associated with sexually coercive behavior. I have also offered a general model of sexual coercion and have proposed specific pathways through which insecure attachment promotes sexual coercion. Moreover, I have shown that attachment style affects every component of the model. Finally, I have argued, with some evidence, that anxiety and avoidance promote coercion through separate but overlapping pathways. Unfortunately, research to date has not tested all of these specific propositions. Research with offender populations has involved very small and nonrandom samples and has not distinguished between the specific instigators, targets, and circumstances of coercion necessary to test the model. On the other hand, studies of college student samples have involved larger numbers but likewise have not examined the important distinctions. In light of the potential of the model to elucidate when, how, and under what circumstances anxiety and avoidance can separately and distinctively influence sexually coercive behavior, I hope this chapter will serve as a road map and conceptual framework for future research in this area.

REFERENCES

Abbey, A., Saenz, C., & Buck, P. O. (2005). The cumulative effects of acute alcohol consumption, individual differences and situational perceptions on sexual decision making. *Journal of Studies on Alcohol, 66*, 82–90.

Abbey, A., Zawacki, T., & Buck, P. O. (2005). The effects of past sexual assault perpetration and alcohol consumption on men's reactions to women's mixed signals. *Journal of Social and Clinical Psychology, 24*, 129–155.

Alexander, P. C. (1992). Application of attachment theory to the study of sexual abuse. *Journal of Consulting and Clinical Psychology, 60*, 185–195.

Anders, S. L., & Tucker, J. S. (2000). Adult attachment style, interpersonal communication competence, and social support. *Personal Relationships, 7*, 379–389.

Baker, E., & Beach, A. R. (2004). Dissociation and variability of adult attachment dimensions and early maladaptive schemas in sexual and violent offenders. *Journal of Interpersonal Violence, 19*, 1119–1136.

Baron, M., & Ortiz, J. (2002). Apego y satisfaccion afectivo sexual en la pareja [Love and satisfaction with sex in the couple]. *Psicothema, 14*, 469–475.

Bartholomew, K. (1990). Avoidance of intimacy: An attachment perspective. *Journal of Social and Personal Relationships, 7*, 147–178.

Bartholomew, K., & Horowitz, L. M. (1991). Attachment styles among young adults: A test of a four-category model. *Journal of Personality and Social Psychology, 61*, 226–244.

Baumeister, R. F., Catanese, K. R., & Wallace, H. M. (2002). Conquest by force: A narcissistic reactance theory of rape and sexual coercion. *Review of General Psychology, 6*, 92–135.

Baumeister, R. F., & Tice, D. M. (2000). *The social dimension of sex*. Boston: Allyn & Bacon.

Baumeister, R. F., & Vohs, K. D. (Eds.). (2004). *Handbook of self-regulation: Research, theory, and applications*. New York: Guilford Press.

Black, K. A., Jaeger, E., McCartney, K., & Crittenden, P. M. (2000). Attachment models, peer interaction behavior, and feelings about the self: Indications of maladjustment in dismissing/preoccupied (Ds/E) adolescents. In P. M. Crittenden & A. H. Claussen (Eds.), *Organization of attachment relationships: Maturation, culture, and context* (pp. 300–324). New York: Cambridge University Press.

Bowlby, J. (1973). *Attachment and loss: Vol. 2. Separation: Anxiety and anger.* New York: Basic Books.

Bowlby, J. (1982). *Attachment and loss: Vol. 1. Attachment*. New York: Basic Books. (Original work published 1969)

Bradford, S. A., Feeney, J. A., & Campbell, L. (2002). Links between attachment orientations and dispositional and diary-based measures of disclosure in dating couples: A study of actor and partner effects. *Personal Relationships, 9*, 491–506.

Brehm, J. W. (1966). *A theory of psychological reactance*. New York: Academic Press.

Brehm, S. S., & Brehm, J. W. (1981). *Psychological reactance: A theory of freedom and control*. New York: Academic Press.

Brennan, K. A., & Bosson, J. K. (1998). Attachment-style differences in attitudes toward and reactions to feedback from romantic partners: An exploration of the relational bases of self-esteem. *Personality and Social Psychology Bulletin, 24*, 699–714.

Brennan, K. A., & Morris, K. A. (1997). Attachment styles, self-esteem, and patterns of seeking feedback from romantic partners. *Personality and Social Psychology Bulletin, 23*, 23–31.

Brennan, K. A., & Shaver, P. R. (1995). Dimensions of adult attachment, affect regulation, and romantic relationship functioning. *Personality and Social Psychology Bulletin, 21*, 267–283.

Burk, L. R., & Burkhart, B. R. (2003). Disorganized attachment as a diathesis for sexual deviance: Developmental experience and the motivation for sexual offending. *Aggression and Violent Behavior, 8*, 487–511.

Bushman, B. J., & Baumeister, R. F. (1998). Threatened egotism, narcissism, self-esteem, and direct and displaced aggression: Does self-love or self-hate lead to violence? *Journal of Personality and Social Psychology, 75*, 219–229.

Bushman, B. J., Bonacci, A. M., van Dijk, M., & Baumeister, R. F. (2003). Narcissism, sexual refusal, and aggression: Testing a narcissistic reactance model of sexual coercion. *Journal of Personality and Social Psychology, 84*, 1027–1040.

Calkins, S. D. (2004). Early attachment processes and the development of emotional self-regulation. In R. F. Baumeister & K. D. Vohs (Eds.), *Handbook of self-regulation: Research, theory, and applications* (pp. 324–339). New York: Guilford Press.

Collins, N. L. (1996). Working models of attachment: Implications for explanation, emotions and behavior. *Journal of Personality and Social Psychology, 571*, 1053–1073.

Collins, N. L., & Feeney, B. (2000). A safe haven: An attachment theory perspective on support seeing and caregiving in intimate relationships. *Journal of Personality and Social Psychology, 78*, 1053–1073.

Collins, N. L., & Read, S. J. (1990). Adult attachment, working models, and relationship quality in dating couples. *Journal of Personality and Social Psychology, 58*, 644–663.

Cooper, M. L., Shaver, P. R., & Collins, N. L. (1998). Attachment styles, emotion regulation, and adjustment in adolescence. *Journal of Personality and Social Psychology, 74*, 1380–1397.

Craissati, J., McClurg, G., & Browne, K. (2002). The parental bonding experiences of sex offenders: A comparison between child molesters and rapists. *Child Abuse and Neglect*, 26, 909–921.

Creasey, G. (2002). Associations between working models of attachment and conflict management behavior in romantic couples. *Journal of Counseling Psychology, 49*, 365–375.

Creasey, G., & Hesson-McInnis, M. (2001). Affective responses, cognitive appraisals, and conflict tactics in late adolescent romantic relationships: Associations with attachment orientations. *Journal of Counseling Psychology, 48*, 85–96.

Crittenden, P. M. (1992). Quality of attachment in the preschool years. *Development and Psychopathology, 4*, 209–241.

Crittenden, P. M. (1997). Patterns of attachment and sexual behavior: Risk of dysfunction versus opportunity for creative integration. In L. Atkinson & K. J. Zucker (Eds.), *Attachment and psychopathology* (pp. 47–93). New York: Guilford Press.

Crowell, N. A., & Burgess, A. W. (Eds.). (1996). *Understanding violence against women*. Washington, DC: National Academy Press.

Davila, J., Karney, B. R., & Bradbury, T. N. (1999). Attachment change processes in the early years of marriage. *Journal of Personality and Social Psychology, 76*, 783–802.

Davis, D. (2004, October). *Sex in service of attachment and caregiving*. Paper presented at Dynamics of romantic love: Attachment, caregiving, and sex [conference], Davis, CA.

Davis, D., Carlen, L., & Gallio, J. (2006, May). *Attachment, rape supportive attitudes, perceived validity of claims in three rape scenarios*. Paper presented at the meeting of the American Psychological Society, New York.

Davis, D., & Follette, W. C. (2000a, April). *Attachment style and emotional expression in close relationships.* Paper presented at the meeting of the Western Psychological Association, Portland, OR.

Davis, D., & Follette, W. C. (2000b, April). *Attachment, marital interaction: The four horsemen and their first cousins.* Paper presented at the meeting of the Western Psychological Association, Portland, OR.

Davis, D., Follette, W. C., Vernon, M. L., & Shaver, P. R. (2001, May). *Adult attachment style, extent and manner of expression of sexual needs.* Paper presented at the meeting of the Western Psychological Association, Maui, Hawaii.

Davis, D., Follette, W. C., & Vernon, M. L. (2001, May). *Adult attachment style and the experience of unwanted sex.* Paper presented at the meeting of the Western Psychological Association, Maui, Hawaii.

Davis, D., & Loftus, E. F. (2004). What's good for the goose cooks the gander: Inconsistencies between the law and psychology of voluntary intoxication and sexual assault. In W. T. O'Donohue & E. Levensky (Eds.), *Handbook of forensic psychology* (pp. 997–1032). San Diego: Elsevier Academic Press.

Davis, D., Shaver, P. R., & Vernon, M. L. (2003). Physical, emotional and behavioral reactions to breaking up: The roles of gender, age and attachment style. *Personality and Social Psychology Bulletin, 29,* 871–884.

Davis, D., Shaver, P. R., & Vernon, M. L. (2004). Attachment style and subjective motivations for sex. *Personality and Social Psychology Bulletin, 30,* 1076–1090.

Davis, D., Shaver, P. R., Widaman, K., Vernon, M. L., Beitz, K., & Follette, W. C. (in press). "I can't get no satisfaction": Insecure attachment, inhibited sexual communication, and dissatisfaction. *Personal Relationships.*

Davis, D., & Vernon, M. L.(2002). Sculpting the body beautiful: Attachment style, neuroticism, and use of cosmetic surgeries. *Sex Roles, 47,* 129–138.

Davis, K. E. (1999). What attachment styles and love styles add to the understanding of relationship commitment and stability. In J. M. Adams & W. H. Jones (Eds.), *Handbook of interpersonal commitment and relationship stability* (pp. 221–237). Dordrecht, Netherlands: Kluwer Academic.

Davis, K. E., Ace, A., & Andra, M. (2002). Stalking perpetrators and psychological maltreatment of partners: Anger-jealousy, attachment insecurity, need for control, and break-up context. In K. E. Davis & I. H. Frieze (Eds.), *Stalking: Perspectives on victims and perpetrators* (pp. 237–264). New York: Springer.

Davis, K. E., Frieze, I. H., & Maiuro, R. D. (2002). *Stalking: Perspectives on victims and perpetrators.* New York: Springer.

Davis, K. E., Kirkpatrick, L. A., & Levy, M. B. (1994). Stalking the elusive love style: Attachment styles, love styles, and relationship development. In R. Erber & R. Gilmour (Eds.), *Theoretical frameworks for personal relationships* (pp. 179–210). Hillsdale, NJ: Erlbaum.

Downey, G., Freitas, A. L., Michaelis, B., & Khouri, H. (1998). The self-fulfilling prophecy in close relationships: Rejection sensitivity and rejection by romantic partners. *Journal of Personality and Social Psychology, 75,* 545–560.

Dutton, D. G. (1999). *The abusive personality: Violence and control in intimate relationships.* New York: Guilford Press.

Elizur, Y., & Mintzer, A. (2001). A framework for the formation of gay male identity: Processes associated with adult attachment style and support from family and friends. *Archives of Sexual Behavior, 30,* 143–167.

Feeney, B. C., & Collins, N. L. (2001). Predictors of caregiving in adult intimate relationships: An attachment theoretical perspective. *Journal of Personality and Social Psychology, 80*, 972–994.

Feeney, B. C., & Collins, N. L. (2003). Motivations for caregiving in adult intimate relationships: Influences on caregiving behavior and relationship functioning. *Personality and Social Psychology Bulletin, 29*, 950–968.

Feeney, J. A. (1999). Adult romantic attachment and couple relationships. In J. Cassidy & P. R. Shaver (Eds.), *Handbook of attachment: Theory, research, and clinical applications* (pp. 355–377). New York: Guilford Press.

Feeney, J. A. (2002). Attachment, marital interaction, and relationship satisfaction: A diary study. *Personal Relationships, 9*, 39–55.

Feeney, J. A., Kelly, L., Gallois, C., Peterson, C., & Terry, D. J. (1999). Attachment style, assertive communication, and safer-sex behavior. *Journal of Applied Social Psychology, 29*, 1964–1983.

Feeney, J. A., & Noller, P. (1990). Attachment style as a predictor of adult romantic relationships. *Journal of Personality and Social Psychology, 58*, 281–291.

Feeney, J. A., & Noller, P. (2004). Attachment and sexuality in close relationships. In J. H. Harvey, A. Wenzel, & S. Sprecher (Eds.), *Handbook of sexuality in close relationships* (pp. 183–201). Mahwah, NJ: Erlbaum.

Feeney, J. A., Noller, P., & Callan, V. J. (1994). Attachment style, communication and satisfaction in the early years of marriage. In K. Bartholomew & D. Perlman (Eds.), *Advances in personal relationships: Vol. 5. Attachment processes in adulthood* (pp. 269–308). London: Kingsley.

Feeney, J. A., Noller, P., & Patty, J. (1993). Adolescents' interactions with the opposite sex: Influence of attachment style and gender. *Journal of Adolescence, 16*, 169–186.

Feeney, J. A., Peterson, C., Gallois, C., & Terry, D. J. (2000). Attachment style as a predictor of sexual attitudes and behavior in late adolescence. *Psychology and Health, 14*, 1105–1122.

Feiring, C., Deblinger, E., Hoch-Espada, A., & Haworth, T. (2002). Romantic relationship aggression and attitudes in high school students: The role of gender, grade, and attachment and emotional styles. *Journal of Youth and Adolescence, 31*, 373–385.

Follingstad, D. R., Bradley, R. G., Helff, C. M., & Laughlin, J. E. (2002). A model for predicting dating violence: Anxious attachment, angry temperament, and need for relationship control. *Violence and Victims, 17*, 35–47.

Fonagy, P. (1999). Male perpetrators of violence against women: An attachment theory perspective. *Journal of Applied Psychoanalytic Studies, 1*, 7–27.

Fonagy, P., & Target, M. (1997). Attachment and reflective function: Their role in self-organization. *Development and Psychopathology, 9*, 679–700.

Forgas, J. P., & East, R. (2003). Affective influences on social judgments and decisions: Implicit and explicit processes. In J. P. Forgas & K. D. Williams (Eds.), *Social judgments: Implicit and explicit processes* (pp. 198–226). New York: Cambridge University Press.

Frei, J. R., & Shaver, P. R. (2002). Respect in close relationships: Prototype definition, self-report assessment, and initial correlates. *Personal Relationships, 9*, 121–139.

Fricker, J., & Moore, S. (2002). Relationship satisfaction: The role of love styles and attachment styles. *Current Research in Social Psychology, 7*, 182–205.

George, W. H., & Stoner, S. A. (2000). Understanding acute alcohol effects on sexual behavior. *Annual Review of Sex Research, 11*, 92–124.

Gillath, O., Bunge, S. A., Shaver, P. R., Wendelken, C., & Mikulincer, M., (in press). Attachment-style differences and the ability to suppress negative thoughts: Exploring the neural correlates. *NeuroImage.*

Groth, A. N. (1979). *Men who rape: The psychology of the offender.* New York: Plenum.

Hall, G. C. N., & Hirschman, R. (1991). Towards a theory of sexual aggression: A quadripartite model. *Journal of Consulting and Clinical Psychology, 59*, 662–669.

Hamilton, M., & Yee, J. (1990). Rape knowledge and propensity to rape. *Journal of Research in Personality, 24*, 111–122.

Harlow, H. F. (1961). The development of affectional patterns in infant monkeys. In B. M. Foss (Ed.), *Determinants of infant behavior* (pp. 17–52). London: Methuen.

Hendrick, C., & Hendrick, S. S. (1989). Research on love: Does it measure up? *Journal of Personality and Social Psychology, 56*, 784–794.

Hendrick, S. S., & Hendrick, C. (1987). Love and sexual attitudes, self-disclosure and sensation seeking. *Journal of Social and Personal Relationships, 4*, 281–297.

Henningsen, D. D. (2004). Flirting with meaning: An examination of miscommunication in flirting interactions. *Sex Roles, 50*, 481–489.

Higgins, E. T., & Spiegel, S. (2004). Promotion and prevention strategies for self-regulation: A motivated cognition perspective. In R. F. Baumeister & K. D. Vohs (Eds.), *Handbook of self-regulation: Research, theory, and applications* (pp. 171–187). New York: Guilford Press.

Holtzen, D. W., Kenny, M. E., & Mahalik, J. R. (1995). Contributions of parental attachment to gay or lesbian disclosure to parents and dysfunctional cognitive processes. *Journal of Counseling Psychology, 42*, 350–355.

Hudson, S. M., & Ward, T. (1997). Intimacy, loneliness, and attachment style in sexual offenders. *Journal of Interpersonal Violence, 12*, 323–339.

Hudson, S. M., & Ward, T. (2000). Interpersonal competency in sex offenders. *Behavior Modification, 24*, 494–527.

Hudson, S. M., Ward, T., & McCormack, J. C. (1999). Offense pathways in sexual offenders. *Journal of Interpersonal Violence, 14*, 779–798.

Hull, J. G., & Slone, L. B. (2004). Alcohol and self-regulation. In R. F. Baumeister & K. D. Vohs (Eds.), *Handbook of self-regulation: Research, theory, and applications* (pp. 466–491). New York: Guilford Press.

Impett, E. A., & Peplau, L. A. (2002). Why some women consent to unwanted sex with a dating partner: Insights from attachment theory. *Psychology of Women Quarterly, 26*, 360–370.

Johnston, L., & Ward, T. (1996). Social cognition and sexual offending: A theoretical framework. *Sexual Abuse: Journal of Research and Treatment, 8*, 55–80.

Kalichman, S. C., Sarwer, D. B., & Johnson, J. R. (1993). Sexually coercive behavior and love styles: A replication and extension. *Journal of Psychology and Human Sexuality, 6*, 93–106.

Kanin, E. J. (1965). Male sex aggression and three psychiatric hypotheses. *Journal of Sex Research, 1*, 221–231.

Kanin, E. J. (1969). Selected dyadic aspects of male sex aggression. *Journal of Sex Research, 5*, 148–161.

Kanin, E. J. (1971). Sexually aggressive college males. *Journal of College Student Personnel*, *12*, 107–110.

Kanin, E. J. (1985). Date rapists: Differential sexual socialization and relative deprivation. *Archives of Sexual Behavior*, *14*, 219–231.

Karney, B. R., & Bradbury, T. N. (1995). The longitudinal course of marital quality and stability: A review of theory, methods, and research. *Psychological Bulletin*, *118*, 3–34.

Keenan, T., & Ward, T. (2000). A theory of mind perspective on cognitive, affective, and intimacy deficits in child sexual offenders. *Sexual Abuse: Journal of Research and Treatment*, *12*, 49–60.

Kirkpatrick, L. A., & Davis, K. E. (1994). Attachment style, gender, and relationship stability: A longitudinal analysis. *Journal of Personality and Social Psychology*, *66*, 502–512.

Koss, M. P. (1998). Hidden rape: Sexual aggression and victimization in a national sample of students in higher education. In M. E. Odem & J. Clay-Warner (Eds.), *Confronting rape and sexual assault* (pp. 51–69). Wilmington, DE: SR Books.

Lalumière, M. L., Chalmers, L. J., Quinsey, V. L., & Seto, M. C. (1996). A test of the mate deprivation hypothesis of sexual coercion. *Ethology and Sociobiology*, *17*, 299–318.

Lalumière, M. L., Harris, G. T., Quinsey, V. L., & Rice, M. E. (2005). *The causes of rape*. Washington, DC: American Psychological Association.

Laumann, E. O., Gagnon, J. H., Michael, R. T., & Michaels, S. (1994). *The social organization of sexuality: Sexual practices in the United States*. Chicago: University of Chicago Press.

Levy, M. B., & Davis, K. E. (1988). Lovestyles and attachment styles compared: Their relations to each other and to various relationship characteristics. *Journal of Social and Personal Relationships*, *5*, 439–471.

Lisak, D., & Ivan, C. (1995). Deficits in intimacy and empathy in sexually aggressive men. *Journal of Interpersonal Violence*, *10*, 296–308.

Lisak, D., & Roth, S. (1988). Motivational factors in nonincarcerated sexually aggressive men. *Journal of Personality and Social Psychology*, *55*, 795–802.

Lyn, T. S., & Burton, D. L. (2004). Adult attachment and sexual offender status. *American Journal of Orthopsychiatry*, *74*, 150–159.

Lyons-Ruth, K. (1996). Attachment relationships among children with aggressive behavior problems: The role of disorganized early attachment patterns. *Journal of Consulting and Clinical Psychology*, *64*, 64–73.

Mahoney, E. R., Shively, M. D., & Traw, M. (1986). Sexual coercion and assault: Male socialization and female risk. *Sexual Coercion and Assault*, *1*, 2–8.

Main, M. (1990). Parental aversion to infant-initiated contact is correlated with the parent's own rejection during childhood. In K. E. Barnard & T. B. Brazleton (Eds.), *Touch: The foundation of experience* (pp. 461–495). Madison, CT: International Universities Press.

Main, M., & Hesse, E. (1990). Parents' unresolved traumatic experiences are related to infant disorganized attachment status: Is frightened and/or frightening parental behavior the linking mechanism? In M. Greenberg, D. Cicchetti & M. Cummings (Eds.), *Attachment in the preschool years* (pp. 161–182). Chicago: University of Chicago Press.

Malamuth, N. M. (1988). Predicting laboratory aggression against female and male targets: implications for sexual aggression. *Journal of Research in Personality, 22*, 123–132.

Malamuth, N. M., Heavey, C. L., & Linz, D. (1993). Predicting men's antisocial behavior against women: The interaction model of sexual aggression. In G. C. N. Hall, R. Hirschman, J. R. Graham, & M. S. Zaragoza (Eds.), *Sexual aggression: Issues in etiology, assessment and treatment* (pp. 63–97). Washington, DC: Taylor & Francis.

Marshall, W. L. (1989). Intimacy, loneliness and sexual offenders. *Behaviour Research and Therapy, 27*, 491–503.

Marshall, W. L. (1993). The role of attachments, intimacy, and loneliness in the etiology and maintenance of sexual offending. *Sexual and Marital Therapy, 8*, 109–121.

Marshall, W. L., & Barbaree, H. E. (1990). An integrated theory of the etiology of sexual offending. In W. L. Marshall, D. R. Laws, & H. E. Barbaree (Eds.), *Handbook of sexual assault: Issues, theories, and treatment of the offender* (pp. 257–275). New York: Plenum.

Marshall, W. L., Hudson, S. M., & Hodkinson, S. (1993). The importance of attachment bonds in the development of juvenile sex offending. In H. E. Barbaree, W. L. Marshall, & S. M. Hudson (Eds.), *The juvenile sex offender* (pp. 164–181). New York: Guilford Press.

Marshall, W. L., Hudson, S. M., Jones, R. J., & Fernandez, Y. M. (1995). Empathy in sex offenders. *Clinical Psychology Review, 15*, 99–113.

Marx, G. P., & Gross, A. M. (1995). Date rape: An analysis of two contextual variables. *Behavior Modification, 19*, 451–463.

McCormack, J., Hudson, S. M., & Ward, T. (2002). Sexual offenders' perceptions of their early interpersonal relationships: An attachment perspective. *Journal of Sex Research, 39*, 85–93.

McDonel, E. C., & McFall, R. M. (1991). Construct validity of two heterosocial perception skill measures for assessing rape proclivity. *Violence and Victims*, 6, 17–30.

Mikulincer, M. (1998a). Attachment style and affect regulation: Strategic variations in self-appraisals. *Journal of Personality and Social Psychology, 75*, 420–435.

Mikulincer, M. (1998b). Attachment working models and the sense of trust: An exploration of interaction goals and affect regulation. *Journal of Personality and Social Psychology, 74*, 1209–1224.

Mikulincer, M., & Arad, D. (1999). Attachment, working models, and cognitive openness in close relationships: A test of chronic and temporary accessibility effects. *Journal of Personality and Social Psychology, 77*, 710–725.

Mikulincer, M., & Florian, V. (1998). The relationship between adult attachment styles and emotional and cognitive reactions to stressful events. In J. A. Simpson & W. S. Rholes (Eds.), *Attachment theory and close relationships* (pp. 143–165). New York: Guilford Press.

Mikulincer, M., Gillath, O., Halevy, V., Avihow, N., Avidan, S., & Eshkoli, N. (2001). Attachment theory and reactions to others' needs: Evidence that activation of the sense of attachment security promotes empathic responses. *Journal of Personality and Social Psychology, 81*, 1205–1224.

Mikulincer, M., & Nachshon, O. (1991). Attachment styles and patterns of self-disclosure. *Journal of Personality and Social Psychology, 61*, 321–332.

Mikulincer, M., & Shaver, P. R. (2003). The attachment behavioral system in adulthood: Activation, psychodynamics, and interpersonal processes. In M. P. Zanna

(Ed.), *Advances in experimental social psychology* (Vol. 35, pp. 53–152). New York: Academic Press.

Mikulincer, M., & Shaver, P. R. (2005). Attachment theory and emotions in close relationships: Exploring the attachment-related dynamics of emotional reactions to relational events. *Personal Relationships, 12*, 149–168.

Mikulincer, M., Shaver, P. R., & Pereg, D. (2003). Attachment theory and affect regulation: The dynamics, development, and cognitive consequences of attachment-related strategies. *Motivation and Emotion, 27*, 77–102.

Mohr, J. J., & Fassinger, R. E. (2003). Self-acceptance and self-disclosure of sexual orientation in lesbian, gay, and bisexual adults: An attachment perspective. *Journal of Counseling Psychology, 50*, 482–495.

Morf, C. C., & Rhodewalt, F. (2001). Unraveling the paradoxes of narcissism: A dynamic self-regulatory processing model. *Psychological Inquiry, 12*, 177–196.

Muehlenhard, C. L., & Hollabaugh, L. C. (1988). Do women sometimes say no when they mean yes? The prevalence and correlates of women's token resistance to sex. *Journal of Personality and Social Psychology, 23*, 241–259.

Neumann, E., & Bierhoff, H. W. (2004). Egotism versus love in romantic relationships: Narcissism related to attachment and love styles. *Zeitschrift für Sozialpsychologie, 35*, 33–44.

Norris, J., George, W. H., Davis, K. C., Martell, J., & Leonesio, R. J. (1999). Alcohol and hypermasculinity as determinants of men's empathic responses to violent pornography. *Journal of Interpersonal Violence, 14*, 683–700.

O'Donohue, W., Yeater, E. A., & Fannetti, M. (2003). Rape prevention with college males: The roles of rape myth acceptance, victim empathy, and outcome expectancies. *Journal of Interpersonal Violence, 18*, 513–531.

Ognibene, T. C., & Collins, N. L. (1998). Adult attachment styles, perceived social support and coping strategies. *Journal of Social and Personal Relationships, 15*, 323–345.

O'Sullivan, L. F., Byers, E., & Finkelman, L. (1998). A comparison of male and female college students' experiences of sexual coercion. *Psychology of Women Quarterly, 22*, 177–195.

Park, L. E., Crocker, J., & Mickelson, K. D. (2004). Attachment styles and contingencies of self-worth. *Personality and Social Psychology Bulletin, 30*, 1243–1254.

Pistole, M. C. (1989). Attachment in adult romantic relationships: Style of conflict resolution and relationship satisfaction. *Journal of Social and Personal Relationships, 6*, 505–510.

Pistole, M. C. (1993). Attachment relationships: Self-disclosure and trust. *Journal of Mental Health Counseling, 15*, 94–106.

Pistole, M. C., & Arricale, F. (2003). Understanding attachment beliefs about conflict. *Journal of Counseling and Development, 81*, 318–328.

Priel, B., & Shamai, D. (1995). Attachment style and perceived social support: Effects on affect regulation. *Personality and Individual Differences, 19*, 235–241.

Psychological Inquiry. (1999). Special issue, *10*(1).

Psychological Inquiry. (2002). Special issue, *13*(1).

Ridge, S. R., & Feeney, J. A. (1998). Relationship history and relationship attitudes in gay males and lesbians: Attachment style and gender differences. *Australian and New Zealand Journal of Psychiatry, 32*, 848–859.

Roberts, N., & Noller, P. (1998). The associations between adult attachment and couple violence. In J. A. Simpson & W. S. Rholes (Eds.), *Attachment theory and close relationships* (pp. 317–350). New York: Guilford Press.

Safer, M. A., Christianson, S.-Å., & Autry, M. W. (1998). Tunnel memory for traumatic events. *Applied Cognitive Psychology, 12*, 99–117.

Schachner, D. A., & Shaver, P. R. (2002). Attachment style and human mate poaching. *New Review of Social Psychology, 1*, 122–129.

Schachner, D. A., & Shaver, P. R. (2004). Attachment dimensions and sexual motives. *Personal Relationships, 11*, 179–195.

Scully, D. (1990). *Understanding sexual violence*. London: HarperCollins Academic.

Shaver, P. R., & Hazan, C. (1988). A biased overview of a study of love. *Journal of Social and Personal Relationships, 5*, 473–501.

Shi, L. (2003). The association between adult attachment styles and conflict resolution in romantic relationships. *American Journal of Family Therapy, 31*, 143–157.

Simpson, J. A. (1990). Influence of attachment styles on romantic relationships. *Journal of Personality and Social Psychology, 59*, 971–980.

Simpson, J. A., Rholes, W. S., & Nelligan, J. S. (1992). Support seeking and support giving within couples in an anxiety-provoking situation. *Journal of Personality and Social Psychology, 71*, 434–446.

Simpson, J. A., Rholes, W. S., & Orina, M. M. (2002). Working models of attachment, support giving, and support seeking in a stressful situation. *Personality and Social Psychology Bulletin, 28*, 598–608.

Simpson, J. A., Rholes, W. S., & Phillips, D. (1996). Conflict in close relationships: An attachment perspective. *Journal of Personality and Social Psychology, 71*, 899–914.

Smallbone, S. W., & Dadds, M. R. (1998). Childhood attachment and adult attachment in incarcerated adult male sex offenders. *Journal of Interpersonal Violence, 13*, 555–573.

Smallbone, S. W., & Dadds, M. R. (2000). Attachment and sexually coercive behavior. *Sexual Abuse: Journal of Treatment and Research, 12*, 3–15.

Smallbone, S. W., & Dadds, M. R. (2001). Further evidence for a relationship between attachment insecurity and coercive sexual behavior in nonoffenders. *Journal of Interpersonal Violence, 16*, 22–35.

Sprecher, S., Hatfield, E., Cortese, A., Potapova, E., & Levitskaya, A. (1994). Token resistance to sexual intercourse and consent to unwanted intercourse: College students' dating experiences in three countries. *Journal of Sex Research, 31*, 125–132.

Steele, C. M., & Josephs, R. A. (1990). Alcohol myopia: Its prized and dangerous effects. *American Psychologist, 45*, 921–933.

Thornhill, R., & Palmer, C. T. (2000). *A natural history of rape: Biological bases of sexual coercion*. Cambridge, MA: MIT Press.

Tracy, J. L., Shaver, P. R., Albino, A. W., & Cooper, M. L. (2003). Attachment styles and adolescent sexuality. In P. Florsheim (Ed.), *Adolescent romance and sexual behavior: Theory, research, and practical implications* (pp. 137–159). Mahwah, NJ: Erlbaum.

Treboux, D., Crowell, J. A., & Waters, E. (2004). When "new" meets "old": Configurations of adult attachment representations and their implications for marital functioning. *Developmental Psychology, 40*, 295–314.

Vohs, K. D., & Ciarocco, N. J. (2004). Interpersonal functioning requires self-regulation.

In R. F. Baumeister & K. D. Vohs (Eds.), *Handbook of self-regulation: Research, theory, and applications* (pp. 392–410). New York: Guilford Press.

Vrij, A., Paterson, B., Nunkoosing, K., Soukara, S., & Oosterwegel, A. (2003). Perceived advantages and disadvantages of secrets disclosure. *Personality and Individual Differences, 35*, 593–602.

Ward, C. A. (1995). *Attitudes toward rape: Feminist and social psychological perspectives*. Thousand Oaks, CA: Sage.

Ward, T. (2000). Sexual offenders' cognitive distortions as implicit theories. *Aggression and Violent Behavior, 5*, 491–507.

Ward, T., Hudson, S. M., Johnston, L., & Marshall, W. L. (1997). Cognitive distortions in sex offenders: An integrative review. *Clinical Psychology Review, 17*, 479–507.

Ward, T., Hudson, S. M., & Keenan, T. (1998). A self-regulation model of the sexual offense process. *Sexual Abuse: Journal of Research and Treatment, 10*, 141–157.

Ward, T., Hudson, S. M., & Marshall, W. L. (1996). Attachment style in sex offenders: A preliminary study. *Journal of Sex Research, 33*, 17–26.

Ward, T., Hudson, S. M., Marshall, W. L., & Siegert, R. J. (1995). Attachment style and intimacy deficits in sexual offenders: A theoretical framework. *Sexual Abuse: Journal of Research and Treatment, 7*, 317–335.

Ward, T., Hudson, S. M., & McCormack, J. (1997). Attachment style, intimacy deficits, and sexual offending. In B. K. Schwartz & H. R. Cellini (Eds.), *The sex offender: New insights, treatment innovations, and legal developments* (Vol. 2, pp. 2.1–2.11). Kingston, NJ: Civic Research Institute.

Ward, T., Keenan, T., & Hudson, S. M. (2000). Understanding cognitive, affective, and intimacy deficits in sexual offenders: A developmental perspective. *Aggression and Violent Behavior, 5*, 41–62.

Ward, T., McCormack, J., & Hudson, S. M. (1997). Sex offenders' perceptions of their intimate relationships. *Sexual Abuse, 9*, 57–74.

Ward, T., Polaschek, D., & Beech, A. (2005). *Theories of sexual offending*. New York: Wiley.

Weinfield, N. S., Stroufe, L. A., Egeland, B., & Carlson, E. A. (1999). The nature of individual differences in infant–caregiver attachment. In J. Cassidy & P. R. Shaver (Eds.), *Handbook of attachment: Theory, research, and clinical applications* (pp. 68–111). New York: Guilford Press.

Wekerle, C., & Wolfe, D. A. (1998). The role of child maltreatment and attachment style in adolescent relationship violence. *Development and Psychopathology, 10*, 571–586.

Wiederman, M. W. (2004). Self-control and sexual behavior. In R. F. Baumeister & K. D. Vohs (Eds.), *Handbook of self-regulation: Research, theory, and applications* (pp. 525–536). New York: Guilford Press.

Worobey, J. (2001). Associations between temperament and love attitudes in a college sample. *Personality and Individual Differences, 31*, 461–469.

13

How Do Sexuality and Attachment Interrelate?

Goals, Motives, and Strategies

OMRI GILLATH and DORY A. SCHACHNER

There is an extensive body of research on sexual attitudes and behavior (reviewed, e.g., by Hyde & DeLamater, 2003) but almost nothing on the sexual behavioral system itself (its goals, activating triggers, and functions) or on the ways in which its activation interacts with the attachment system to affect adult pair bonding. Although these two behavioral systems (sexual behavioral system and attachment), along with caregiving, have been theorized to underlie adult romantic love or pair bonding (e.g., Fraley & Shaver, 2000; Shaver, Hazan, & Bradshaw, 1988), their interplay has received little attention.

Hazan and Shaver (1987; Shaver et al., 1988) were the first to apply Bowlby's (1969/1982) attachment theory to adult romantic and sexual relationships. Since then, a large body of research has shown that individual differences in attachment anxiety and avoidance predict differences in the ways people experience romantic relationships. However, much less research has been conducted on the relations between attachment style and sexual motives and behaviors, and almost no experimental research has been done on the effects that activating one of these systems has on the operation of the other.

In our recent research we have considered the sexual behavioral system, particularly its goals and motives, within the framework of attachment theory. We have examined how the activation of one behavioral system (attachment or sex) affects the other, and how the two systems interact to affect adult pair bonding. This chapter summarizes some of this research, beginning with an overview of the literature on attachment and sexuality. We next present findings from our correlational studies examining associations between attachment style and sexual behaviors and motives. We then discuss two sets of experiments, one in which the sexual system was activated (or primed) and the effects on relationship- or attachment-related variables were examined and one in which the attachment system was activated and the effects on sex-related variables were examined.

ATTACHMENT THEORY: A BRIEF OVERVIEW

In the epilogue to an influential book titled *The Psychology of Love*, Ellen Berscheid (1988) said: "If someone held a gun to my head and asked me what romantic love was, I would have to say: It's about 90% sexual desire as yet not sated" (p. 373). In the same book, Shaver, Hazan, and Bradshaw (1988) argued that romantic love can be conceptualized as a confluence or integration of three innate behavioral systems discussed by Bowlby (1969/1982): attachment, caregiving, and sex.

Of the three behavioral systems discussed by Shaver et al. (1988), the attachment system has received the overwhelming bulk of researchers' attention (see reviews by Fraley & Shaver, 2000, and Mikulincer & Shaver, 2003). A few studies have related attachment style to forms of caregiving (e.g., supportive, intrusive, or controlling; Feeney & Collins, 2004; Kunce & Shaver, 1994; Gillath, Shaver, et al., 2005) and to certain kinds of sexual behavior (e.g., Brennan & Shaver, 1995; Feeney, Noller, & Patty, 1993; for a review, see Feeney & Noller, 2004). In most of these studies, the investigators have interpreted their results as indicating that individual differences in attachment history affect the way a person cares for others and uses sex to meet a variety of attachment-related needs. It has yet to be revealed whether and how individual differences in sexual attitudes and schemas affect attachment-related behavior and how activation of one behavioral system affects the functioning of the other.

Although both the conceptualization and measurement of attachment style have varied across researchers and disciplines (see Crowell, Fraley, & Shaver, 1999, and Shaver & Mikulincer, 2002, for reviews), most investigators who use self-report and interview measures of attachment style in the context of romantic and marital relationships agree that two primary dimensions are involved. They have been called attachment-related anxiety and avoidance by Brennan, Clark, and Shaver (1998) and self model and other model by Bartholomew and Horowitz (1991). The first dimension (anxiety, or self model) is concerned with fear of rejection and abandonment by romantic partners; the second (avoidance, or other model) is concerned with the degree to which a person feels uncomfortable trusting, depending on, and being close to (i.e., psychologically intimate with) others.

Bartholomew and Horowitz (1991) distinguished among four categories defined by the two dimensions: *secure* (low on both the anxiety and avoidance dimensions), *preoccupied* (high on anxiety but low on avoidance), *dismissing* (high on avoidance but low on anxiety), and *fearful* (high on both anxiety and avoidance). Brennan et al. (1998) and Fraley and Waller (1998) found no psychometric justification for conceptualizing attachment style in terms of natural categories; instead, they concluded that attachment style is better conceptualized as a person's location in a continuous two-dimensional space defined by degrees of anxiety and avoidance. Although there are no clearly defined real categories, Bartholomew and Horowitz's (1991) names for the four quadrants of the two-dimensional space are still useful in describing and interpreting individual-difference findings, and we occasionally use them for that purpose here.

ATTACHMENT AND SEXUAL RELATIONSHIPS

Individual differences on the anxiety and avoidance dimensions accurately predict differences in the way people experience romantic and sexual relationships. People who are securely attached (i.e., are low on anxiety and avoidance) tend to have long, stable, and satisfying relationships characterized by high investment, trust, and friendship (Collins & Read, 1990; Simpson, 1990). They describe their style of love as selfless and devoid of game playing. In the sexual realm, they are open to sexual exploration and enjoy a variety of sexual activities, including mutual initiation of sexual activity and enjoyment of physical contact, usually in the context of a long-term relationship (Hazan, Zeifman, & Middleton, 1994). Secure adolescents engage in dating and romantic relationships, are more likely than insecure adolescents to be involved in long-term relationships, and report a greater frequency of sexual intercourse than avoidant adolescents (Tracy, Shaver, Albino, & Cooper, 2003). Additionally, secure adolescents enjoy sex more than their anxious and avoidant peers do. As summarized by Tracy et al. (2003), attachment security is conducive to intimacy, considerate communication, and openness to sexual exploration.

People who are insecurely attached in different ways behave differently in romantic and sexual relationships. Those high on the anxiety dimension and low on the avoidance dimension tend to become obsessed with their romantic partners (Hazan & Shaver, 1987) and experience low relationship satisfaction and a high breakup rate (Carnelley, Pietromonaco, & Jaffe,

1996; Collins, 1996; Collins & Read, 1990). They are more likely than secure or avoidant people to experience passionate love (Hatfield, Brinton, & Cornelius, 1989) and exhibit an obsessive, dependent style of love (Collins & Read, 1990; Feeney & Noller, 1990; Shaver & Hazan, 1988). On average they display a stronger preference for the affectionate and intimate aspects of sexuality (hugging and cuddling) than for the genital aspects (e.g., vaginal or anal intercourse; Hazan et al., 1994). Attachment anxiety is also associated with concern about one's own sexual attractiveness and acceptability—an extension of anxious individuals' general concern with rejection and abandonment (Hazan et al., 1994; Tracy et al., 2003). In a recent study of mate poaching (i.e., stealing someone else's mate or having one's own mate taken by someone else; Schmitt & Buss, 2001), attachment anxiety was related to believing that one's partner could easily be poached (Schachner & Shaver, 2002, Study 1).

In contrast, relatively avoidant people are less interested than those who are not avoidant in romantic/sexual relationships, especially long and committed ones (Shaver & Brennan, 1992). Like the relationships of people high in anxiety, theirs are characterized by low satisfaction and a high breakup rate (Hazan & Shaver, 1987; Kirkpatrick & Davis, 1994) but also by low intimacy (Levy & Davis, 1988). More avoidant people are less likely than their counterparts to fall in love (Hatfield et al., 1989), and their love style is characterized by game playing (Shaver & Hazan, 1988). According to Tracy et al. (2003), "attachment avoidance interferes with intimate, relaxed sexuality because sex inherently calls for physical closeness and psychological intimacy, a major source of discomfort for avoidant individuals" (p. 141). Thus avoidant people show a greater preference for nonintimate sex (i.e., anal or oral intercourse without extensive holding, caressing, or cuddling) over intimate sex (Hazan et al., 1994).

As adolescents, avoidant individuals tend to avoid sexual relationships altogether. Tracy et al. (2003) found that avoidant adolescents were less likely than their anxious or secure peers to have had a date or to have had sexual intercourse or any sort of sexual experience, and avoidant virgins scored high on measures of erotophobia. When avoidant adolescents do begin having sexual relations, they seem to do so "to lose their virginity," and they report experiencing less positive emotion in the process. They are also more likely than secure or anxious individuals to drink or use drugs prior to having sex (Tracy et al., 2003), which may be another indication of their discomfort with sexual intimacy.

Together, these findings suggest that adolescents who score high on the avoidance dimension are relatively afraid of sex and tend not to enjoy it. Yet, paradoxically, avoidant adults score high on measures of sociosexuality (willingness to have sex outside a long-term, intimate relationship; Simpson & Gangestad, 1991) and promiscuity (Schachner & Shaver, 2002). Avoidant adults express dislike for much of sexuality, especially its affectionate and intimate aspects (Hazan et al., 1994), yet they also adopt more accepting attitudes toward casual sex and tend to have more "one-night stand" sexual encounters than secure or anxious people (Brennan & Shaver, 1995; Feeney et al., 1993; Fraley, Davis, & Shaver, 1998). In the previously mentioned study of mate poaching (Schachner & Shaver, 2002, Study 1), relatively avoidant individuals were particularly likely to attempt to poach someone else's mate, but only for the purpose of short-term sex (e.g., a one-night stand). Interestingly, a second study found that avoidant adults' promiscuity could not be explained by a stronger sex drive (Schachner & Shaver, 2002, Study 2).

ATTACHMENT AND SEXUAL MOTIVES

Only a few studies have examined sexual *motives* in relation to attachment style. A recent study by Davis, Shaver, and Vernon (2004) used an Internet survey technique to investigate the relations between attachment-style dimensions and subjective motivations for sex. Davis et al. (2004) examined specific sexual motives or goals, such as emotional closeness, reassurance, self-esteem enhancement, stress reduction, partner manipulation, and physical pleasure. Attachment anxiety was positively associated with most of the motives except physical pleasure, whereas avoidance was strongly negatively related to having sex to foster emotional closeness and gain reassurance, and it was unrelated to the other motives. Davis and colleagues (2004) concluded that sexual motivation, which powers the sexual behavioral system, is shaped by the attachment and caregiving behavioral systems. They also concluded that sexual motives are activated by conditions known also to activate attachment-related behaviors (e.g., threats that activate proximity seeking).

As an example, among highly anxious individuals, sexual behavior, like its analogue, proximity seeking, is activated when partner availability seems threatened (Davis, Shaver, & Vernon, 2003). Similarly, attachment avoidance includes aversion to emotional closeness and independence, and in the Davis et al. (2004) study, high scores on this dimension were negatively associated with seeking emotional closeness and reassurance through sex.

Whereas this and a few other studies (e.g., Davis & Lesbo, 2000) reveal which motives are negatively associated with avoidance, they fail to identify any sexual motives that are *positively* associated with avoidance. They leave open the question of what motivates avoidant individuals to engage in sex at all. This issue is especially important because, as already noted, avoidant individuals are afraid of sex as adolescents and claim not to enjoy it very much as adults. Davis et al.'s (2004) study examined motives associated specifically with the couple relationship itself (e.g., having sex to nurture one's partner). However, Tracy et al.'s (2003) discovery that relatively avoidant adolescents initially had sex to lose their virginity (which might have allowed them to brag that they had lost it) suggested that their motives for having sex might be related to concerns with self-enhancement and public reputation.

This implication is compatible with other evidence concerning avoidant attachment and self-inflation. For example, Mikulincer (1998) found in a series of studies that avoidance is associated with suppression or denial of negative traits and exaggeration of positive traits following threatening experiences. He interpreted this as indicating a need to convince others of one's autonomous strength and capacity for self-reliance. In a related study, Rice and Mirzadeh (2000) found that avoidant attachment was related to perfectionism (i.e., maintaining a perfect and powerful self). Despite these enticing hints concerning avoidant individuals' sexual motives, there was still a great deal to be learned about relations between attachment styles and sexual motivation.

To delve further into these issues we followed up Davis et al.'s (2004) research, measuring attachment and an array of sexual motives, including ones based specifically on attachment theory (Schachner & Shaver, 2004). Two general hypotheses were proposed linking attachment-style dimensions with motives for having sex, and both hypotheses were largely supported. Findings showed that people who scored high on the avoidance dimension, regardless of gender, had sex for reasons other than ones concerned with their relationship with their sexual partners. Relatively avoidant individuals, particularly those who engaged in casual sex, were likely to have sex to fit in with their social group, to comply with peer pressure, to be able to brag about it, and for other such reasons. They specifically did not have sex to increase intimacy or to express any warm, loving feelings for their partners. In short, avoidant people seem to have sex to gain social power and status.

In contrast, relatively anxious people, regardless of gender, have sex for reasons associated with insecurity and a desire for intense intimacy. They have sex because they want to feel valued and overpowered (perhaps intensely attended to) by their partners and to induce their partners to love them more. Their main purpose seems to be not to enjoy sex per se but rather to achieve a sense of affirmation and allay fears of abandonment. Anxious people, much like avoidant people, use sex to meet needs that are only indirectly related to the sexual behavioral system per se. For avoidant people, status seems to be the main motive; for anxious people, it is proximity, reassurance, attention, and love.

Theoretically, our results are compatible with the notion that some components of the sexual system are associated with, and perhaps even shaped by, the other two systems (attachment and caregiving). This is what we would expect given that the attachment system appears first in development (in the first year of life), followed at a fairly early age by the caregiving system. (Empathy for an injured or needy person, for example, appears as early as age 2 or 3 and is related to attachment security; Kestenbaum, Farber, & Sroufe, 1989.) These two systems are well developed and, in some cases, systematically distorted by insecurities by the time overt sexuality emerges at puberty. The finding that relatively avoidant individuals have sex for reasons other than intimacy and attachment fits with both Bowlby's (1969/1982) idea that the two behavioral systems have separable functions and Diamond's theory (Diamond, 2003; Chapter 11, this volume) that the processes underlying sexual desire and affectional bonding are functionally distinct. Thus, although attachment orientations influence the way sexuality is experienced and expressed, it would be a mistake simply to assimilate sexuality to attachment (see also Berscheid, Chapter 16, this volume).

ACTIVATION OF THE SEXUAL BEHAVIORAL SYSTEM

According to evolutionary psychology (e.g., Buss & Schmitt, 1993), sexuality is associated with a behavioral system that evolved over millions of years, with the ultimate goal being genetic reproduction. Achieving this ultimate goal means having offspring. For offspring to be born, several other events must usually occur, including, in the case of human beings, two people meeting, developing some kind of relationship, and having sexual intercourse. If indeed the function of the sexual system is to achieve this ultimate goal, a person should be motivated to take the required steps when the system is activated. Those steps are: (1) initiating a couple relationship—that is, finding and forming a relationship with a sexual partner; (2) sustaining motivation to have sex with that partner (to ensure the repetition of sexual intercourse, so that even if one copulation does not result in pregnancy, more attempts will occur and the likelihood for fertilization will be high); and (3) maintaining the couple relationship so that offspring have a supportive environment for successful development (see also Brumbaugh & Fraley, Chapter 4, this volume). These steps can be conceptualized as subgoals of the sexual behavioral system.

If indeed these subgoals are part of the sexual system, activation of the system should trigger them and guide behavior toward their fulfillment. Until now, however, there has been no attempt to examine hypotheses regarding activation of sexual-system subgoals. Here, we describe a set of studies in which the sexual behavioral system was experimentally activated and the effects on relationship variables related to the proposed subgoals were assessed.

When conceptualizing the sexual system in this way, the relevance of the sexual subgoals and their fulfillment for the functioning of the attachment and caregiving systems is clearly high. Specifically, fulfillment of the relationship-maintenance subgoal would facilitate parallel goals of the attachment system (maintaining proximity to a relationship partner) and the caregiving system (caring for one's partner and offspring). On the other hand, failure to fulfill sexual subgoals might interfere with optimal functioning of the attachment and caregiving systems.

If our theory about the subgoals of the sexual system is correct, activation of the system should cause a person to become more interested in initiating a romantic/sexual relationship, more interested in having sexual intercourse, and more interested in sustaining a relationship that provides a foundation for continued sexual intercourse and reliable care for offspring. Therefore, we wanted to examine the extent to which sexual stimuli (e.g., nude pictures of age-appropriate members of the opposite sex) activate the three subgoals of the sexual behavioral system and influence thoughts and behavior. Because we assume that personal history shapes aspects of the sexual system, just as attachment history affects adult attachment style, we also wanted to examine individual differences in sexual schemas and their relation to subgoals of the sexual system.

In all, we conducted 11 studies. The first 4 involved selecting and evaluating stimuli that might activate the sexual system. In the next 3, we created a measure of sexual system subgoals (the Sexual Behavioral System Subgoals scale, or SBSS; Birnbaum & Gillath, in press). The SBSS measures individual differences in the levels of participants' agreement with the use of sex as a means of attaining each of the subgoals. The measure consists of four subscales, one focusing on initiation of relationships using sex (e.g., "Having sex is a way to begin romantic relationships"), one focusing on maintaining a relationship by having sex (e.g., "Having sex helps me maintain a romantic relationship"), and finally two subscales focusing on sexual activities as a motivator for having more sex. These two subscales focus on the hedonically positive and negative sides of sex ("Sexual intercourse is great fun"; "I feel bored while having sex"). The final four studies tested specific hypotheses. Each study included an experimental factor—subliminal exposure to a sexual stimulus, or sexual priming—and an individual-difference factor (identification with or endorsement of a particular sexual system subgoal). A different dependent variable was used in each study and was selected to represent one of the sexual system subgoals.

Because of space limitations, we describe only one of the hypothesis-testing studies here (for a complete description of the project, see Gillath, Mikulincer, Birnbaum, & Shaver, 2005). This study focused on one subgoal, using sex to initiate a romantic relationship, which we operationalized in terms of the tendency to self-disclose. This inclination was selected because previous research had documented an association between self-disclosure tendencies and desire to initiate a close relationship (Dindia, 2002). We predicted that a subliminal sexual prime would increase a person's tendency to self-disclose. We were unsure whether a supraliminal sexual prime would have the same effect, because a person's beliefs and attitudes concerning sexuality (the residue of the person's sexual socialization) might alter the effects of the sexual stimulus.

We compared sexual and neutral stimuli in sub- and supraliminal priming conditions, which resulted in four conditions nested within each gender group: subliminal sexual prime, supraliminal sexual prime, subliminal neutral prime, and supraliminal neutral prime. One hundred and eighty-one university students took part in the study. The priming procedure occurred within a computerized judgment task in which participants rated the degree of similarity between two pieces of furniture. In between stimulus pairs, participants were exposed to the sexual or neutral prime. Immediately after the judgment task, participants completed a questionnaire assessing willingness to self-disclose (Miller, Berg, & Archer, 1983), which was followed by a distractor questionnaire. Finally, participants completed the SBSS and provided demographic information.

We obtained a significant interaction between type of stimulus (sexual, neutral) and kind of priming (subliminal, supraliminal), such that only subliminal sexual stimuli caused an increase in willingness to self-disclose. There was also an interaction between identification with the relevant sexual subgoal (measured via the SBSS scale) and stimulus type. People who endorsed the use of sex to initiate relationships, as measured by the SBSS, self-disclosed more after being exposed subliminally, but not supraliminally, to sexual stimuli. In general, then, the hypotheses were confirmed: Subliminal sexual priming, as compared with neutral priming, produced a stronger tendency to self-disclose, and the effect was amplified for people who scored high on the relevant subgoal (using sex to initiate a relationship).

The other three experiments yielded similar results: After exposure to a subliminal sexual prime, participants used more positive than negative strategies for conflict resolution, had better memory for intimacy-related words, and reported greater liking for previously neutral stimuli (a diffusion of positive affect that, when applied to sexual partners, might cause them to be perceived as more likeable). Additionally, in most cases, differences in participants' identification with the relevant sexual system subgoal moderated the association between subliminal sexual priming and the corresponding dependent measure in each study. We therefore concluded that identification with a particular subgoal is not necessary for the sexual prime to affect the sexual behavioral system, but its presence amplifies the effect of the sexual prime. In all of the studies, men and women displayed similar patterns of reactions to subliminal sexual priming, suggesting that, at least at a subconscious level, the sexual behavioral system is universal in nature.

A more general conclusion can be drawn from our research concerning the interplay between the sexual and attachment systems. When the sexual system is activated, and people are sexually aroused, their behavior seems to be guided not only by the motivation to reproduce their genes but also, for example, by the motivation to strengthen their current relationship. A person's identification with a particular sexual subgoal at a given time (e.g., higher identification with the initiation subgoal than with the preservation subgoal), as well as the level of activation of each behavioral system at that moment (e.g., sexuality, attachment, or caregiving), influences the person's behavior. Thus, whereas an attractive sexual stimulus is expected always to activate the sexual system, it can have different consequences depending on an individual's identification with the different sexual system subgoals and a person's attachment orientation. Our initial studies provide preliminary support for the idea that the three systems (sex, attachment, and caregiving) function in tandem and jointly determine relational motives and behaviors.

PRIMING THE ATTACHMENT SYSTEM

Having described some ways in which activation of the sexual system affects attachment-related processes (e.g., self-disclosure and constructive resolution of conflicts with a romantic partner), we turn to a set of studies in which the attachment system was primed and the effects on sexual strategies were measured. The term "sexual strategies" was suggested by David Buss (1989; Buss & Schmitt, 1993) in his evolutionary psychological theory of human mating. Both men and women are hypothesized to have evolved psychological mechanisms that underlie short-term and long-term mating strategies. According to Buss, one can prefer either a short- or a long-term strategy at any particular moment, in addition to possessing a general tendency toward one or the other. There is a gender difference in this preference because men and women in the environments of evolutionary adaptation confronted different adaptive problems in short-term as compared with long-term mating contexts.

Based on previous attachment research, some of which we cited earlier in this chapter, we predicted that attachment security would be associated with preference for a long-term sexual mating strategy (i.e., establishing and maintaining a committed relationship), whereas avoidant attachment would be associated with preference for a short-term, uncommitted sexual strategy. The effect of attachment anxiety on sexual strategies was harder to predict. To the extent that an attachment-anxious person wants to get psychologically close to a partner and be protected and taken care of, anxiety might be associated with a long-term mating strategy. However, to the extent that attachment anxiety causes a person to long for attention, recognition, affection, and so on, an anxious person might be willing to engage in short-term sex simply to make contact with a partner rather than remain alone. Thus we left open the question of the direction of any association between attachment anxiety and mating strategies.

As in the previously reported studies of sexual priming, we included both an experimental manipulation of attachment security or insecurity and dispositional measures of attachment anxiety and avoidance. We expected dispositional and manipulated attachment patterns to have similar effects.

Our objectives were to (1) examine the extent to which activation of the attachment system (priming) affects interest in short- and long-term mating strategies, and (2) examine how dispositional differences in attachment style relate to preferences for the two kinds of sexual strategies. We conducted three studies, in all of which attachment security was manipulated and compared with either neutral (non-attachment-related) or insecure attachment conditions. In all three studies, chronic attachment style was measured with the Experience in Close Relationships (ECR) scales (Brennan et al., 1998), and the dependent measures assessed endorsement of short-term and long-term sexual strategies, measured separately. That is, instead of looking at sexual strategies as alternatives requiring a forced choice, we decided to assess both short- and long-term strategies as two continua. This allowed us to examine shifts in the level of interest in long- and short-term strategies as a function of attachment-related priming.

In the first study, half of the participants received a previously used attachment security prime (WHOTO; Fraley & Davis, 1997, which involves thinking about security-providing attachment figures—the people to whom one turns for help, support, and sharing of successes), whereas the other half received a neutral prime (thinking about mundane daily activities). Following the priming procedure, participants completed a sexual strategies questionnaire. The questionnaire consisted of five items that tapped favorability toward a long-term strategy (e.g., "I'm looking for a potential spouse and hope to get married before too long") and five items that tapped favorability toward a short-term strategy (e.g., "I have no objection to 'casual' sex, as long as I like the person I'm having sex with"). Attachment scores were computed from data collected weeks earlier.

The results included a main effect of dispositional attachment avoidance, such that avoidance was negatively associated with interest in the long-term sexual strategy. A main effect was also obtained for type of prime, such that the attachment-security prime (compared with the neutral prime) led to greater interest in the long-term strategy. Exposure to the attachment-security prime (compared with the neutral prime) also led to lower interest in the short-term strategy. Finally, there was a significant interaction between priming condition and attachment anxiety: The security prime decreased interest in the short-term strategy (i.e., having sex outside the confines of a long-term relationship) mainly among less anxious people.

This finding suggests that although the security prime was generally associated with reduced interest in the short-term strategy, among highly anxious people it was not. It is possible that the WHOTO "security" prime reminded some anxious participants of disappointing relationships. Previous studies have repeatedly revealed correlations between attachment anxiety and negative attachment-related memories, schemas, and beliefs. Perhaps this negativity interfered with what we intended to be a strong dose of imagined security.

Although generally compatible with our predictions, the results of Study 1 can be accepted only with caution, because they might have been due in part to a prime that was both social and secure in nature, whereas the control prime was neither security inducing nor social. We therefore conducted a second experiment in which one-third of the participants were exposed to an attachment-security prime (thinking about a previous secure relationship), whereas another third were asked to think about doing a daily chore *with their partners*, and another third were asked to think about doing a daily chore *by themselves* (similar to the control condition in Study 1).

Once again, exposure to the attachment-security prime (compared with the neutral prime, thinking about doing chores alone) led to greater interest in the long-term sexual strategy. There were no significant differences between the "chores with partner" condition and the other two conditions. One possible explanation for this unpredicted lack of difference between conditions may be that thinking about any activity with a partner, even one as mundane as doing chores, was enough to elicit positive thoughts about relationships and thus a preference for long-term strategies. Perhaps for some people, doing household tasks together is pleasurable and indicative of the cooperation involved in a successful long-term relationship (as opposed to doing chores alone or not doing them at all). Perhaps the shared-chores prime activated thoughts of sharing and collaborating, rather than being neutral.

Exposure to the attachment-security prime (again compared with the neutral prime, thinking about doing chores alone) led to lower interest in the short-term sexual strategy. In addition, attachment avoidance was negatively associated with interest in the long-term strategy and positively associated with interest in the short-term strategy, whereas attachment anxiety was positively associated with interest in the long-term strategy. Although the findings were generally supportive of our hypotheses in both Studies 1 and 2, we wanted to be even more confident that the effects were due to a sense of security and not simply to thinking about the *relationship* with one's partner (especially in light of the lack of a difference between the security prime and the neutral but relational prime, thinking about doing daily tasks with one's partner). Thus we conducted a third experiment in which all of the primes were relationship-related but differed in their associations with security and insecurity.

A third of the participants in Study 3 received an attachment-security prime used in previous studies conducted by our research group (thinking about a relationship in which one felt secure), a third received an attachment-avoidance prime (thinking about a relationship in which they felt avoidant), and the remaining third received an attachment-anxiety prime (thinking about a relationship in which they felt anxious). For example, the instructions for the avoidant condition were: "Try to remember a close relationship in which you did not feel comfortable getting close to your partner, you had difficulty trusting your partner completely and had difficulty being dependent on your partner, a relationship in which you felt tense when your partner got too close, and often felt as though your partner wanted a relationship more intimate than you were ready for."

Results indicated that exposure to the attachment-security prime (compared with the avoidance prime) led to greater interest in the long-term sexual strategy and that exposure to the avoidance prime (compared with the security and anxiety primes), on the other hand, led to greater interest in the short-term sexual strategy. The results also revealed that dispositional attachment avoidance was negatively associated with interest in the long-term strategy, whereas dispositional attachment anxiety was positively associated with interest in the long-term strategy. Finally, there were two interactions between priming condition and attachment anxiety. In the first interaction, the effect of the avoidance prime on interest in the long-term strategy was significant only when chronic attachment anxiety was low. In other words, thinking about a past relationship in which one felt relatively avoidant decreased interest in a long-term mating strategy only among relatively nonanxious people. In the second interaction, the effect of the anxiety prime on interest in the long-term strategy was significant only when chronic attachment anxiety was low. In other words, thinking about a past relationship in which one felt relatively anxious decreased interest in a long-term mating strategy only among relatively non-anxious people.

Together these interactions suggest that highly anxious individuals are interested in a long-term mating strategy regardless of being especially reminded of times in the past when they felt relatively anxious or avoidant. Only among participants who scored relatively low on the anxiety dimension did reminding them of times when they felt relatively anxious or avoidant (in contrast with a group of people who had been reminded of times when they felt secure) cause them, presumably only for a short time, to feel less sure that they wanted to invest in a long-term relationship.

In conclusion, avoidance, whether dispositional or manipulated, was related, as expected, to preference for a short-term sexual strategy. This fits with previous findings showing that avoidant people are less interested in a lasting relationship (e.g., Kirkpatrick & Hazan, 1994). Hazan and Shaver (1987) and Feeney and Noller (1990) found that avoidant adults were more likely to say they did not believe in romantic love and had never really experienced it. They viewed other people as overly eager for commitment and tended to be less committed themselves (Morgan & Shaver, 1999; Pistole & Vocaturo, 1999). They were open to poaching someone else's partner, and when their relationships ended, they tended to experience less distress than anxious or secure people (Schachner & Shaver, 2002; Simpson, 1990). Avoidant people also tend to be more promiscuous, to have more short-term partners, and to hold positive attitudes toward casual sex (Davis et al., 2004; Tracey et al., 2003). All of these findings fit with ours and confirm that avoidant individuals prefer short-term mating strategies.

Attachment anxiety, in contrast, was related to preference for a long-term mating strategy, presumably because of a desire for reliable love and acceptance. Indeed, anxious people have sometimes been found to have relationships as long as those of secure individuals (Kirkpatrick & Hazan, 1994) and to be as committed to their partners as are secure individuals (Pistole & Vocaturo, 1999). However, it is also not uncommon for anxious people to be rejected as a result of pressuring their partners for more love and greater intimacy (e.g., Simpson, 1990). Indeed, in some studies with large *n*s, anxious people's relationship breakup rate was found to be higher than that of secure individuals. Moreover, anxious people tend to break up with and then get back together with the same partner (Davis et al., 2003; Hazan & Shaver, 1987). This tendency to drive partners away may explain the interaction we found between the security prime and level of anxiety. People who are high on anxiety may feel threatened when primed with an attachment-related prime, even a security prime, if it reminds them of negative thoughts and experiences in close relationships. This possibility, as mentioned earlier, fits with previous findings associating anxiety with negative attitudes, activation of negative memories, and negative schemas related to attachment (Mikulincer & Orbach, 1995; Pereg & Mikulincer, 2004).

Finally, we repeatedly found that a sense of security increases people's preference for a long-term mating strategy, as expected based on previous findings linking attachment security with stability and commitment (e.g., Duemmler & Kobak, 2001; Morgan & Shaver, 1999). Relatively secure individuals report positive early family relationships and trusting attitudes toward people in general (e.g., Hazan & Shaver, 1987; Simpson, 1990). Moreover, other studies have shown that security priming increases the cognitive accessibility of a sense of communion (Bartz & Lydon, 2004), benevolence, and altruistic values and behaviors (Gillath, Shaver, & Mikulincer, 2005; Mikulincer et al., 2001; Mikulincer et al., 2003). Our own previous studies have also demonstrated positive effects of security primes on the caregiving system (Mikulincer et al., 2001; Mikulincer et al., 2003). Thus, having one's sense of security primed, even subliminally, seems to reduce most people's insecurity and wariness, opening them to both more humane behavior toward others and greater interest in a long-term, intimate, and committed romantic/sexual relationship. The exceptions to this rule seem to be some of the anxious individuals in our studies, but even for them the evidence suggests that subliminal security primes might be effective.

CONCLUDING REMARKS

The studies summarized in this chapter are compatible with the idea, advanced by Hazan and Shaver (1987) and Shaver et al. (1988), that human sexual pair bonding involves three behavioral systems postulated by Bowlby (1969/1982)—attachment, caregiving, and sex. When two adults come together in a sexual relationship, they are likely to be carrying with them motives and personal agendas related to attachment and caregiving, as well as sexuality. They are likely to be moved by their need for, as well as defenses against, attachment, caregiving, and sex. Our studies also seem compatible with the possibility (Davis et al., 2004) that the attachment and sexual behavioral systems not only affect each other but also sometimes serve each other's ends. Although each of the behavioral systems has its own function, primary goal and subgoals, triggers, and behavioral repertoires, they can influence each other, interfere with each other (as when attachment anxiety or avoidance interferes with caregiving or comfortable, intimate sexuality), or serve each other's purposes. Psychologists from Freud's time forward have realized that love is complex and quite different from the simple "attitude" or "cognitive label" it was thought by social psychologists to be 30 years ago (e.g., Berscheid & Walster, 1974; Rubin, 1970; although see Berscheid's explanation of her part in this history in Chapter 16 of this volume). Romantic love involves at least three behavioral systems that can support or interfere with each other, and all three can be affected in complex ways by a person's relational history. We are still only on the threshold of characterizing these systems in detail, mapping their interrelations, and determining how we might ameliorate or overcome their dysfunctions.

REFERENCES

Bartholomew, K., & Horowitz, L. M. (1991). Attachment styles among young adults: A test of a four-category model. *Journal of Personality and Social Psychology, 61*, 226–244.

Bartz, J. A., & Lydon, J. E. (2004). Close relationships and the working self-concept: Implicit and explicit effects of priming attachment on agency and communion. *Personality and Social Psychology Bulletin, 30*, 1389–1401.

Berscheid, E. (1988). Some comments on love's anatomy: Or, whatever happened to old-fashioned lust? In R. J. Sternberg & M. L. Barnes (Eds.), *The psychology of love* (pp. 359–374). New Haven, CT: Yale University Press.

Berscheid, E., & Walster, E. (1974). A little bit about love. In T. L. Huston (Ed.), *Foundations of interpersonal attraction* (pp. 355–381). New York: Academic Press.

Birnbaum, E. G., & Gillath, O. (in press). Measuring subgoals of the sexual behavioral system: What is sex good for? *Journal of Social and Personal Relationships.*

Bowlby, J. (1982). *Attachment and loss: Vol. 1. Attachment* (2nd ed.). New York: Basic Books. (Original edition published 1969)

Brennan, K. A., Clark, C. L., & Shaver, P. R. (1998). Self-report measurement of adult attachment: An integrative overview. In J. A. Simpson & W. S. Rholes (Eds.), *Attachment theory and close relationships* (pp. 46–76). New York: Guilford Press.

Brennan, K. A., & Shaver, P. R. (1995). Dimensions of adult attachment, affect regulation, and romantic relationship functioning. *Personality and Social Psychology Bulletin, 21*, 267–283.

Buss, D. M. (1989). Conflict between the sexes: Strategic interference and evocation of anger and upset. *Journal of Personality and Social Psychology, 56*, 735–747.

Buss, D. M., & Schmitt, D. P. (1993). Sexual strategies theory: An evolutionary perspective on human mating. *Psychological Review, 100*, 204–232.

Carnelley, K. B., Pietromonaco, P. R., & Jaffe, K. (1996). Attachment, caregiving, and relationship functioning in couples: Effects of self and partner. *Personal Relationships, 3*, 257–277.

Collins, N. L. (1996). Working models of attachment: Implications for explanation, emotion, and behavior. *Journal of Personality and Social Psychology, 71*, 810–832.

Collins, N. L., & Read, S. J. (1990). Adult attachment, working models, and relationship quality in dating couples. *Journal of Personality and Social Psychology, 58*, 644–663.

Crowell, J. A., Fraley, R. C., & Shaver, P. R. (1999). Measurement of individual differences in adolescent and adult attachment. In J. Cassidy & P. R. Shaver (Eds.), *Handbook of attachment: Theory, research, and clinical applications* (pp. 434–465). New York: Guilford Press.

Davis, D., & Lesbo, M. (2000, April). *Gender, attachment and subjective motivations for sex.* Paper presented at the meeting of the Western Psychological Association, Portland, OR.

Davis, D., Shaver, P. R., & Vernon, M. L. (2003). Physical, emotional, and behavioral reactions to breaking up: The roles of gender, age, emotional involvement, and attachment style. *Personality and Social Psychology Bulletin, 29*, 871–884.

Davis, D., Shaver, P. R., & Vernon, M. L. (2004). Attachment style and subjective motivations for sex. *Personality and Social Psychology Bulletin, 30*, 1076–1090.

Diamond, L. M. (2003). What does sexual orientation orient? A biobehavioral model distinguishing romantic love and sexual desire. *Psychological Review, 110*, 173–192.

Dindia, K. (2002). Self-disclosure research: Knowledge through meta-analysis. In M. Allen, R. W. Preiss, B. M. Gayle, & N. A. Burrell (Eds.), *Interpersonal communication research: Advances through meta-analysis* (pp. 169–185). Mahwah, NJ: Erlbaum.

Duemmler, S. L., & Kobak, R. (2001). The development of commitment and attachment in dating relationships: Attachment security as a relationship construct. *Journal of Adolescence, 24*, 401–415.

Feeney, B. C., & Collins, N. L. (2004). Interpersonal safe haven and secure base caregiving processes in adulthood. In W. S. Rholes & J. A. Simpson (Eds.), *Adult attachment: Theory, research, and clinical implications* (pp. 300–338). New York: Guilford Press.

Feeney, J. A., & Noller, P. (1990). Attachment style as a predictor of adult romantic relationships. *Journal of Personality and Social Psychology, 58*, 281–291.

Feeney, J. A., & Noller, P. (2004). Attachment and sexuality in close relationships. In J.

Harvey, A. Wenzel, & S. Sprecher (Eds.), *Handbook of sexuality in close relationships* (pp. 183–202). Hillsdale, NJ: Erlbaum.

Feeney, J. A., Noller, P., & Patty, J. (1993). Adolescents' interactions with the opposite sex: Influence of attachment style and gender. *Journal of Adolescence*, *16*, 169–186.

Fraley, R. C., & Davis, K. E. (1997). Attachment formation and transfer in young adults' close friendships and romantic relationships. *Personal Relationships*, *4*, 131–144.

Fraley, R. C., Davis, K. E., & Shaver, P. R. (1998). Dismissing-avoidance and the defensive organization of emotion, cognition, and behavior. In J. A. Simpson & W. S. Rholes (Eds.), *Attachment theory and close relationships* (pp. 249–279). New York: Guilford Press.

Fraley, R. C., & Shaver, P. R. (2000). Adult romantic attachment: Theoretical developments, emerging controversies, and unanswered questions. *Review of General Psychology*, *4*, 132–154.

Fraley, R. C., & Waller, N. G. (1998). Adult attachment patterns: A test of the typological model. In J. A. Simpson & W. S. Rholes (Eds.), *Attachment theory and close relationships* (pp. 77–114). New York: Guilford Press.

Gillath, O., Mikulincer, M., Birnbaum, G. E., & Shaver, R. P. (2005). *Priming the sexual system: How activation of the sexual system affects relationship goals*. Manuscript under review.

Gillath, O., Shaver, P. R., & Mikulincer, M. (2005). An attachment-theoretical approach to compassion and altruism. In P. Gilbert (Ed.), *Compassion: Conceptualizations, research, and use in psychotherapy* (pp. 121–147). London: Brunner-Routledge.

Gillath, O., Shaver, P. R., Mikulincer, M., Nitzberg, R. E., Erez, A., & van IJzendoorn, M. H. (2005). Attachment, caregiving, and volunteering: Placing volunteerism in an attachment-theoretical framework. *Personal Relationships*, *12*, 425–446.

Hatfield, E., Brinton, C., & Cornelius, J. (1989). Passionate love and anxiety in young adolescents. *Motivation and Emotion*, *13*, 271–289.

Hazan, C., & Shaver, P. R. (1987). Romantic love conceptualized as an attachment process. *Journal of Personality and Social Psychology*, *52*, 511–524.

Hazan, C., Zeifman, D., & Middleton, K. (1994, July). *Adult romantic attachment, affection, and sex*. Paper presented at the International Conference on Personal Relationships, Groningen, Netherlands.

Hyde, J. S., & DeLamater. J. (2003). *Understanding human sexuality* (8th ed.). Boston: McGraw-Hill.

Kestenbaum, R., Farber, E. A., & Sroufe, L. A. (1989). Individual differences in empathy among preschoolers: Relation to attachment history. *New Directions for Child Development*, *44*, 51–64.

Kirkpatrick, L. A., & Davis, K. E. (1994). Attachment style, gender, and relationship stability: A longitudinal analysis. *Journal of Personality and Social Psychology*, *66*, 502–512.

Kirkpatrick, L. A., & Hazan, C. (1994). Attachment styles and close relationships: A four-year prospective study. *Personal Relationships*, *1*, 123–142.

Kunce, L. J., & Shaver, P. R. (1994). An attachment-theoretical approach to caregiving in romantic relationships. In K. Bartholomew & D. Perlman (Eds.), *Advances in personal relationships: Vol. 5. Attachment processes in adulthood* (pp. 205–237). London: Kingsley.

Levy, M., & Davis, K. (1988). Lovestyles and attachment styles compared: Their relations to each other and to various relationship characteristics. *Journal of Social and Personal Relationships, 5*, 439–471.

Mikulincer, M. (1998). Adult attachment style and affect regulation: Strategic variations in self-appraisals. *Journal of Personality and Social Psychology, 75*, 420–435.

Mikulincer, M., Gillath, O., Halevy, V., Avihou, N., Avidan, S., & Eshkoli, N. (2001). Attachment theory and reactions to others' needs: Evidence that activation of the sense of attachment security promotes empathic responses. *Journal of Personality and Social Psychology, 81*, 1205–1224.

Mikulincer, M., Gillath, O., Sapir-Lavid, Y., Yaakobi, E., Arias, K., Tal-Aloni, L., & Bor, G. (2003). Attachment theory and concern for others' welfare: Evidence that activation of the sense of secure base promotes endorsement of self-transcendence values. *Basic and Applied Social Psychology, 25*, 299–312.

Mikulincer, M., & Orbach, I. (1995). Attachment styles and repressive defensiveness: The accessibility and architecture of affective memories. *Journal of Personality and Social Psychology, 68*, 917–925.

Mikulincer, M., & Shaver, P. R. (2003). The attachment behavioral system in adulthood: Activation, psychodynamics, and interpersonal processes. In M. P. Zanna (Ed.), *Advances in experimental social psychology* (Vol. 35, pp. 53–152). New York: Academic Press.

Miller, L. C., Berg, J. H., & Archer, R. L. (1983). Openers: Individuals who elicit intimate self-disclosure. *Journal of Personality and Social Psychology, 44*, 1234–1244.

Morgan, H. J., & Shaver, P. R. (1999). Attachment processes and commitment to romantic relationships. In J. M. Adams & W. H. Jones (Eds.), *Handbook of interpersonal commitment and relationship stability* (pp. 109–124). Dordrecht, Netherlands: Kluwer Academic.

Pereg, D., & Mikulincer, M. (2004). Attachment style and the regulation of negative affect: Exploring individual differences in mood congruency effects on memory and judgment. *Personality and Social Psychology Bulletin, 30*, 67–80.

Pistole, M. C., & Vocaturo, L. C. (1999). Attachment and commitment in college students' romantic relationships. *Journal of College Student Development, 40*, 710–720.

Rice, K. G., & Mirzadeh, S. A. (2000). Perfectionism, attachment, and adjustment. *Journal of Counseling Psychology, 47*, 238–250.

Rubin, Z. (1970). Measurement of romantic love. *Journal of Personality and Social Psychology, 16*, 265–273.

Schachner, D. A., & Shaver, P. R. (2002). Attachment style and human mate poaching. *New Review of Social Psychology, 1*, 122–129.

Schachner, D. A., & Shaver, P. R. (2004). Attachment dimensions and sexual motives. *Personal Relationships, 11*, 179–195.

Schmitt, D. P., & Buss, D. M. (2001). Human mate poaching: Tactics and temptations for infiltrating existing mateships. *Journal of Personality and Social Psychology, 80*, 894–917.

Shaver, P. R., & Brennan, K. A. (1992). Attachment styles and the "Big Five" personality traits: Their connections with each other and with romantic relationship outcomes. *Personality and Social Psychology Bulletin, 18*, 536–545.

Shaver, P. R., & Hazan, C. (1988). A biased overview of the study of love. *Journal of Social and Personal Relationships, 5*, 473–501.

Shaver, P. R., Hazan, C., & Bradshaw, D. (1988). Love as attachment: The integration of three behavioral systems. In R. J. Sternberg & M. Barnes (Eds.), *The psychology of love* (pp. 68–99). New Haven, CT: Yale University Press.

Shaver, P. R., & Mikulincer, M. (2002). Attachment-related psychodynamics. *Attachment and Human Development, 4*, 133–161.

Simpson, J. A. (1990). Influence of attachment styles on romantic relationships. *Journal of Personality and Social Psychology, 59*, 971–980.

Simpson, J. A., & Gangestad, S. W. (1991). Individual differences in sociosexuality: Evidence for convergent and discriminant validity. *Journal of Personality and Social Psychology, 60*, 870–883.

Tracy, J. L., Shaver, P. R., Albino, A. W., & Cooper, M. L. (2003). Attachment styles and adolescent sexuality. In P. Florsheim (Ed.), *Adolescent romance and sexual behavior: Theory, research, and practical implications* (pp. 137–159). Mahwah, NJ: Erlbaum.

Part V

Interfaces between Attachment Theory and Other Perspectives on Romantic Love

14

Romantic Relationships from the Perspectives of the Self-Expansion Model and Attachment Theory

Partially Overlapping Circles

ARTHUR ARON and ELAINE N. ARON

This chapter briefly summarizes our self-expansion model of romantic love and some of the research that supports it, describes links with attachment theory, and considers some similarities and differences between the self-expansion and attachment perspectives and the implications of these differences. We also offer some ideas regarding future directions and a brief note from a Jungian perspective.

THE SELF-EXPANSION MODEL AND ROMANTIC LOVE

The self-expansion model (Aron & Aron, 1986; Aron, Aron, & Norman, 2001) is based on two fundamental principles:

1. *Motivational principle.* People seek to expand their potential efficacy—that is, the model posits that a major human motive is what has

previously been described as exploration, effectance, curiosity, or competence.

2. *Inclusion-of-other-in-the-self principle.* One way in which people seek to expand the self is through close relationships, because in a close relationship the other's resources, perspectives, and identities are experienced, to some extent, as one's own (i.e., the other is to some extent "included in the self").

We first consider the motivational aspect and then turn to the inclusion-of-other aspect.

Self-Expansion Motivation

Aron et al. (2001; see also Aron, Norman, & Aron, 1998) suggest that a central human motive is the desire to expand the self—to acquire resources, perspectives, and identities that enhance one's ability to accomplish goals. This is part of a general motive to enhance one's potential efficacy, which has been postulated in other well-known models of competence motivation, self-efficacy, and intrinsic motivation (e.g., Bandura, 1977; Gecas, 1989; Ryan & Deci, 2000; White, 1959). Similarly, Taylor, Neter, and Wayment (1995) proposed that self-improvement, an idea much like self-expansion, may be an important self-related motive. Like other self-related motives, self-expansion is not necessarily a conscious process. That is, it should not be confused with a conscious plan to "use" others for one's own purposes. Feeling expanded may often be a conscious state (though not necessarily labeled self-expansion, of course). Seeking self-expansion is not generally a conscious motive, although specific acts that will serve that motive may be conscious and chosen with that motive underlying the choice.

Rapid expansion of the self, as often occurs when forming a new romantic relationship, is posited to result in high levels of excited positive affect. This notion is consistent with Carver and Scheier's (1990) analysis of the impact on affective state of rapid movement toward a goal. The model also implies a correspondingly intense negative affect when there is rapid "de-expansion" of the self (i.e., when there is a rapid loss of perceived potential efficacy, as might occur, for example, with the sudden death of a spouse).

These abstract ideas can be made more concrete by considering a measure developed by Lewandowski and Aron (2002) to assess the degree of experienced self-expansion in close relationships. The Self-Expansion Questionnaire (SEQ) consists of 14 items assessing the extent to which a person experiences a relationship partner as facilitating increased knowledge, skill, abilities, mate value, positive life changes, and novel experiences. Example items include "How much does your partner help to expand your sense of the kind of person you are?", "How much does your partner provide a source of exciting experiences?", "How much has knowing your partner made you a better person?", and "How much do you see your partner as a way to expand your own capabilities?" The SEQ is internally consistent and unifactorial, suggesting that these various experiences represent a coherent construct. The SEQ has also demonstrated discriminant and convergent validity in relation to other relationship variables, as well as showing specific theoretically consistent mediational patterns with such variables.

A number of research programs lend support to hypotheses generated from the self-expansion-motivation aspect of the model in the context of romantic love. We briefly review four of them here. First, one implication of the proposed self-expansion motivation in the context of close relationships is that developing a new relationship expands the self. To examine this idea, Aron, Paris, and Aron (1995, Study 1) tested 325 students five times, once every 2½ weeks over a 10-week period. At each testing the participants answered a number of other questions, including items indicating whether they had fallen in love since the last testing. At each testing they also completed a timed task in which they listed as many self-descriptive words or phrases as came to mind during a 3-minute period in response to the question, "Who are you today?" Their responses were coded for 19 content domains, such as family roles, occupations, and various emotions. (Judges were blind to participants' responses about falling in love, as well as to the entire purpose of the research and to any information about the participant.) As predicted, there was a significantly greater increase in number of self-content domains in the self-descriptions from before to after falling in love, as compared with the average changes from before to after other testing sessions for those who fell in love or as compared with typical between-test changes for participants who did not fall in love. In a sense, then, a literal expansion of self took place.

A second study was conducted (Aron et al., 1995, Study 2), with a new sample of 529 participants in which scales were used to measure self-efficacy and self-esteem every 2½ weeks. As predicted, there was a significantly greater increase in these variables from before to after falling in love, as compared with the average changes from before to after other testing sessions for those who fell in love or as compared with typical testing-to-testing changes for those who did not fall in love. In both of these studies, the effects on the self were maintained when measures of mood change were controlled statistically.

Based on this same line of thinking, Lewandowski, Aron, Bassis, and Kunak (in press) hypothesized that the more expansion provided by a relationship before its dissolution, the greater the contraction of the working self-concept after its dissolution, and that this pattern would remain when controlling for predissolution closeness. These hypotheses were tested in two questionnaire studies and a priming experiment. In the questionnaire studies, individuals who had recently experienced a breakup were asked to rate predissolution self-expansion on the SEQ (described earlier), as well as predissolution closeness. Diminished self-concept after dissolution was assessed in one of the questionnaire studies by a direct self-report item, "To what extent did you feel as though you lost part of who you are, as a result of the breakup?" In the other questionnaire study, diminished self-concept was assessed by content analysis for number of negative minus number of positive thoughts in response to the open-ended question, "How were you affected by the breakup of your relationship?" In both of these studies, predissolution self-expansion predicted more diminished self-concept, a result that remained after controlling for recalled predissolution closeness.

In the priming experiment, individuals first completed a task that increased the salience of either highly self-expanding or non-self-expanding aspects of their current relationships and then were led through a guided imagery task in which they imagined breaking up with their partners. For example, the salience manipulation in the self-expansion condition involved the participant spending several minutes thinking about a time in which his or her partner "added to your sense of who you are. That is, the skills and abilities that your partner possessed helped you to improve who you are as a person. As a result of the relationship with your partner, the amount of things you could accomplish, enjoy, and experience increased." At the start and end of the study, all participants completed the open-ended measure of spontaneous self-concept used in the Aron et al. (1995) falling-in-love study, which was coded for number of self-concept domains, as described earlier. The result was a significantly greater decline in the diversity of the content of the self-concept from before to after imagining the breakup for those in the high-self-expansion primed condition compared with those in the low-self-expansion primed condition. This result is exactly parallel (in the opposite direction) to what was found in Aron et al. (1995) for change in diversity of self-concept for individuals who fell in love compared with those who did not fall in love.

Another key implication of the motivational aspect of the model, and one that has generated a number of studies, is based on the idea that the *process* of rapid expansion is affectively positive. That is, rapid self-expansion produces strong positive affect (so long as the rate of expansion is not so great as to be stressful). Because this rapid expansion is pleasurable, in addition to a desire to be expanded (to possess high levels of potential efficacy), a key motivator is the desire to experience the process of expanding, to feel oneself increasing rapidly in potential self-efficacy. This notion is similar to Carver and Scheier's (1990) conception of self-regulatory process, noted earlier, in which people are portrayed as monitoring the rate at which they are making progress toward goals and as experiencing positive affect when the perceived rate exceeds an expected rate. Indeed, they propose that accelerations in the rate cause feelings of exhilaration. Our notion of being motivated to experience the expanding process is also similar to Pyszczynski,

Greenberg, and Solomon's (1997) "self-expansive motives" (p. 6). They argue that people desire the feeling that goes with enhancing their abilities and knowledge and that it is this *process* of expanding that gives rise to this exhilaration.

The major line of work developed from and supporting our principle of self-expansion as a motivator is a set of studies focusing on a predicted increase in satisfaction in long-term relationships from joint participation in self-expanding activities. This work emerged from a consideration of the well-documented typical decline in relationship satisfaction after the "honeymoon period" in a romantic relationship, a lowered level that is typically maintained over subsequent years (e.g., Tucker & Aron, 1993). When two people first enter a relationship, there is usually an initial, exhilarating period in which the couple spends hours talking, engaging in intense risk taking and self-disclosure. From the perspective of the self-expansion model, this initial exhilarating period is one in which the partners are expanding their selves at a rapid rate by virtue of the intense exchange. Once they know each other fairly well, opportunities for further rapid expansion of this sort inevitably decrease. When rapid expansion occurs, they experience a high degree of satisfaction; when expansion is slow or nonexistent, they experience little emotion, or perhaps even boredom. If slow expansion follows a period of rapid expansion, the loss of enjoyable emotion may be disappointing and attributed to deficiencies in the relationship.

To examine this idea, we conducted several survey studies, field experiments, and laboratory studies. In one series of laboratory experiments (e.g., Aron, Norman, Aron, McKenna, & Heyman, 2000, Studies 3–5) dating and married couples from the community came to our lab for what they believed was an assessment session involving questionnaires and being videotaped while interacting. Indeed, when they came, that is what happened—they completed questionnaires, participated together in a task that was videotaped, and then completed more questionnaires. However, from our perspective, the questionnaires before the task served as a pretest and those after as a posttest, and the task itself was experimentally manipulated so that some couples engaged in an expanding activity (one that was novel and challenging) and those in the control condition engaged in a more mundane activity. In the expanding activity, the couple was tied together on one side at the wrists and ankles and then took part in a task in which they crawled together on mats for 12 meters, climbing over a barrier at one point, while pushing a foam cylinder with their heads. The task was timed and the couple received a prize if they beat a time limit, but the situation was rigged so that they almost made it within the time limit on the first two tries and then just barely made it on the third try. In all three studies, as predicted, there was a significantly greater increase in relationship satisfaction for the couples in the expanding condition. The first study demonstrated the basic effect; the second included a no-activity control condition and found that the effect was indeed due to increased satisfaction in the self-expansion condition (and not to decreased satisfaction in the mundane condition); the third study included a short videotaped discussion of a standardized topic before and after the interaction task and replicated the basic finding of increased relationship quality using measures based on blind coding of the videotaped interactions.

The implications of these findings have been further clarified in two additional laboratory experiments (summarized in Aron et al., 2001). In one study, one member of each couple carried out approximately the same crawling task as described earlier by him- or herself, but in one condition the partner was or was not made salient. (The instructions for which way to push the foam cylinder with the head were given in a lit arrow that was directly beneath a TV monitor. In the partner-salient condition, the monitor itself was "accidentally" left on and showed the partner filling out a questionnaire; in the control condition, the monitor was turned off.) The result was a greater increase in satisfaction for those in the partner-salient condition compared with those in the control condition. This suggests that the effect of self-expanding activities on relationships requires that the partner be salient; otherwise, the impact of doing self-expanding activities does not generalize to the relationship. The other additional experiment had couples do tasks that were systematically constructed to be either high or low in novelty/challenge or, independently, high and low in arousal (in a 2 × 2 factorial design). The results showed significant effects for high versus low novelty and challenge but no significant effect for high versus low arousal. (Interestingly, a parallel 2 × 2 study that used the same tasks to study romantic attraction between strangers at initial meeting showed significant effects for high versus low arousal, but not for high versus low novelty/challenge; Lewandowski & Aron, 2004).

Yet another line of work emerging from the motivational aspect of the model focuses on the nature of romantic love. Specifically, we hypothesized (Aron & Aron, 1991) that passionate love is best conceptualized as a goal-oriented motivational state in which the individual is experiencing an intense desire to merge with the partner. That is, we conceive of passionate love as the experience that corresponds to the intense desire to expand the self by including another person in the self. Thus passionate love is not a distinct emotion in its own right (such as sadness or happiness) but rather can evoke a variety of emotions according to whether and how the desire is fulfilled or frustrated. This view contrasts with views of passionate love that consider it an emotion in its own right (e.g., Gonzaga, Keltner, Londahl, & Smith, 2001; Shaver, Morgan, & Wu, 1996; Shaver, Schwartz, Kirson, & O'Connor, 1987). The status of love as a specific emotion has been controversial in the affect literature. On the one hand, it is highly emotional (indeed, Shaver et al., 1987, found that "love" is the first response individuals give when asked to list a prototypic emotion) and functions in many ways like other emotions and thus has been included even as a "primary emotion" in many emotion schemes. On the other hand, passionate love differs from most specific emotions in that it tends to be hard to control, is not associated with any specific facial expression, and is focused on a very specific reward. Thus some emotion researchers, such as Ekman (1992), have pointedly not included it among the basic emotions.

Our own research on this topic has taken three forms. First, in one series of studies (Acevedo & Aron, 2004), participants were asked to check the emotions they feel (from a list of about 150 taken from Shaver et al., 1987) when they experience love or one of several emotions. The basic finding is that many more emotions are checked in relation to feeling love than in relation to feeling sadness, anger, fear, or happiness. Most interestingly, people check many more negative valence items than for happiness or other positive emotions used in these studies. These results have held up using a variety of procedures.

A second line of research (Acevedo, Aron, & Gross, 2006) focuses on the up- and down-regulation of emotion. Preliminary results from interviews and questionnaires suggest that people can down-regulate feelings of passionate love about as easily as they can emotions such as anger, fear, and happiness; however, they find that it is much more difficult to up-regulate (increase) feelings of passionate love than emotions.

A third line of research has examined the neural correlates of passionate love (Aron et al., 2005). Here the hypothesis is that feelings of passionate love should consistently engage brain regions associated with intense reward (such as the caudate nucleus and associated dopamine system) but should be much less consistent across participants in engaging brain regions associated with specific emotions (such as orbital frontal cortex, anterior cingulate cortex, and amygdala). Thus we (Aron et al., 2005) conducted a functional magnetic resonance imaging (fMRI) study with 17 participants who were all very intensely, and very recently, "in love" (as verified by interviews and questionnaire responses). While in the scanner, participants viewed images of their beloveds and of familiar neutral individuals of the same sex and age as their partners. Consistent with predictions, a significantly greater consistent activation appeared across participants in reward areas (but not in emotion areas) when viewing the images of their beloveds than when viewing the control images. Further, the degree of greater activation when viewing the image of the beloved was strongly correlated with a self-report measure of intensity of passionate love, in spite of the considerably restricted range of scores.

Taken together, we think the findings from these three lines of work (greater diversity of emotions associated with passionate love than with particular emotions, greater difficulty up-regulating passionate love than emotions, and passionate love engaging common reward areas, but not common emotion areas, across participants) lend considerable support to the self-expansion model hypothesis that passionate love should be considered a goal-oriented state rather than a specific emotion. This hypothesis derives from the central idea in the self-expansion model that people seek close relationships in order to expand the self by including others in the self and that romantic love represents the experience of a perceived opportunity for very rapid expansion of this kind.

In sum, the motivational aspect of the self-expansion model proposes that a major human motive, which occurs in diverse contexts that includes close relationships, is the desire to expand one's ability to accomplish goals. We have here described four lines of research examining implications of this idea in the context of romantic love: studies of changes in self-concept associated with (1) falling in love and (2) with relationship dissolution; (3) studies of the effect on satisfaction in long-term relationships of shared participation in self-expanding activities; and (4) studies attempting to determine whether passionate love is better conceptualized as a motivational state or as a specific emotion. In each case, we believe the research confirmed predictions from the model, as well as demonstrating the heuristic value of the model for generating novel hypotheses relevant to important theoretical and practical issues.

Including Others in the Self

According to the self-expansion model, this general motivation to expand the self often leads to a desire to enter and maintain a particular close relationship, in part because close relationships are an especially satisfying, useful, and human means to self-expansion. (Although we continue to use the term "*self*-expansion," in the relationship context, typically each partner includes the other in the self, so that the inclusion and resulting expansion is mutual.) Specifically, in a close relationship, each includes to some extent in his or her self the other's resources, perspectives, and identities. Here we briefly elaborate what we mean by each of these aspects of inclusion and how they relate to the self-expansion motivational process. People also self-expand in ways besides including others in the self, a point to which we return at the end of the chapter. But for most human beings, the inclusion of another person in the self is a particularly important opportunity for self-expansion because of the complexity and richness of another human being and because social linkages are so important in our species.

Resources

With regard to the "resources" of the other that are potentially included in the self, we are referring to material, knowledge-related (conceptual/informational/procedural), and social assets that can facilitate the achievement of goals. Perceiving oneself as including a relationship partner's resources refers to perceiving oneself as having access to those resources, as if, to some extent, the other's resources were one's own (e.g., "I can do this because my partner will show me how"). This perceived inclusion of another's resources is particularly central from a motivational point of view because it means that the outcomes (rewards and costs) the other incurs are to some extent experienced as one's own. Thus, for example, helping the other is helping the self; interfering with the other is interfering with the self (e.g., "I'll be quiet while my partner reads the instructions"). This analysis also implies that the other's acquisition and loss of resources are experienced to some extent as if they were happening to one's own resources.

One implication of this idea is that we treat to some extent a close other's outcomes as if they were our own. In the first direct test of this principle (Aron, Aron, Tudor, & Nelson, 1991, Experiment 1 and follow-ups 1 and 2), participants took part in an allocation game in which they made a series of decisions allocating money to self, best friend, or another person or persons. In the first two of these studies, the allocations were made in a between-subject design in which participants were or were not led to believe that the other person would know of their allocations (that is, some participants thought that, although their allocations would affect the other, the other would not know that the participant was responsible for that effect). In the third study (follow-up 2), only the other-will-not-know condition was included. We found that allocations to best friend were consistently similar to those for self, but allocations to others who were not close consistently favored oneself. Importantly, these results held up whether or not the other would know who was responsible for the allocations. Several other studies using a variety of paradigms and theoretical orientations support the prediction from the model that people react to a close other's outcomes as if the outcomes were their own (e.g., Beach et al., 1998; De La Ronde & Swann, 1998; Gardner, Gabriel, & Hochschild, 2002; McFarland, Buehler, & MacKay, 2001; Medvene, Teal, & Slavich, 2000).

Perspectives

The perspective aspect of inclusion refers to experiencing (consciously or unconsciously) the world to some extent from the partner's point of view. For example, when a long-term married individual attends a ballet, the ballet may be experienced not only through the individual's own eyes but also, as it were, through the spouse's eyes. Thus our model implies that when another person is included in the self, various self-related attributional and cognitive biases should also apply with regard to that other person.

Regarding attributional biases, consistent with the predictions of the model, several studies have revealed that the usual actor–observer difference in the tendency to make situational versus dispositional attributions (Jones & Nisbett, 1971) is smaller when the other is someone close to oneself, such as a best friend or romantic partner (Aron et al., 1991, Aron & Fraley, 1999; Sande, Goethals, & Radloff, 1988). These studies were all based on a paradigm originally developed by Sande et al. in which participants rate each of a series of 11 trait pairs (e.g., "serious–carefree") for whether the first, the second, neither, or both are true of a target person. Choosing "both" indicates a tendency to make situational attributions for that person. Consistent with the usual bias, people made more situational ("both") choices when rating themselves than when rating other people in general. However, consistent with the model of inclusion of close others in the self, Sande et al. (1988) found that this difference between self and other was greatly reduced when the other was a liked, familiar person. Focusing specifically on *close* others, Aron et al. (1991, introduction to Experiment 1) found that participants rated "both" for 4.5 traits for self, 3.46 for best friend, and 2.71 for non-close other (friend vs. non-close other, $p < .01$). Further, Aron and Fraley (1999) found that the extent to which participants used "both" when rating a romantic partner was significantly positively correlated with subjectively rated "closeness" to the partner ($r = .21$) and that it significantly predicted whether the couple was still together 3 months later ($r = .30$).

Perhaps a more dramatic illustration of including a close other's perspective in the self is a series of studies adapting a paradigm developed by Lord (1980, 1987). This paradigm focuses on the conceptual perspective of seeing oneself as "background" to experience while seeing other people as "figural." Participants are presented with a series of 60 nouns, for each of which they are to form a vivid, elaborated image of a particular person (self or someone else) interacting with the object the noun represents. Later, participants are given a free-recall test for the nouns. As predicted from his model of self as background to experience, Lord (1980) found consistently *fewer* nouns recalled that were imaged with self as compared with nouns imaged with media personalities. In our studies using this paradigm (Aron et al., 1991; Experiment 2 and follow-up), in addition to self and familiar non-close others, participants also imaged nouns with a close other, their mothers. Our results replicated Lord's (1980) for self and non-close other. But *also*, as predicted from our inclusion-of-other-in-the-self model, we found that nouns imaged with the *close* other were recalled at about the same rate as those imaged with self. This result was found both when the non-close other was an entertainment personality and in a replication in which the non-close other was the mother's best friend. Further, in the replication study we included a measure of closeness to mother. This degree of the effect (the mother-minus-mother's-friend difference) correlated strongly ($r = .56$) with the measure of closeness. (We also assessed similarity and familiarity with the mother, and neither correlated significantly with the effect.) We tentatively concluded from these studies that just as one's own perspective is a background to experience, one's perspective gained through close others is also experienced as a background to experience; and the closer the others are, the more this is the case.

Identity

The identity aspect, as we are using the term, refers to features that distinguish one person from other people and objects—primarily the characteristics, memories, and other features that locate the person in social and physical space. Thus, for example, our model implies that people may easily confuse their own traits or memories with those of a close other. In relation to the cognitive aspects in general (that is, perspectives and identities), we have described our model as implying shared cognitive elements of self and close others (Aron & Fraley, 1999). Referring specifically to the shared-traits aspect, Smith, Coats, and Walling (1999) proposed a localist connectionist model of this principle.

Some general support for the notion that in close relationships we include close others in the self can be gleaned from research on the "self-reference effect," an advantage in terms of memory and response time for self-relevant versus other-relevant processing. For example, in a meta-analysis of 126 articles and book chapters on just the memory aspect of the effect, Symons and Johnson (1997) reported a consistent overall better memory for words studied in relation to self than for words studied in relation to other persons. However, consistent with the inclusion-of-other-in-the-self model, they found that the *degree* to which self-referent and other-referent memory differed was moderated by the relationship to the other. Across the 65 relevant studies, Symons and Johnson (1997) found significantly smaller differences between self-reference memory facilitation and other-reference memory facilitation when the other was someone who was close to the self. Thus being in a close relationship does seem to subvert the seemingly fundamental cognitive distinction between self and other.

However, our model also posits that this apparent subversion by close relationships of the self–other distinction is due, specifically, to the other becoming "part of the self"—to the very structure of the self changing, such that the self includes the other in its very makeup. For example, the model implies that one's own and a close other's traits may actually be confused or interfere with each other. To test this idea, we evaluated the patterns of response latencies in making "me/not me" decisions (that is, "does the trait describe me?") about traits previously rated for their descriptiveness of self and of spouse (Aron et al., 1991, Experiment 3 and follow-up). We found that for traits on which the self matched the partner (the trait was true of both or false of both), "me/not-me" responses were faster and had fewer errors than for traits were mismatched for self and partner (was true for one but false for the other). Further, Aron and Fraley (1999) found that the degree of this match–mismatch response-time effect (serving as a measure of overlap of self and other) correlates significantly with self-report measures of relationship quality and significantly predicts increases in subjective closeness over a 3-month period. Using this same response-time paradigm, Smith et al. (1999) replicated both the overall difference between close and non-close others and the correlation with the magnitude of self-reported closeness to the close other. Smith and colleagues eloquently articulated the reason such patterns may result: "If mental representations of two persons . . . overlap so that they are effectively a single representation, reports on attributes of one will be facilitated or inhibited by matches and mismatches with the second" (1999, p. 873).

Another series of studies (Mashek, Aron, & Boncimino, 2003) focused on the model's prediction that people especially confuse information associated with self with information associated with close others. In these studies, participants rated one set of traits for self, a different set of traits for a close other, and still other traits for one or more familiar non-close others. Participants were then administered a surprise recognition task in which participants were presented with each trait and asked to indicate for which person they had rated it. The focus of the analysis was on confusions—traits the participant remembered having rated for one person when it had actually been rated for a different person. The results were consistent with predictions. For example, if participants did not correctly recognize a trait as having been originally rated for the self, they were significantly more likely to remember it as having been rated for the partner than as having been rated for a media personality. Similarly, if participants did not correctly recognize a trait as having been originally rated for the partner, they were significantly more likely to remember it as having been rated for the self than as having been rated for the media personality. These results were replicated in two follow-up studies and held up after controlling for a variety of potential confounds, such as a greater tendency to see traits in general as having been rated for self, valence and extremity of ratings, and familiarity with and similarity to the close other.

Finally, focusing on the issue of the perceived overlap of one's identity with a relationship partner, we asked participants to describe their closest relationship using the Inclusion of Other in the Self (IOS) Scale (Aron, Aron, & Smollan, 1992). The IOS Scale consists of seven pairs of circles overlapping to different degrees, from which the respondent selects the pair (the degree of overlap) that best describes his or her relationship with a particular person. The scale has been shown to have high levels of reliability, as well as of discriminant, convergent, and predictive validity—levels that match or exceed those of other measures of closeness, measures that are typically more complex and lengthy. Since its development, the scale has been used effectively in a number of studies of relationships (for a review, see Agnew, Loving, Le, & Goodfriend, 2004) and correlates with such nonobvious measures as the effect size in the match–mismatch response-time paradigm (e.g., Aron & Fraley, 1999) and the number of plural pronouns such as "we" and "us" used spontaneously in descriptions of one's relationship with the close other (Agnew, Van Lange, Rusbult, & Langston, 1998). Perhaps this measure has been so successful because the metaphor of overlapping circles representing self and other corresponds to how people actually process information about self and other in relationships.

Most recently, we have also obtained preliminary data suggesting an overlap of the neural systems related to self and close others (Aron, Whitfield, & Lichty, in press) in an fMRI study. In this study, participants heard their own names, the name of a familiar other (such as a sibling or friendly acquaintance), and common names that did not refer to people well known to the participant. Participants also indicated their closeness to the familiar other on a questionnaire. The finding of present interest was that the degree of rated closeness to the familiar other predicted significantly greater similarity in the overall pattern of brain activation when hearing one's own name and when hearing the familiar other's name as compared with the similarity in the overall pattern of brain activation when hearing one's own name and when hearing a common name of a stranger.

In sum, the inclusion-of-other-in-the-self aspect of the model posits that in a close relationship each treats the other's resources, perspectives, and identities to some extent as one's own. These ideas have been supported in a number of studies using diverse methods, including self-reports, allocation tasks, memory and response-time procedures, and neuroimaging.

SOME LINKS OF THE SELF-EXPANSION MODEL WITH ATTACHMENT THEORY

Links with Self-Expansion Motivation

We note that Bowlby's (1969) basic idea, as expressed in the secure-base scenario, assumes an exploration motive that we would describe as self-expansion. Further, the different mental models that are developed can be understood as different solutions to the need for self-expansion, given an individual's attachment experience. A secure model is one in which a person is confident of support during self-expansion. An avoidant model is one in which one has learned that intimate others cannot be counted on to provide a secure base for self-expansion (although self-expansion can still proceed by "bracketing" the need for intimate others and substituting for them nonintimate others, who can be safely used for self-expansion). A preoccupied or anxious–ambivalent model is one in which the person has learned that the availability of a secure base is tentative and can be withdrawn at any time (so that self-expansion proceeds through continued efforts to develop a secure base and acquire the support and approval of some intimate other to permit further self-expansion).

There are two relevant studies that bear on these issues. First, Aron, Aron, and Allen (1998) conducted a large questionnaire study focusing on unreciprocated love. Based on the self-expansion model, they hypothesized that intensity of unrequited love would be predicted by three motivational factors: (1) perceived desirability of the partner and a relationship with that partner (e.g., "How perfect is this person in your eyes?"), (2) desirability of the state of being in love even if it is unrequited (e.g., "There is a saying 'Better to have loved in vain than never to have loved at all.' To what extent to do you agree with this?"), and (3) perceived probability at the time of falling in love that a relationship would eventually develop ("Even though you don't feel this person loves you as much as you would like, to what extent has this person done things that would make most people think he or she loves you?"). As predicted, each of these factors was a significant unique predictor of intensity of unrequited love.

In the present context, what is most interesting is that we also predicted that the relative importance of these motivational factors would differ as a function of attachment style. First, we predicted that although desirability of the specific partner/relationship would be most important for everyone, it would be especially important for attachment-anxious individuals because their parents' and/or previous romantic partners' inconsistent caregiving provided random reinforcement that led to strong idealization of the other, especially when the other was not available. This prediction was strongly supported (standardized estimates in the structural equation model that included all three predictors from desirability of partner/relationship to love intensity were .95 for anxious participants compared with .42 and .32, respectively, for secure and avoidant participants). Second, we predicted that desirability of the state of being in unrequited love would be especially important for avoidant individuals, who would be expected to have little desire actually to have a relationship. Thus their reason for being in unrequited love would be more likely to be due to wanting the excitement and role of being in love without actually having to be in a relationship. This prediction was also supported (.35 for avoidant participants vs. .06 and –.26, respectively, for secure and anxious participants). The prediction for probability was not supported (secures were not significantly more likely to be in unrequited love because they initially mistakenly believed love was reciprocated).

Also consistent with our general line of thinking, the proportion of the sample that had experienced unreciprocated love differed significantly across attachment styles in the predicted way: It was highest for anxious participants (89%), second highest for avoidant participants (78%), and lowest for secure participants (74%). (The reason we had expected avoidant individuals to have levels of unrequited love as high or higher than secure individuals was that unrequited love provides avoidant people an opportunity to experience the culturally valued state of being in love without actual fear of a relationship.)

A second line of research linking self-expansion motivation to attachment theory is an exploratory analysis we conducted (in collaboration with Shaver and Mikulincer; Aron et al., 2004) on differences in brain activation as a function of attachment dimensions in the fMRI passionate-love study described earlier (Aron et al., 2005). The main finding was that avoidant attachment, after controlling for the negative association of avoidance with overall intensity of love, predicted activation in visual areas when viewing one's beloved. Our interpretation of this result was that when avoidant people experience intense love, because it is less likely to be motivated by the desire for personal merger, it is instead motivated by the physical appearance of the partner. Thus if an avoidant person and a nonavoidant person experience equal levels of intense love, the avoidant person is likely to be attending more to physical appearance.

Links with Including Others in the Self

As suggested by the preceding finding, we believe that attachment styles affect how much the inclusion of another in the self is used as a means of self-expansion. We expect secure individuals to be comfortable including others in the self. Avoidant individuals would find other ways to expand the self, and anxious individuals, in the interest of solidifying an inconsistently secure base, would be most motivated to include another.

One relevant result is from a study (Aron, Melinat, Aron, Vallone, & Bator, 1997) in which we randomly assigned 152 individuals to pairings representing different attachment style combinations. Each pair then participated in a 45-minute series of relationship-building activities that we have found in several studies to generate high levels of closeness among most participants, including high levels of including the task partner in the self. This was also true in the 1997 study. However, consistent with the reasoning outlined earlier, the degree of inclusion of the partner in the self was moderated by attachment style. Pairs of avoidant individuals became substantially less close and included other in the self substantially less than any of the other pairings. When anxious individuals were paired with secure partners, they did not differ very much from secure individuals in how close they became with their partners, but they were much less satisfied with this degree of closeness than were either secure or avoidant people. That is, anxious people substantially included their partners in the self, but they were dissatisfied that they had not included even more of the partner in the self. One other finding from this study is relevant to the present context: All groups showed an overall decrease in avoidance from before to after the closeness-generating task, and this decline was especially strong for people who scored relatively high on avoidance at the outset. Consistent with studies of the effects of security priming on people with different attachment styles (summarized by Gillath, Shaver, & Mikulincer, 2005), this suggests that even short-term experiences that increase or prime security can create at least temporary changes in adult relationship orientations.

Some New Possibilities

Thinking about links between the self-expansion model and attachment theory in developing this chapter suggested several potentially fruitful directions for attachment theorists that arise when attachment is considered in the context of the self-expansion model. (There are also new ways of thinking that arise for self-expansion theorists when considering attachment, some of which led to some of the studies described earlier. However, the focus of this volume is on attachment theory, and thus this chapter's aim is to show how the self-expansion model may contribute to attachment theory.)

One such possibility concerns the emphasis that attachment theorists have placed on attachment figures as providing a secure base for exploring the world. From the perspective of the self-expansion model, we suggest that it may be fruitful to think of the most important exploration (and self-expansion) being not of the world in general but into and with the attachment figure. That is, including the attachment figure in the self is at least as important for self-expansion as exploring the environment.

Another possibility is that attachment theory traditionally emphasizes that insecure attachment undermines relationships and inhibits exploration and is thus maladaptive. From the perspective of the self-expansion model, we suggest that sometimes avoidance, in particular, may represent a greater desire or perceived opportunity for self-expansion through nonrelationship domains. That is, some individuals with special talents or interests may discover that other avenues of self-expansion, such as art or science or political action, are available, enjoyable, and perhaps preferred over self-expansion through close relationships.

A FINAL, JUNGIAN NOTE

In an effort to expand attachment theory, we discuss what may be its Jungian "shadow." Discussions of the shadow are not meant to focus on flaws or failings but to bring back into consciousness what has been ignored or repressed. After all, a concept's "unthinkable" opposite, relegated to the unconscious, is often the surest path to its further development, as when Einstein found answers in Newton's unthinkable thoughts and Bohr found them in Einstein's. Knowing the shadow helps us "hold the tension of the opposites," as Jungians like to say, until a new conscious position breaks through, providing a significant change in perspective (see Jung, 1979, under "opposites, tension of").

Thus in a spirit of helpfulness we have wondered, when reading reports comparing secure and insecure adults, whether the secure adults are seen in such a positive light, almost bordering on deification, that a long shadow is indeed cast. Actually, Jungians would argue that the deity is not an adult but the archetype of the Divine Child, which always casts two shadows: first, its perfection at birth; and second, the glorification of childhood over adulthood as the prime developmental period.

Why would we as a culture want a Divine Child? Such a child has always been the redeemer of mankind, the eventual innocent sacrifice for the sins of ruined adults. In our own culture, how good it would be to have a leader unalienated from nature and free of lies, cynicism, overemphasized intellect, and convoluted political plots. Part of the myth of the Divine Child, the Redeemer, is that he is born perfect, only needing to be raised by humble, devoted caregivers who do not obstruct the unfolding of his divine nature. With time and nothing else, this secure child will become the wise, heroic, compassionate adult we need. Another part of the myth is that an archetypal evil, in the form of a child-killing king, is always waiting in the wings: Jesus had Mary and Joseph to hide him from the child-killing King Herod; Moses had the pharoah's daughter to hide him from the child-killing pharoah; Krishna had Yasoda and Nanda to hide him from the child-killing King Kamsa. One Jungian, Guggenbuhl-Craig (1990), described how this myth plays out in our culture's complex about child sexual abuse and incest, in which our pure, innocent Divine Child is threatened by near or actual satanic child abusers. Perhaps attachment theory is more sophisticated in that we are hoping our redeemers will be raised by the good parent in all of us, saved from the child killer in all of us that could lead to insecure, disorganized attachments through our own inconsistency, neglect, and abuse of the inner and outer child, in whatever way was done to us by our parents.

In whatever form, the myth of the Divine Child, with the idyllic childhood sheltered from the lurking child-killer king, is what has been constellated—that is, the idea has gathered unconscious collective energy, becoming a collective complex—whenever humans seek redemption through an emphasis on a child's development. In a scientific community the resulting adult is described in scientific terms, of course, but still rings of the redemptive savior. Here is an example:

> Studies have shown that individuals classified as securely attached displayed less emotional distress and negative affect . . . , fewer physical symptoms . . . , and lower fear of death. . . . With respect to interpersonal functioning, people who report more secure attachments have been found to be more willing to seek support when needed . . . and to have relation-

> ships characterized by more positive affect . . . and more stability . . . as well as by greater trust, commitment, satisfaction, and interdependence. . . . Indeed, the benefits of attachment security among adults are so widespread that . . . consider it a general resilience factor across the life span. (La Guardia, Ryan, Couchman, & Deci, 2000, p. 367)

Returning to the first "shadow" cast by the Divine Child on attachment theory, we see an implication that if caregivers provide the right conditions, a child's personality blossoms like the ideal flower, a flower always of the same species (although some variations due to local conditions are granted). But in fact, there are numerous species of flowers—the different temperaments that infants evidence at birth, some of them very difficult or at least a poor fit with their parents, who might be secure and otherwise competent caregivers. A highly reactive infant, screaming because of the slightest rough handling, or a toddler blossoming into a child with ADHD is not our image of the Divine Child, but these children are also born and have to be raised, too.

Further, the vision of the perfect infant unfolding under the watchful eye of humble, sensitive parents protecting the child from human evil also overlooks the fact, from a psychodynamic as well as a "new unconscious" point of view, that all children are exposed to and internalize their caregivers' unconscious complexes (implicit emotional schemas) because all humans have them. These complexes and schemas are not inherently "bad." Rather, they are the building blocks of personality. But they create wonderful variation, as well as sometimes causing astounding trouble when we deny their existence. Specifically, one complex that even the most secure adult must have is organized around attachment—fears of loss, betrayal, abandonment. (Indeed, priming research suggests that an insecure mental model is available to everyone.) Certainly their secure children eventually acquire this complex of insecurity, along with their parents' more or less mature coping strategies, just as children learn from their parents to believe and then not to believe in Santa Claus. But there are many other complexes that pass from generation to generation, like fleas jumping from a mother rat onto her pups as they emerge from the womb. Thus the human Divine Child is made entirely mortal, even if also as able as the parent to bite at or ignore its fleas.

Jungians, however, would see this lack of perfection in even the most secure adult as a blessing of sorts. Identification of oneself or of others with an archetype such as the Divine Child invariably leads to dangerous inflation or deflation—worship or crucifixion. Moreover, something important, the potential wholeness of life, is left out of the perfectly secure life. We would not wish onto any child the terror, rage, despair, hate, and other scars that come from having been neglected, not seen, rejected, betrayed, or abused. But they are part of a universal, archetypal experience, and thinking in alchemical terms, as Jungians do, the making of the philosopher's stone always begins with the grossest possible material.

Jung liked to point out that the only attribute missing in perfection is wholeness, because wholeness must include imperfection (e.g., Jung, 1970, paragraph 616). The danger of the pursuit of perfection is self-righteousness and the dangerous one-sidedness that usually leads, eventually, to psychotic-like behaviors. People who cannot see their own shadows, their imperfections, are also incredibly boring. So we do not want, hiding between the lines of our results sections, a bias against those potentially more whole adults who have or could have struggled with their insecure attachments and distorted mental models until, during that process, they acquired some wholeness of consciousness.

To us, some of this problem of attachment theory's underappreciation of the person less perfect but more whole is resolved by the idea of the somewhat mysterious "earned secure"—those "discordant" adults who report unsupportive early attachments yet score high on security (Berlin & Cassidy, 1999). Various explanations for their existence have been offered, including Mary Main's (1991) idea that they may have been resilient due to strong, innate metacognitive skills. In informal conversations, we have found that many attachment researchers seem to view the earned-secure individuals they have known as products of psychotherapy or some very unusually therapeutic relationship with a secure partner. That is, most of them were consciously involved in a lengthy process of testing and revising their mental models because of another person who gave them the security they had lacked before. Indeed, we find that these consciously earned-secure individuals, however they became that way, can have a level of depth and insight rarely found in those who have been continuously secure. We might imagine that it is because they are less perfect but more whole.

Of course, no one is whole, any more than they are perfect, but there are reasons for imagining that earned-secure individuals merit more attention and respect besides that they are interesting. Becoming secure by definition implies a project undertaken in adulthood, which leads us to the second problem with the Divine Child archetype: It reduces the value of adulthood, especially in the second half of life, when all things childish do or should fall away. The potential for adult influences on attachment has been emphasized from the start of adult attachment research. Hazan and Shaver (1987) noted that "attachment theory includes the idea that social development involves the continual construction, revision, integration, and abstraction of mental models. This idea, which is similar to the notion of scripts and schemas in cognitive social psychology . . . is compatible with the possibility of change based on new information and experiences" (p. 523). However, our impression is that this emphasis has been honored mainly in the breach.

Only humans live half of their lives after their drive to carry on their

DNA has either ceased (females) or waned (males). Jung (1969) seems to be right in saying that the creation of culture "is the meaning and purpose of the second half of life" (p. 400, paragraph 787; see also Jung, 1979, under "life, stages of, afternoon/second half of"). It is the time when the personality almost insists on reversing itself, turning inward rather than outward, emphasizing the growth of inner character over outer achievement. Those who are unable to make this turn, according to Jung, "prefer to be hypochondriacs, niggards, pedants, applauders of the past, or else eternal adolescents—all lamentable substitutes for the illumination of the self, but inevitable consequences of the delusion that the second half of life must be governed by the principles of the first" (1969, p. 399, paragraph 785). It seems highly unlikely that the first 2 years of life completely determine success in the last 40 or 50 years of life. Indeed, it would be interesting to test whether insecure people are even slightly more motivated than secure people to achieve some "illumination of the self" in the second half of life, being compelled to find meaning in their psychological symptoms, relationship failures, negative emotions, and general suffering. (The scientist being honored by this volume might be a case in point.)

If the purpose of the human's long second half of life is that it allows for cultural evolution (probably made possible by our use of language), it is likely that this cultural evolution will be decisive for the species. Most primates, and humans in the first half of life, seem to have a strong predilection to engage in aggressive dominance seeking for themselves and their ingroup. (Others have noted that a nation's ultimate weapon need not be nuclear—a radio station will do, convincing their young men, armed only with knives, that the enemy must be destroyed.) Research on primates and humans suggests that those with insecure attachments in childhood, besides suffering and causing others to suffer, will be unusually cruel toward others or else unusually submissive. Both "natural" and learned aggressive behaviors contribute to more social disruption, as well as another generation of insecure offspring. It seems that this mayhem could be best controlled through the influence of those who are older and therefore less involved, as well as more conscious of the consequences. But such control can come only through continuing experience with developing insecure people into wise, mature earned-secure people. Thus it may be that, compared with the mean contribution of continuously secure adults, insecure adults who manage to become earned-secure adults and can reflect on their development (or whose development we can reflect on) may have the most to offer civilization.

SUMMARY AND CONCLUSION

In this chapter, we first briefly summarized the two main themes of the self-expansion model—self-expansion motivation and including other in the self—as they apply to romantic love. We also summarized the body of research supporting these two aspects of the model. On this foundation, we then considered links between the two themes of this model and attachment theory, in each case exploring relevant research findings, as well as offering some possible but as yet relatively unexplored directions for attachment theory that are suggested by the self-expansion perspective. Finally, we included some ideas and cautions suggested by a Jungian perspective. Our hope is that all of us who study romantic love, including those who focus on attachment and those who focus on self-expansion processes, will expand by including what is most useful in each other's theoretical approaches into our own theoretical selves.

REFERENCES

Acevedo, B., & Aron, A. (2004, January). *Love: More than just a feeling?* Paper presented at the annual meeting of the Society for Personality and Social Psychology, Austin, TX.

Acevedo, B., Gross, J., & Aron, A. (2006, January). *Up-regulation and down-regulation of emotions and passionate love.* Paper presented at the annual meeting of the Society for Personality and Social Psychology, Palm Springs, CA.

Agnew, C. R., Loving, T. J., Le, B., & Goodfriend, W. (2004). Thinking close: Measuring relational closeness as perceived self-other inclusion. In D. Mashek & A. Aron (Eds.), *Handbook of closeness and intimacy* (pp. 103–115). Mahwah, NJ: Erlbaum.

Agnew, C. R., Van Lange, P. A. M., Rusbult, C. E., & Langston, C. A. (1998). Cognitive interdependence: Commitment and the mental representation of close relationships. *Journal of Personality and Social Psychology, 74*, 939–954.

Aron, A., & Aron, E. N. (1986). *Love as the expansion of self: Understanding attraction and satisfaction.* New York: Hemisphere.

Aron, A., & Aron, E. N. (1991). Love and sexuality. In K. McKinney & S. Sprecher (Eds.), *Sexuality in close relationships* (pp. 25–48). Hillsdale, NJ: Erlbaum.

Aron, A., Aron, E. N., & Allen, J. (1998). Motivations for unreciprocated love. *Personality and Social Psychology Bulletin, 24*, 787–796.

Aron, A., Aron, E. N., & Norman, C. (2001). The self-expansion model of motivation and cognition in close relationships and beyond. In M. Clark & G. Fletcher (Eds.), *Blackwell handbook of social psychology: Vol. 2. Interpersonal processes* (pp. 478–501). Oxford, UK: Blackwell.

Aron, A., Aron, E. N., & Smollan, D. (1992). Inclusion of Other in the Self Scale and the structure of interpersonal closeness. *Journal of Personality and Social Psychology, 63*, 596–612.

Aron, A., Aron, E. N., Tudor, M., & Nelson, G. (1991). Close relationships as including other in the self. *Journal of Personality and Social Psychology, 60*, 241–253.

Aron, A., Fisher, H., Mashek, D., Strong, G., Li, H., & Brown, L. (2005). Reward, motivation and emotion systems associated with early-stage intense romantic love. *Journal of Neurophysiology, 94*, 327–337.

Aron, A., Fisher, H. E., Mashek, D., Strong, G., Shaver, P. R., Mikulincer, M., Li, H., & Brown, L. L. (2004, October). *Attachment anxiety and attachment avoidance in romantic love: An fMRI study.* Paper presented at the meeting of the Society for Neuroscience, San Diego, CA.

Aron, A., & Fraley, B. (1999). Relationship closeness as including other in the self: Cognitive underpinnings and measures. *Social Cognition, 17*, 140–160.

Aron, A., Melinat, E., Aron, E. N., Vallone, R., & Bator, R. (1997).The experimental generation of interpersonal closeness: A procedure and some preliminary findings. *Personality and Social Psychology Bulletin, 23*, 363–377.

Aron, A., Norman, C. C., & Aron, E. N. (1998). The self-expansion model and motivation. *Representative Research in Social Psychology, 22*, 1–13.

Aron, A., Norman, C. C., Aron, E. N., McKenna, C., & Heyman, R. (2000). Couples' shared participation in novel and arousing activities and experienced relationship quality. *Journal of Personality and Social Psychology, 78*, 273–283.

Aron, A., Paris, M., & Aron, E. N. (1995). Falling in love: Prospective studies of self-concept change. *Journal of Personality and Social Psychology, 69*, 1102–1112.

Aron, A., Whitfield, S., & Lichty, W. (in press). Whole brain correlations: Examining similarity across conditions of overall patterns of neural activation in fMRI. In S. Sawilowsky (Ed.), *Real data analysis.* Washington, DC: American Educational Research Association.

Bandura, A. (1977). Self-efficacy: Toward a unifying theory of behavioral change. *Psychological Review, 84*, 191–215.

Beach, S. R., Tesser, A., Fincham, F. D., Jones, D. J., Johnson, D., & Whitaker, D. J. (1998). Pleasure and pain in doing well, together: An investigation of performance-related affect in close relationships. *Journal of Personality and Social Psychology, 74*, 923–938.

Berlin, L. J., & Cassidy, J. (1999). Relations among relationships: Contributions from attachment theory and research. In J. Cassidy & P. R. Shaver (Eds.), *Handbook of attachment: Theory, research, and clinical applications* (pp. 688–712). New York: Guilford Press.

Bowlby, J. (1969). *Attachment and loss: Vol. 1. Attachment.* New York: Basic Books.

Carver, C., & Scheier, M. (1990). Principles of self-regulation, action, and emotion. In E. T. Higgins & R. M. Sorrentino (Eds.), *Handbook of motivation and cognition: Vol. 2. Foundations of social behavior* (pp. 3–52). New York: Guilford Press.

De La Ronde, C., & Swann, W. B., Jr. (1998). Partner verification: Restoring shattered images of our intimates. *Journal of Personality and Social Psychology, 75*, 374–382.

Ekman, P. (1992). An argument for basic emotions. *Cognition and Emotion, 6*, 169–200.

Gardner, W. L., Gabriel, S., & Hochschild, L. (2002). When you and I are "we", you are not threatening: The role of self-expansion in social comparison. *Journal of Personality and Social Psychology, 82*, 239–251.

Gecas, V. (1989). Social psychology of self-efficacy. *American Sociological Review, 15*, 291–316.

Gillath, O., Shaver, P. R., & Mikulincer, M. (2005). An attachment-theoretical approach to compassion and altruism. In P. Gilbert (Ed.), *Compassion: Conceptualizations, research, and use in psychotherapy* (pp. 121–147). London: Brunner-Routledge.

Gonzaga, G. C., Keltner, D., Londahl, E. A., & Smith, M. D. (2001). Love and the commitment problem in romantic relations and friendship. *Journal of Personality and Social Psychology, 81*, 247–262.

Guggenbuhl-Craig, A. (1990, November). *The collective interest in sexual child abuse and incest.* Paper presented at C. G. Jung Institute Public Programs of San Francisco.

Hazan, C., & Shaver, P. R. (1987). Romantic love conceptualized as an attachment process. *Journal of Personality and Social Psychology, 52*, 511–524.

Jones, E. E., & Nisbett, R. (1971). The actor and the observer: Divergent perceptions of the causes of behavior. In E. E. Jones et al. (Eds.), *Attribution: Perceiving the causes of behavior* (pp. 79–94). Morristown, NJ: General Learning Press.

Jung, C. G. (1969). *The structure and dynamics of the psyche* (2nd ed., R. F. C. Hull, Trans.). Princeton, NJ: Princeton University Press.

Jung, C. G. (1970). Mysterium coniunctionis: An inquiry into the separation and synthesis of psychic opposites in alchemy (2nd ed., R. F. C. Hull, Trans.). Princeton, NJ: Princeton University Press.

Jung, C. G. (1979). *General index to the collected works of C. G. Jung* (B. Forryan & J. M. Glover, Compilers). Princeton, NJ: Princeton University Press.

La Guardia, J. G., Ryan, R. M., Couchman, C. E., & Deci, E. L. (2000). Within-person variation in security of attachment: A self-determination theory perspective on attachment, need fulfillment, and well-being. *Journal of Personality and Social Psychology, 79*, 367–384.

Lewandowski, G. W., & Aron, A. (2002, February). *The Self-Expansion Scale.* Paper presented at the annual meeting of the Society for Personality and Social Psychology, Savannah, GA.

Lewandowski, G. W., & Aron, A. P. (2004). Distinguishing arousal from novelty and challenge in initial romantic attraction. *Social Behavior and Personality, 32*, 361–372.

Lewandowski, G. W., Aron, A. P., Bassis, S., & Kunak, J. (in press). Losing a self-expanding relationship: Implications for the self-concept. *Personal Relationships.*

Lord, C. G. (1980). Schemas and images as memory aids: Two modes of processing social information. *Journal of Personality and Social Psychology, 38*, 257–269.

Lord, C. G. (1987). Imagining self and others: Reply to Brown, Keenan, and Potts. *Journal of Personality and Social Psychology, 53*, 445–450.

Main, M. (1991). Metacognitive knowledge, metacognitive monitoring, and singular (coherent) versus multiple (incoherent) models of attachment. In C. M. Parkes, J. Stevenson-Hinde, & P. Marris (Eds.), *Attachment across the life cycle* (pp. 407–474). Hillsdale, NJ: Analytic Press.

Mashek, D. J., Aron, A., & Boncimino, M. (2003). Confusions of self and close others. *Personality and Social Psychology Bulletin, 29*, 382–392.

McFarland, C., Buehler, R., & MacKay, L. (2001). Affective responses to social comparisons with extremely close others. *Social Cognition, 19*, 547–586.

Medvene, L. J., Teal, C. R., & Slavich, S. (2000). Including the other in self: Implications for judgments of equity and satisfaction in close relationships. *Journal of Social and Clinical Psychology, 19*, 396–419.

Pyszczynski, T. A., Greenberg, J., & Solomon, S. (1997). Why do we need what we need? A terror management perspective on the roots of human social motivation. *Psychological Inquiry, 8*, 1–20.

Ryan, R. M., & Deci, E. L. (2000). Self-determination theory and the facilitation of intrinsic motivation, social development, and well-being. *American Psychologist, 55*, 68–78.

Sande, G. N., Goethals, G. R., & Radloff, C. E. (1988). Perceiving one's own traits and others': The multifaceted self. *Journal of Personality and Social Psychology, 54*, 13–20.

Shaver, P. R., Morgan, H. J., & Wu, S. (1996). Is love a "basic" emotion? *Personal Relationships, 3*, 81–96.

Shaver, P. R., Schwartz, J., Kirson, D., & O'Connor, C. (1987). Emotion knowledge: Further exploration of a prototype approach. *Journal of Personality and Social Psychology, 52*, 1061–1086.

Smith, E., Coats, S., & Walling, D. (1999). Overlapping mental representations of self, in-group, and partner: Further response time evidence and a connectionist model. *Personality and Social Psychology Bulletin, 25*, 873–882.

Symons, C. S., & Johnson, B. T. (1997). The self-reference effect in memory: A meta-analysis. *Psychological Bulletin, 121*(3), 371–394.

Taylor, S. E., Neter, E., & Wayment, H. A. (1995). Self-evaluative processes. *Personality and Social Psychology Bulletin, 21*, 1278–1287.

Tucker, P., & Aron, A. (1993). Passionate love and marital satisfaction at key transition points in the family life cycle. *Journal of Social and Clinical Psychology, 12*, 135–147.

White, R. W. (1959). Motivation reconsidered: The concept of competence. *Psychological Review, 66*, 297–333.

15

Implications of Attachment Theory for Research on Intimacy

HARRY T. REIS

Intimacy has been an enduring interest among relationship scientists. Although the term "relationship science" is of recent vintage, scientific inquiry into the processes that govern close relationships has a longer history, emerging during the 1950s and early 1960s, when scholars in the fields of social psychology, human communication, and experimental sociology focused attention on human social interaction. Intimacy and its component processes were among the first topics these pioneers pursued; for example, Jourard's self-disclosure research (1971), Altman and Taylor's experiments on the social penetration process (1973), and studies of expressive exchanges and nonverbal immediacy by several investigators (e.g., Capella, 1981; Mehrabian, 1972; Noller, 1984; Patterson, 1976). That researchers interested in exploring fundamental questions about social interaction and its role in human social life would gravitate toward intimacy as a point of departure is not extraordinary. When the early grand theorists of psychosocial development, such as Erich Fromm and Harry Stack Sullivan, theorized about close relationships, their key concepts were remarkably similar to what we today mean by intimacy. Likewise, and not coincidentally, when ordinary people are asked about their relationship goals, intimacy and its related elements invariably rank at or near the top of the list (Reis,

1990; Sanderson, 2004). As William James (1920) put it, "Human beings are born into this little span of life of which the best thing is its friendships and intimacies" (p. 109).

Early attachment theorists and researchers paid little attention to adult intimacy, except insofar as the general idea of intimacy was used to characterize the adult terminus of a series of relationships influenced by attachment experiences "from the cradle to the grave," Bowlby's (1979, p. 129) well-known phrase concerning the lifelong applicability of his theory. To be sure, Bowlby had thought about the adult results of successful attachment experiences: As he expressed it, "the capacity to make intimate emotional bonds with other individuals . . . is regarded as a principal feature of effective personality functioning and mental health" (1988, p. 121). Nevertheless, neither in Bowlby's writings nor anywhere else was there much elaboration of the specific relational properties underlying this dictum nor of the processes regulating "intimate emotional bonds" in the unique context of close adult relationships. Fortunately, more than two decades worth of adult attachment research, spawned by the seminal contributions of Phil Shaver and his students and colleagues (reflected in part in the other chapters in this volume), has begun to provide answers to important questions about the nature of intimacy, its origin in early-life relationships, and its consequences for relational well-being and personal health. In fact, as I argue throughout this chapter, adult attachment theory and research have been singularly helpful in imposing theoretical coherence on the myriad phenomena traditionally subsumed under the heading "intimacy." In so doing, attachment theory has led directly to important advances in our understanding of intimacy.

If theories are useful because of the questions they suggest, attachment theory may be the most useful theory in relationship science. This is because attachment theory has led researchers to ask novel and diverse questions about many different relationship phenomena, not just those directly concerned with attachment. In this chapter, my goal is to illustrate this generativity in a particular domain, showing how insights derived from attachment theory have led directly to important advances in research on intimacy. In some instances, these insights were not available in alternative theoretical approaches; in other cases, attachment theory suggested different, more compelling perspectives on established findings. In yet other instances, attachment theory led researchers to posit and probe novel hypotheses. Broadly speaking, attachment theory provides a set of mechanisms and principles that link intimacy in a coherent and integrated way with important developmental, psychodynamic, and biological processes. Stated another way, if adult attachment theory were not available, intimacy research would be impoverished for it.

This chapter begins with a brief overview of intimacy theory and research as it existed before adult attachment theory. I then review the Reis and Shaver (1988) process model of intimacy, which provided an initial theoretical framework for integrating insights from attachment theory into research on intimacy. Subsequently, I discuss advances in intimacy research that have occurred in the years since 1988, all of them derived straightforwardly from attachment theory. The chapter concludes with a brief proposal for new directions in intimacy research.

RESEARCH ON INTIMACY AND THE CONTRIBUTIONS OF THE ATTACHMENT PERSPECTIVE

In the 1970s and 1980s, several influential reviews likened intimacy research to the Buddhist parable of the blind men and the elephant (e.g., Acitelli & Duck, 1987). In that fable, each blind man touches a different part of the elephant and thereby reaches a different conclusion about the fundamental nature of the beast. One touches the tusk, concluding that elephants are firm and sharp-ended, like the blade of a plow. Another feels the soft, flexible ear, concluding that elephants are pliant, like a basket. A third focuses on the pillar-like structure of the leg. Each quarrels with the others, arguing that his experience is the most valid one. The point of the parable, of course, is that although each man's perspective is valid, that perspective could identify only a tiny portion of reality. To understand the full entity one had to integrate multiple perspectives. Intimacy, or so the various reviews insisted, was similarly multifaceted. Only by considering and synthesizing multiple and diverse perspectives would we discover the true nature of the beast.

Unfortunately, that integration was described and celebrated mostly for its potential and not as an established reality. Instead, throughout the literature, three strands of research coexisted, side by side but with limited convergence. The first, and most empirically documented, concerned self-disclosure and the manner in which the mutual revelation of personal information contributed to the acquaintance process (e.g., Altman & Taylor, 1973; Jourard, 1971). A second tradition concerned nonverbal immediacy, exploring the ways in which nonverbal factors such as gaze, touch, facial expressions, and seating position regulated interaction intensity. Intimacy, it was proposed, consisted of interactions with a high degree of nonverbal engagement. The third perspective grew out of the immensely popular writings of Erik Erikson. Intimacy was the descriptor he applied to the fifth of eight life stages, namely the stage concerned with establishing a primary, exclusive, and sexual relationship characterized by a sense of openness, trust, and authentic interdependence.

Before the creation of adult attachment theory, although these three perspectives on intimacy had each contributed to researchers' understanding of it, little theoretical integration had been accomplished. Attachment theory changed this. When Shaver and I sat down to develop a process model of intimacy, we found that the various theoretical principles of attachment theory, not only as articulated by Bowlby (1969/1982, 1973, 1980) but also as extended by later researchers and theorists who used attachment as a theoretical centerpiece (e.g., Alan Sroufe; Mary Ainsworth; Inge Bretherton; Robert Hinde), could provide a general framework for integrating the three perspectives on intimacy, not only with one another but also with several additional processes we believed were central to intimate interaction. Attachment theory, in other words, provided elegant principles, deep insights, and an empirically plausible framework that could clarify the complex thoughts, feelings, and behaviors that contribute to intimacy. This is, of course, precisely the sort of theoretical generativity that Bowlby intended and that explains why attachment theory remains a compelling conceptual model more than four decades after its inception.

To highlight the contributions of an attachment-theoretic approach to intimacy, I list seven principles and ideas concerning aspects of the intimacy process that will be explicated more fully in the remainder of this chapter.

1. That internalized mental representations of the self and close relationship partners influence perceptions of, and responses to, those partners.
2. That these representations are developmentally significant; that is, they are shaped in early interactions with caregivers and then affect the development of later relationships with significant others.
3. That emotion is central to the regulation of intimacy.
4. That the "self" in self-disclosure most fundamentally consists not simply of self-related information or facts but also of affectively significant desires, fears, beliefs, affects, and goals regarding the self in relation to others.
5. That although intimate interactions are influenced significantly by the individual's internal mental representations, at a fundamental level intimacy is grounded in the reality of actual interactions.
6. That intimacy depends less on patterns of self-disclosure than on the perceived responsiveness of partners to the self.
7. That the satisfaction of intimacy needs contributes to well-being and personal growth.

These principles came together in the intimacy process model that Shaver and I published in 1988 (Reis & Shaver, 1988; later updated by Reis & Patrick, 1996). A slightly revised version of that model is depicted in Figure 15.1. Because I use this model to organize discussion of specific principles and research findings, a brief overview is presented first.

The model conceptualizes intimacy as a dynamic process that unfolds during interaction (as opposed to a set of beliefs about existing relation-

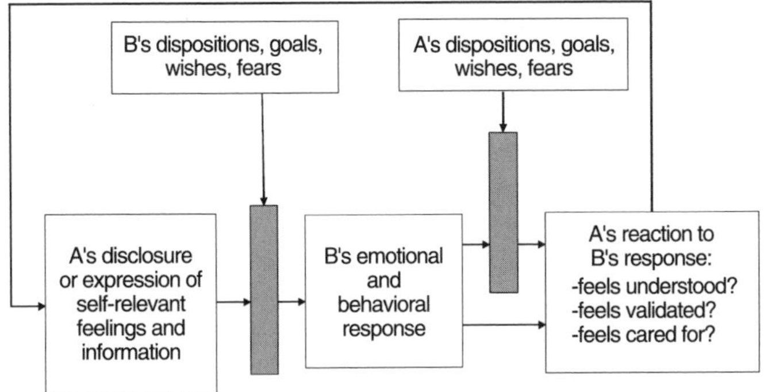

FIGURE 15.1. The intimacy process model.

ships). This unfolding begins when one person reveals personally significant aspects of the self to a partner. Although typically verbal, nonverbal factors such as facial expressions and body posture figure prominently in these self-revelations, as do behaviors. (For example, traveling cross-country for a longtime friend's 60th birthday party conveys important information about the self and one's values.) The closer the revealed material is to core aspects of the self, which are typically but not exclusively affective in nature, the greater is the potential of the ensuing interaction to become intimate. Next, the process is shaped by the partner's response. A supportive, encouraging response is likely to facilitate the development of intimacy, whereas a distant, uninterested, or disparaging response is likely to dampen, if not shut down, the process entirely. Effective responses are characterized by three feelings engendered in the self-revealer: a feeling of being understood (that is, that the partner has "got the facts right" and perceives what is important to the self), a feeling of being validated (that is, that the partner appreciates and respects the self), and a feeling of caring (that is, that the partner is concerned about one's welfare and will act in a manner responsive to one's needs).

This process is both reciprocal and iterative (Gable & Reis, in press). That is, contributing to the process as a responsive listener is likely to facilitate one's willingness to exchange roles, with the listener beginning a process of self-revelation to which the original self-revealer now serves as respondent. This is because the feelings of understanding, validation, and caring undergird a sense of trust in partners. Another important feature of the model, shown in the "dispositions, goals, wishes, and fears" boxes of Figure 15.1, concerns the influence of what in 1988 we called interpretive filters. These filters indicate that preexisting mental representations of the self in close relationships influence all stages of the process: willingness to reveal oneself to another; how another's self-revelations are interpreted and responded to; and how attempts at responsive feedback are experienced.

In the remaining sections of this chapter, I select particular features of this model that have been the focus of research in our lab and elsewhere. These particular features have been chosen because they illustrate the generativity of attachment-theoretic ideas for developing a theoretically rich understanding of adult intimacy.

The Affective Core of Intimate Self-Revelation

First proposed during an era in which affect and emotion were treated as taboo topics in psychology, attachment theory points directly to the cardinal role of affect and affect regulation in close relationships. As Magai (1999) illustrates, many of the central processes of attachment are fundamentally affective. For example, emotions and emotional signals regulate the experience of attachment-related needs (e.g., distress, fear, despair, contentment, love) and their expression (e.g., crying, soothing, hypervigilance, and deactivation). Similarly, Mikulincer and Shaver (2005a) show that emotional reactions to interpersonal events are the hallmark of adult attachment styles. Thus it is clear that the attachment relationship is an emotionally significant bond (as the title of Bowlby's 1979 collection of essays makes plain: "The Making and Breaking of Affectional Bonds").

In the original formulations, self-disclosure theories featured privacy regulation and the transmission of normatively private information from one individual to another. An attachment-theoretic view suggests a somewhat different emphasis: on the fact that emotionally significant information has the greatest relevance to the development of intimacy, and, furthermore, that emotional displays that accompany verbal interaction contribute to this process. Contemporary research has generally supported this inference. For example, independent diary studies by Lin (1992) and by Laurenceau, Barrett, and Pietromonaco (1998) revealed that emotional self-disclosure during social interaction was a stronger predictor of intimacy than was factual self-disclosure. Similar studies by Lippert and Prager (2001) and by Laurenceau, Barrett, and Rovine (2005) have shown that emotional self-disclosure predicts interaction intimacy among married and dating couples, respectively. Not surprisingly, then, studies of marital communication and intimacy have shown that nonverbal expressions of affect, both hostile and affectionate, provide the most diagnostic and influential information about couple well-being (see Heyman, 2001; Johnson, 2004, for overviews).

Spurred by these and many other studies, contemporary theories of intimacy now stress the importance of emotion and emotional expression. Reis and Patrick (1996) and Markus and Cross (1990) theorize that because the self has a fundamentally affective core, close interpersonal bonds (of which intimacy is one type) involve affective interdependence. Beach and Tesser (1988) argue that intimate experiences require emotional intensity, because "deep" self-disclosures and responses to them are necessarily novel, risky, and arousing, conditions that foster strong emotions. Clark, Fitness, and Brissette (2001) theorize that emotional expression provides a vehicle for communicating important personal needs to partners, a process by which partners display responsiveness and mutual support for each other's needs. Consistent with these theories, emotionally focused couple therapy stresses the interactive nature of perceived betrayal by one partner and subsequent self-protective responses by the other, a pattern that restricts emotional openness in couples and thereby inhibits the development of intimacy (Firestone & Catlett, 1999). For example, in describing emotionally focused couple therapy, Johnson (2004) states:

> The most appropriate paradigm for adult intimacy is that of an emotional bond. The key issue in marital conflict is the security of this bond. Such bonds are created by accessibility and responsiveness. (p. 51)

These advances in theorizing about intimacy and in treating intimacy problems can be traced, directly or indirectly, to appreciation of the attachment perspective.

Mental Models of Self in Relation to Others

The notion that personal dispositions influence intimate behavior, both in terms of preferences for certain kinds of interaction and in terms of the capacity to enact them, became popular in early research. Although many such studies were conducted, for the most part they were unsystematic in the sense that neither these dispositional predictors nor their association with intimacy were situated within a larger network of theoretical principles. In other words, although lengthy lists of the dispositional correlates of intimacy were readily generated (see, for example, Derlega, Metts, Petronio, & Margulis, 1993), integration of these lists into a coherent conceptual framework was not so easily accomplished. Furthermore, intimacy research did little to specify the origin of these dispositional predictions. This is, of course, a major strength of the attachment theoretic approach.

The psychometrics of adult attachment predispositions have received more attention than any other similar traits. Sophisticated psychometric studies indicate that two dimensions underlie many of the dispositional processes embodied in attachment theory (Crowell, Fraley & Shaver, 1999; Fraley, Waller, & Brennan, 2000). One dimension, commonly labeled anxiety, for attachment-related anxiety, embodies the extent to which individuals worry about their connections with partners and fear abandonment or rejection; the second dimension, called avoidance, represents the extent to which individuals feel comfortable with closeness and interdependence or instead prefer distance and self-reliance. Attachment security is captured by the simultaneous absence of both anxiety and avoidance.

This two-dimensional conceptualization helps integrate the many individual correlates of intimacy. For example, lower levels of intimacy have been associated with fear of exploitation in close relationships, with lower levels of trust and openness, with private self-consciousness, with fear of intimacy, with weaker intimacy motivation, with fewer intimacy goals, with low levels of empathic concern for others, with unmitigated agency (a trait that represents hypermasculinity), with self-reliant coping styles, and, of course, with avoidant attachment (see Reis & Patrick, 1996, for detailed references). In other words, a broad array of variables indicative of distance from others and discomfort with emotionally focused relating is meaningfully and consistently associated with the absence and avoidance of intimacy.

With regard to attachment anxiety, the picture is more complex. Whereas individuals high in attachment anxiety profoundly desire intimate connections with partners, when such connections are attained, anxious persons often become preoccupied with the possibility of abandonment, leading to behaviors that may undermine intimacy. For example, Downey and colleagues have shown that individuals high in rejection sensitivity (a tendency toward heightened concern about and expectancy of rejection) may, when feeling unsupported or rebuffed by partners, react in a provocative manner that, in much the manner of a self-fulfilling prophecy, elicits the very rejection that was feared (Downey, Freitas, Michaelis, & Khouri, 1998; Pietrzak, Downey, & Ayduk, 2005). It is noteworthy that this pattern—heightened desire for intimacy coupled with anxiety-induced relationship deterioration once intimacy is attained—appears characteristic of several related constructs describing people's perceptions about the availability and trustworthiness of significant others. Among these are reassurance seeking (the tendency to seek validation about one's worth from others), self-esteem (perceived worth of the self and, in so-called "sociometer theories," perceived acceptance of the self by others), unmitigated communion (excessive concern about meeting the needs of others), and relationally contingent self-esteem (deriving perceptions of self-worth from current relational events). (Reis, Clark, & Holmes, 2004, elaborate on what may be a common conceptual core among these traits.) For present purposes, I note that the tendency to pursue intimacy while ironically contributing to its deterioration is readily accounted for in terms of attachment theorists' and researchers' work on the dynamics of anxious preoccupation (Mikulincer & Shaver, 2003).

A further contribution of the attachment theoretic approach to intimacy research involves the role of attachment-related dispositions in predicting social interaction behaviors such as empathy, supportiveness, and love. Numerous studies of attachment dynamics demonstrate how working models of attachment affect perceptions of a partner's behavior and shape the nature of one's response to that behavior (see Mikulincer and Shaver, 2005a, for a review). These various mechanisms likely apply to intimacy as well, although to date little research has directly evaluated this possibility.

The Key Role of Partner Responsiveness

Reflecting its roots in studies of the self-disclosure process, most intimacy research has focused on the behavior of one or both partners in initiating intimate exchanges rather than on the partner's response to the initiator's overture. In marked contrast, attachment theory teaches that the partner's response to the self may be the more critical step. After all, the child's emerging sense of security is predicated less on the child's displays of distress and need and more on the availability and responsiveness of an emotionally sensitive caregiver (Bowlby, 1973), which, over the course of development, become internalized as working models of the self in relation to others. In adulthood, the availability and responsiveness of attachment partners is similarly central to secure representations of that relationship (e.g., Collins & Feeney, 2000, 2004; Simpson, Rholes, & Phillips, 1996). In other words, partner responsiveness underlies the formation of secure attachment bonds, both developmentally and in particular adult relationships.

Recent studies generalizing from this principle indicate that responsiveness, rather than self-disclosure, may be the linchpin of adult intimacy. For example, diary studies by Lin (1992) and Laurenceau and colleagues (1998, 2005) indicate that perceptions of a partner's response to self-disclosure accounted for more variance in ratings of intimacy than did the nature or extent of the disclosure itself. In this respect, intimate relationships likely exemplify what Clark and her colleagues meant in distinguishing communal relationships from exchange relationships. The former are characterized by the expectation that partners will be responsive to each other's personal needs, whereas the latter involve no such expectation (e.g., Clark et al., 2001). Similar conclusions may be drawn from the extensive literatures on socially supportive communication and marital interaction, each of which includes extensive evidence demonstrating that supportive, responsive listening encourages emotional openness, feelings of closeness and connection, and personal well-being (see Burleson, 2003; Gottman, 1994, for reviews).

A recent set of studies conducted in our lab or in collaboration with others underscores this general point. In one study of a community sample of 88 married couples, we examined the impact of "positive illusions" (i.e., perceptions of a partner that are more favorable than the partner's self-perceptions), which have been shown to predict both personal and relational well-being (e.g., Murray, Holmes, & Griffin, 1996). Couples in this sample completed daily diaries of relationship-relevant events and feelings, including measures of intimacy and satisfaction. Analyses revealed that the benefits of positive illusions were fully mediated by perceived partner responsiveness to the self. In other words, the benefits of being idealized by a partner were obtained only when partners felt valued by the idealizer (Reis & Carmichael, 2005). In another study, Kumashiro, Rusbult, and Reis (2005) examined the so-called "Michelangelo phenomenon," a process by which partners view and treat each other in a manner consistent with personal ideals and thereby encourage personal growth toward those ideals. As in the Reis and Carmichael (2005) study, this effect was mediated by the perception that partners were responsive to the self's ideals.

Considerable debate has arisen concerning the extent to which perceptions of partner responsiveness are motivated constructions (i.e., distortions) or accurate reflections of interpersonal reality. Much, if not most, intimacy research seems to adopt one or the other position, as if relationship life required them to be mutually exclusive. Attachment theory, of course, incorporates both alternatives, reflecting, in the former case, Bowlby's (1988) insistence that attachment beliefs had to be "tolerably accurate" representations of early experience and, in the latter case, substantial evidence that working models of attachment influence interpretations of contemporaneous experience (Shaver, Collins, & Clark, 1996). Current studies indicate that both tolerable accuracy and what Shaver and I originally called interpretive filters are operative during intimate interaction. For example, Collins and Feeney (2000) coded videotaped laboratory interactions in a support-seeking situation, showing that observable features of interaction behavior, as well as idiosyncratic interpretations of those exchanges, contributed to responsiveness. My colleagues and I used a quasi-signal detection methodology (Gable, Reis, & Downey, 2003) to compare the impact of *hits* (support provided by one partner that is recognized by both partners), *misses* (support provided by one partner but not recognized by the other), and *false alarms* (support reported as received by one partner of which the provider seems unaware). In one recent study, intimacy was facilitated to a greater extent by hits than by false alarms or misses, although false alarms were also influential (Reis & Carmichael, 2005). These and other results led Reis et al. (2004) to conclude that "both reality and social construction matter . . . involving, for example, dynamic associations among dispositional factors, relationship-specific schemas, interaction qualities, and the situational context in which those interactions take place" (p. 214). This conclusion implicates a level of complexity familiar to attachment researchers from which intimacy research (and, for that matter, many other interpersonal theories) has yet to fully profit.

Understanding and Validation

Extensive research has examined the impact of two self-regulatory motives in relationship contexts: self-verification (the desire to receive feedback from partners that confirms self-conceptions) and self-enhancement (the desire to receive positive feedback from partners). Much theorizing has been offered regarding this distinction, and many studies have been conducted, some linked directly to intimacy. For example, Swann, de la Ronde, and Hixon (1994) demonstrated that intimacy in married couples was greatest when self-views and partner views of the self corresponded. On the other hand, other studies have shown that partner positivity predicts intimacy (e.g., Murray, Holmes, & Griffin, 1996; Neff & Karney, 2002), independent of self-views. Although several theorists have attempted to reconcile these positions, by and large the two processes have remained in the research literature as competing predictors of intimacy and closeness.

An attachment theoretic perspective suggests that these two self-regulatory motives may be better conceptualized as coactors than as competitors. In attachment theory terms, the origin of intimacy resides in internalized beliefs that the self is worthy of love and that significant others can be trusted to provide support and comfort when needed (e.g., Sroufe & Fleeson, 1988). Following Bowlby (1969/1982), Bartholomew and Horowitz (1991) referred to these as "model of self" and "model of other," respectively. To them, and to most attachment theorists, security involves positivity of both models. Believing that attachment figures will be available and helpful if needed requires believing that these others accurately and sensitively perceive oneself and one's needs; otherwise, support is likely to be mismatched and/or inappropriate (for example, inadequate or overly intrusive). Thus the concept of mental representations, or internal working models, of attachment relationships incorporates assessments of the positivity of partner feedback (validation), as well as perceptions of the accuracy of that feedback (understanding), without subordinating either to the other.

Partner positivity in the absence of perceived understanding—that is, a partner's positive evaluation that contradicts self-perception without credible rationale—may be expected to be ineffective, inasmuch as the perceived inconsistency with the individual's working model of self would be unlikely to satisfy concerns about trustworthiness and availability. (In fact, positive partner evaluations that are inconsistent with the existing self-model may trigger defensive reactions, such as distancing or wariness.) On the other hand, negative self-perceptions that are too eagerly or uniformly confirmed by a partner also seem unlikely to be characteristic of felt security and secure relationship representations. Generally, the belief that partners neither attend to nor appreciate one's inner self is integral to attachment theoretic models of developmental psychopathology (e.g., Carlson & Sroufe, 1995).

Attachment theory, therefore, leads to the suggestion that positive feedback from a partner will be validating only to the extent that it is perceived as authentic; that is, congruent in large measure with self-perceptions. Positive feedback will enhance intimacy only when also seen as understanding (in the sense of "getting the facts right" about the self). A pair of experiments by Patrick and Reis (1995) support this conjecture. In these experiments, participants in a mock interview situation were given evaluative feedback about their personalities that was positive, negative, or neutral. Simultaneously, the interviewer's comments included details that made clear that he or she either had understood the participant's self-description very well or very poorly. Importantly, accuracy and inaccuracy were manipulated in such a way that neither implied a more positive nor a more negative evaluation. As shown in Figure 15.2, a significant interaction effect was obtained. Positive evaluative feedback increased attraction to the partner when based on accurate understanding; when the feedback indicated misunderstanding, positive feedback actually created lesser attraction to the interviewer. Another way to interpret these data is to note that accuracy in and of itself had no influence on attraction.

Although comprehensive review of this complex issue is beyond the scope of this chapter, there is other evidence that the value of favorable feedback from others depends on the perception of understanding by the source. For example, using social relations analysis, Monsour, Betty, and Kurzweil (1993) showed that metaperspectives (Partner A believing that Partner B understands how A perceives himself or herself) predicted intimacy better than did any of these components in isolation. Schimel, Arndt, Pyszczynski, and Greenberg (2001) demonstrated that validation of the intrinsic self—positive feedback about core aspects of self—led to less defensiveness than praise did. Neff and Karney (2002) suggest that partners may desire accurate feedback on specific traits for which clear self-representations are available, which allows them to accept positive feedback on more ambiguous traits. Murray, Holmes, Bellavia, Griffin, and Dolderman (2002) found that feelings of being understood predicted greater satisfaction in marriage, over and above actual understanding. These ideas support Holmes's

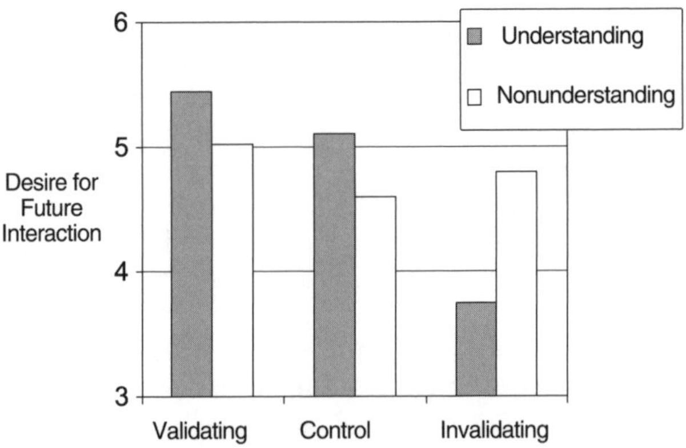

FIGURE 15.2. The role of understanding and validation in a laboratory interaction.

(2005) recent suggestion that expectations about the responsiveness of partners results from both models of the self and of the other—that is, the simultaneous belief that the self is worthy of support and that partners will be willing to provide it. This is consistent with the idea that both perceived understanding and validation are intrinsic to intimacy.

Intimacy Promotes Openness

In experimental research on intimacy and self-disclosure, causality has usually been unidirectional: Higher levels of self-disclosure cause increases in intimacy. Similarly, other variables are typically investigated as causes of intimacy, whereas the reverse pattern, namely that increases in intimacy may lead to increases in other relational behaviors, is rarely investigated. Nevertheless, many prominent intimacy theories propose that the causal links are bidirectional. For example, a key tenet of early research was that increases in intimacy would engender increases in emotional openness (e.g., Jourard, 1971; Rogers, 1961). Thus our theoretical model (shown in Figure 15.1) incorporated links implicating a feedback mechanism whereby the successful unfolding of the intimacy process would facilitate both partners' subsequent willingness to be emotionally open.

Why does intimacy promote openness? Attachment theory provides one good explanation. Developmentally, attachment security is fostered by sensitive, responsive caregiving, and extensive evidence shows that a dispositionally secure attachment style is associated with trust and emotional openness to others (e.g., Grabill & Kerns, 2000; Mikulincer et al., 2001). After all, trust and openness create vulnerability, and without the expectation that caregivers will respond appropriately and sensitively, caution would be the more adaptive orientation. Thus the responsiveness inherent in intimacy promotes the expectation that emotional openness will not be exploited. This effect has contextual, as well as dispositional, antecedents. Experiences of sensitive, responsive caregiving may, at least in the moment, activate representations of security, producing behaviors characteristic of chronic trait security (Mikulincer & Shaver, 2005b). This has been shown, for example, in observational studies of responsive caregiving (e.g., Collins & Feeney, 2004) and in laboratory studies in which attachment security has been activated through experimental priming procedures (e.g., Mikulincer et al., 2001). For example, Mikulincer (1998) demonstrated that experimentally activated attachment security fostered willingness to talk with partners about trust violations, whereas insecurity more characteristically led to ruminative worry or emotional distance from partners, both signs of unwillingness to express emotions directly to that person.

In a pair of multilevel modeling studies, Clark, Reis, Tsai, and Brissette (2005) examined the association between expectations of responsive caregiving and the willingness to express emotions. Participants in both studies were first asked to evaluate a series of relationship partners, ranging from distant (e.g., classmate, neighbor) to close (e.g., sibling, romantic partner), in terms of the expectation that each would go out of his or her way to be responsive to the participant's needs. They were then asked how willing they would be to express various emotions to that partner, whether the emotion had been caused by that person or by someone or something else. The greater the expectation of responsiveness, the more willing participants were to be open about their emotions. This was true for both positive and negative emotions and for emotions caused by the partner or by someone or something else. Interestingly, this effect was stronger for persons high in dispositional security than for avoidant persons, implying that security is characterized by the ability to discriminate appropriate partners for emotional self-disclosure and not just to produce various levels of emotional self-disclosure (see Tidwell, Reis, & Shaver, 1996, for a similar effect in daily emotional experience). This is another area in which security is associated with a kind of interpersonal accuracy rather than a perceptually biasing wish to feel good about the self or confirmed in one's negative self-views.

Intimacy Promotes Effectiveness in Other Life Domains

Intimacy provides a compelling research theme for several reasons, one of which is its hypothesized links to competence and well-being in other domains of life. In Erikson's seminal life-stage theory, for example, successful attainment of intimacy during early adulthood is prerequisite to later generativity, which in his theorizing represents concern for one's legacy to the next generation, spanning diverse activities such as successful parenting, creative endeavors, and productive work (Erikson, 1950). Success in intimate relationships is associated with various interpersonal and personal competencies (Prager, 1995), competencies that are implicated not just in close relationships but in most forms of social connection. Also, intimacy, and particularly self-disclosure, has been associated with emotional well-being, psychosocial adjustment, and physical health across the lifespan (e.g., Pennebaker, 1995; Vaillant, 1977).

Although plausible accounts of these and similar effects are plentiful, missing in much of this work is a broader theoretical explanation of why success in one domain of experience, close interpersonal relationships of an intimate nature, should influence behavior in other life domains. Once again, attachment theory suggests such an explanation in the complementary motives of the attachment behavioral system and the exploration behavioral system. This latter system includes motives, emotions, thoughts, and behavioral tendencies that prompt individuals to explore the environments in which they live, thereby gaining valuable knowledge and mastering important skills. The attachment system serves a more protective function, providing a safe haven when threatening circumstances arise and a secure base when no threats are imminent. Because protection from danger represents a more immediate threat to the individual's survival, the attachment system tends to dominate; in other words, and as numerous theorists have asserted, exploration takes place only when the attachment system senses relatively little risk.

Although attachment and exploration both contribute to human well-being, the latter has received significantly less attention than the former, with most existing research focusing on children's play and peer relationships. In a series of studies, Andrew Elliot and I (Elliot & Reis, 2003) examined exploratory activities in adulthood and their relation to the attachment system. We reasoned that exploration is exemplified in activities that promote the development of skills and abilities that enable a person to investigate, learn from, and adapt to his or her surroundings in an open-minded and confident manner. Drawing an analogy to infant–caregiver research methods (e.g., the well-known Strange Situation devised by Ainsworth, Blehar, Waters, & Wall, 1978), we theorized that secure attachment would foster confident pursuit of mastery goals and achievement and a pleasurable sense of challenge in learning activities. On the other hand, insecure attachment would create fear of failure, anxiety about achievement, and a foreboding sense of threat in the activity. The reason is that a secure base allows a person to explore the environment (in infancy, a playroom with attractive toys; in adulthood, a task with the potential for personal growth) confidently, knowing that supportive partners are available if needed, whereas the absence of a secure base endows exploratory situations with risk, a sense of being out on a limb, and the potential for rejection, activating self-protective mind-sets.

Elliot and Reis (2003) reported four correlational studies demonstrating that secure attachment is associated with stronger achievement motivation, lesser fear of failure in academic settings, a stronger tendency to set mastery-approach goals, and a weaker tendency to set mastery-avoidance and performance-avoidance goals. (Mastery-approach goals are associated with strivings to attain mastery of an important task, whereas performance-avoidance and mastery-avoidance goals are associated with strivings to avoid failing or appearing incompetent, respectively, on important tasks.) Mediational analyses established that these effects were mediated by attachment-related appraisals: An anxious attachment orientation leads people to construe achievement-related settings in terms of potential threats to well-being and perceived competence, whereas avoidance leads people to minimize the possibility of challenge and growth opportunities. Both of these interfere with confident, fully engaged exploration. In a subsequent unpublished laboratory experiment, subliminal priming of secure, anxious, and avoidant attachment led research participants to differentially endorse approach and avoidance goals for the semester (Reis & Tsai, 2003).

Another achievement domain full of possibilities for threat and challenge is athletics. Peter Capranello and I (2006) recently conducted a survey study of a large national sample of university athletes. Once again, attachment security was associated with approach motivation and challenge orientation, whereas insecurity was associated with avoidance motivation and threat orientation.

This research suggests an important new domain for adult attachment researchers. Arguably, love and work are the two most central domains of adult life, but for the most part, they are studied as if they were independent. (See Hazan & Shaver, 1990, for an exception that has not been followed up adequately by subsequent studies.) To be sure, it is often acknowledged that relationships affect one's ability to work with others, but this is usually conceptualized in terms of our abilities to get along in the workplace or to manage relationship stress that spills over from home to work. Our research on attachment and exploration in adulthood suggests a more profound process, however. To the extent that mental models of attachment security influence people's willingness and ability to test their personal competencies and explore environments, a key insight into the importance of the satisfaction of intimacy needs for effective, creative functioning in the adult world will have been established.

CONCLUSION

One can scarcely argue that intimacy, in its fifth decade of research interest, is a hot topic among social psychologists or, for that matter, relationship scientists. Although the topic remains active, new theoretical approaches to intimacy are rare or nonexistent, and new empirical findings tend to make incremental contributions to knowledge rather than advancing research to a new level of understanding. Why might this be the case? The parable of the blind men and the elephant, discussed earlier, suggests that in our commendable zeal to be inclusive of multiple approaches and diverse manifestations of intimacy, we may have overlooked that which is most central to investigation of any behavioral process: a deeply textured theoretical account of the core phenomenon, its ontological roots, and its most characteristic behavioral manifestations. Such a theoretical account would need to be more than descriptive. It would need to be biologically plausible, consistent with available knowledge about cognitive and affective processes in human relationships, capable of representing both dispositional differences and contextual influences, and sufficiently broad to encompass cross-cultural universals and variations. Without being overly censorious, it seems safe to say that existing theories of intimacy have yet to provide such an account.

The premise of this chapter is that the foundation for such a theory is available. Two decades since its migration into social psychology, attachment theory has given strong indications of its potential to supply cardinal principles and important insights about intimate relations. To be sure, attachment and intimacy are not equivalent processes. As attachment theorists correctly point out, an attachment relationship is a very special kind of relationship, geared by evolutionary forces to contend with particular circumstances. Indeed, some might say that the attempt to generalize attachment theory to all manner of social relations, as a casual scan of the literature would suggest, distorts the careful theorizing that was the hallmark of Bowlby's (1969/1982, 1973, 1980) masterwork trilogy. Nevertheless, the attachment relationship represents the prototype of intimacy; the processes that characterize attachment relations are almost surely present, to varying degrees, in all intimate relationships. As a result, there is remarkable overlap between adult attachment and intimacy in terms of their component subprocesses.

Instead of insisting that intimacy be conceptualized from multiple perspectives, then, it may be more fruitful to explore more fully the insights that an attachment theoretic approach can bring to this enduring and important process of human social connection.

REFERENCES

Acitelli, L. K., & Duck, S. W. (1987). Intimacy as the proverbial elephant. In D. Perlman & S. W. Duck (Eds.), *Intimate relationships: Development, dynamics, and deterioration* (pp. 297–308). Newbury Park, CA: Sage.

Ainsworth, M. D. S., Blehar, M. C., Waters, E., & Wall, S. (1978). *Patterns of attachment: A psychological study of the Strange Situation.* Hillsdale, NJ: Erlbaum.

Altman, I., & Taylor, D. A. (1973). *Social penetration: The development of interpersonal relationships.* New York: Holt, Rinehart & Winston.

Bartholomew, K., & Horowitz, L. M. (1991). Attachment styles among young adults: A test of a four-category model. *Journal of Personality and Social Psychology, 61,* 226–244.

Beach, S. R. H., & Tesser, A. (1988). Love in marriage: A cognitive account. In R. J. Sternberg & M. L. Barnes (Eds.), *The psychology of love* (pp. 330–355). New Haven, CT: Yale University Press.

Bowlby, J. (1973). *Attachment and loss: Vol. 2. Separation: Anxiety and anger.* New York: Basic Books.

Bowlby, J. (1979). *The making and breaking of affectional bonds.* London: Tavistock.

Bowlby, J. (1980). *Attachment and loss: Vol. 3. Loss: Sadness and depression.* New York: Basic Books.

Bowlby, J. (1982). *Attachment and loss: Vol. 1. Attachment* (2nd ed.). New York: Basic Books. (Original edition published 1969)

Bowlby, J. (1988). *A secure base: Parent–child attachment and healthy human development.* New York: Basic Books.

Burleson, B. R. (2003). The experience and effects of emotional support: What the study of cultural and gender differences can tell us about close relationships, emotion, and interpersonal communication. *Personal Relationships*, *10*, 1–23.

Cappella, J. N. (1981). Mutual influence in expressive behavior: Adult–adult and infant–adult dyadic interaction. *Psychological Bulletin*, *89*, 101–132.

Capranello, P., & Reis, H. T. (2006). *Attachment security and sports goals*. Unpublished raw data.

Carlson, E. A., & Sroufe, L. A. (1995). Contribution of attachment theory to developmental psychopathology. In D. Cicchetti & D. J. Cohen (Eds.), *Developmental psychopathology: Vol. 1. Theory and methods* (pp. 581–617). Oxford, UK: Wiley.

Clark, M. S., Fitness, J., & Brissette, I. (2001). Understanding people's perceptions of relationships is crucial to understanding their emotional lives. In M. Hewstone & M. Brewer (Eds.), *Blackwell handbook of social psychology: Vol. 2. Interpersonal processes* (pp. 253–278). Oxford, UK: Blackwell.

Clark, M. S., Reis, H. T., Tsai, F. F., & Brissette, I. (2005). *The willingness to express emotions in close relationships*. Manuscript in preparation.

Collins, N. L., & Feeney, B. C. (2000). A safe haven: An attachment theory perspective on support seeking and caregiving in intimate relationships. *Journal of Personality and Social Psychology*, *78*, 1053–1073.

Collins, N. L., & Feeney, B. C. (2004). Working models of attachment shape perceptions of social support: Evidence from experimental and observational studies. *Journal of Personality and Social Psychology*, *87*, 363–383.

Crowell, J. A., Fraley, R. C., & Shaver, P. R. (1999). Measurement of individual differences in adolescent and adult attachment. In J. Cassidy & P. R. Shaver (Eds.), *Handbook of attachment: Theory, research, and clinical applications* (pp. 434–465). New York: Guilford Press.

Derlega, V. J., Metts, S., Petronio, S., & Margulis, S. T. (1993). *Self-disclosure*. Newbury Park, CA: Sage.

Downey, G., Freitas, A. L., Michaelis, B., & Khouri, H. (1998). The self-fulfilling prophecy in close relationships: Rejection sensitivity and rejection by romantic partners. *Journal of Personality and Social Psychology*, *75*, 545–560.

Elliot, A. J., & Reis, H. T. (2003). Attachment and exploration in adulthood. *Journal of Personality and Social Psychology*, *85*, 317–331.

Erikson, E. H. (1950). *Childhood and society*. New York: Norton.

Firestone, R. W., & Catlett, J. (1999). *Fear of intimacy*. Washington, DC: APA Press.

Fraley, R. C., Waller, N. G., & Brennan, K. A. (2000). An item-response theory analysis of self-report measures of adult attachment. *Journal of Personality and Social Psychology*, *78*, 350–365.

Gable, S. L., & Reis, H. T. (in press). Intimacy and the self: An iterative model of the self and close relationships. In J. Feeney & P. Noller (Eds.), *Frontiers in social psychology: Close relationships*. New York: Psychology Press.

Gable, S. L., Reis, H. T., & Downey, G. (2003). He said, she said: A quasi-signal detection analysis of daily interactions between close relationship partners. *Psychological Science*, *14*, 100–105.

Gottman, J. M. (1994). *What predicts divorce? The relationship between marital processes and marital outcomes*. Hillsdale, NJ: Erlbaum.

Grabill, C. M., & Kerns, K. A. (2000). Attachment style and intimacy in friendship. *Personal Relationships*, *7*, 363–378.

Hazan, C., & Shaver, P. R. (1990). Love and work: An attachment-theoretical perspective. *Journal of Personality and Social Psychology, 59*, 270–280.

Heyman, R. E. (2001). Observation of couple conflicts: Clinical assessment applications, stubborn truths, and shaky foundations. *Psychological Assessment, 13*, 5–35.

Holmes, J. G. (2005). An integrative review of theories of interpersonal cognition: An interdependence theory perspective. In M. Baldwin (Ed.), *Interpersonal cognition* (pp. 415–447). New York: Guilford Press.

James, W. (1920). *The letters of William James*. Boston: Atlantic Monthly Press.

Johnson, S. M. (2004). *The practice of emotionally focused couple therapy* (2nd ed.). New York: Taylor & Francis.

Jourard, S. M. (1971). *Self-disclosure: An experimental analysis of the transparent self*. New York: Wiley.

Kumashiro, M., Rusbult, C. E., & Reis, H.T. (2005). *Partner responsiveness and self-regulation*. Manuscript in preparation.

Laurenceau, J. P., Barrett, L. F., & Pietromonaco, P. (1998). Intimacy as an interpersonal process: The importance of self-disclosure, partner disclosure, and perceived partner responsiveness in interpersonal exchanges. *Journal of Personality and Social Psychology, 74*, 1238–1251.

Laurenceau, J. P., Barrett, L. F., & Rovine, M. J. (2005). The interpersonal process model of intimacy in marriage: A daily-diary and multilevel modeling approach. *Journal of Family Psychology, 19*, 314–323.

Lin, Y. C. (1992). *The construction of the sense of intimacy from everyday social interaction*. Unpublished doctoral dissertation, University of Rochester.

Lippert, T., & Prager, K. J. (2001). Daily experiences of intimacy: A study of couples. *Personal Relationships, 8*, 283–298.

Magai, C. (1999). Affect, imagery, and attachment: Working models of interpersonal affect and the socialization of emotion. In J. Cassidy & P. R. Shaver (Eds.), *Handbook of attachment: Theory, research, and clinical applications* (pp. 787–802). New York: Guilford Press.

Markus, H., & Cross, S. (1990). The interpersonal self. In L. A. Pervin (Ed.), *Handbook of personality: Theory and research* (pp. 576–608). New York: Guilford Press.

Mehrabian, A. (1972). *Nonverbal communication*. Chicago: Aldine-Atherton.

Mikulincer, M. (1998). Attachment working models and the sense of trust: An exploration of interaction goals and affect regulation. *Journal of Personality and Social Psychology, 74*, 1209–1224.

Mikulincer, M., Gillath, O., Halevy, V., Avihou, N., Avidan, S., & Eshkoli, N. (2001). Attachment theory and reactions to others' needs: Evidence that activation of the sense of attachment security promotes empathic responses. *Journal of Personality and Social Psychology, 81*, 1205–1224.

Mikulincer, M., & Shaver, P. R. (2003). The attachment behavioral system in adulthood: Activation, psychodynamics, and interpersonal processes. In M. P. Zanna (Ed.), *Advances in experimental social psychology* (Vol. 35, pp. 53–152). San Diego, CA: Academic Press.

Mikulincer, M., & Shaver, P. R. (2005a). Attachment theory and emotions in close relationships: Attachment-related dynamics of emotional reactions to relational events. *Personal Relationships, 12*, 149–168.

Mikulincer, M., & Shaver, P. R. (2005b). Mental representations of attachment security: Theoretical foundation for a positive social psychology. In M. W. Baldwin (Ed.), *Interpersonal cognition* (pp. 233–266). New York: Guilford Press.

Monsour, M., Betty, S., & Kurzweil, N. (1993). Levels of perspectives and the perception of intimacy in cross-sex friendships: A balance theory explanation of shared perceptual reality. *Journal of Social and Personal Relationships*, *10*, 529–550.

Murray, S. L., Holmes, J. G., Bellavia, G., Griffin, D. W., & Dolderman, D. (2002). Kindred spirits? The benefits of egocentrism in close relationships. *Journal of Personality and Social Psychology*, *82*, 563–581.

Murray, S. L., Holmes, J. G., & Griffin, D. (1996). The benefits of positive illusions: Idealization and the construction of satisfaction in close relationships. *Journal of Personality and Social Psychology*, *70*, 79–98.

Neff, L. A., & Karney, B. R. (2002). Judgments of a relationship partner: Specific accuracy but global enhancement. *Journal of Personality*, *70*, 1079–1112.

Noller, P. (1984). *Nonverbal communication and marital interaction*. Elmsford, NY: Pergamon Press.

Patrick, B. C., & Reis, H. T. (1995). *Responsiveness to self-disclosure as a mechanism for intimacy development: The relative effects of interpersonal understanding and validation*. Unpublished manuscript.

Patterson, M. L. (1976). An arousal model of interpersonal intimacy. *Psychological Review*, *83*, 235–245.

Pennebaker, J. W. (1995). Emotion, disclosure, and health. Washington, DC: American Psychological Association.

Pietrzak, J., Downer, G., & Ayduk, O. (2005). Rejection sensitivity as an interpersonal vulnerability. In M. W. Baldwin (Ed.), *Interpersonal cognition* (pp. 62–84). New York: Guilford Press.

Prager, K. (1995). *The psychology of intimacy*. New York: Guilford Press.

Reis, H. T. (1990). The role of intimacy in interpersonal relations. *Journal of Social and Clinical Psychology*, *9*, 15–30.

Reis, H. T., & Carmichael, C. (2005). *Perceived partner regard in close relationships*. Manuscript in preparation.

Reis, H. T., Clark, M. S., & Holmes, J. G. (2004). Perceived partner responsiveness as an organizing construct in the study of intimacy and closeness. In D. Mashek & A. Aron (Eds.), *The handbook of closeness and intimacy* (pp. 201–225). Mahwah, NJ: Erlbaum.

Reis, H. T., & Patrick, B. C. (1996). Attachment and intimacy: Component processes. In E. T. Higgins & A. Kruglanski (Eds.), *Social psychology: Handbook of basic principles* (pp. 523–563). New York: Guilford Press.

Reis, H. T., & Shaver, P. (1988). Intimacy as an interpersonal process. In S. Duck (Ed.), *Handbook of personal relationships* (pp. 367–389). Chichester, UK: Wiley.

Reis, H. T., & Tsai, F. F. (2003). *Priming attachment security and goals*. Unpublished raw data.

Rogers, C. R. (1961). *On becoming a person*. Boston: Houghton Mifflin.

Sanderson, C. A. (2004). The link between the pursuit of intimacy goals and satisfaction in close relationships: An examination of the underlying processes. In D. J. Mashek & A. P. Aron (Eds.), *Handbook of closeness and intimacy* (pp. 247–266). Mahwah, NJ: Erlbaum.

Schimel, J., Arndt, J., Pyszczynski, T., & Greenberg, J. (2001). Being accepted for who we are: Evidence that social validation of the intrinsic self reduces general defensiveness. *Journal of Personality and Social Psychology, 80*, 35–52.

Shaver, P. R., Collins, N., & Clark, C. L. (1996). Attachment styles and internal working models of self and relationship partners. In G. Fletcher & J. Fitness (Eds.), *Knowledge structures and interaction in close relationships: A social psychological approach* (pp. 25–61). Hillsdale, NJ: Erlbaum.

Simpson, J. A., Rholes, W. S., & Phillips, D. (1996). Conflict in close relationships: An attachment perspective. *Journal of Personality and Social Psychology, 71*, 899–914.

Sroufe, L. A., & Fleeson, J. (1988). The coherence of individual relationships. In R. A. Hinde & J. Stevenson-Hinde (Eds.), *Relationships within families: Mutual influences* (pp. 27–47). Oxford, UK: Oxford University Press.

Swann, W. B., Jr., de la Ronde, C., & Hixon, J. G. (1994). Authenticity and positivity strivings in marriage and courtship. *Journal of Personality and Social Psychology, 66*, 857–869.

Tidwell, M. C. O., Reis, H. T., & Shaver, P. R. (1996). Attachment, attractiveness, and social interaction: A diary study. *Journal of Personality and Social Psychology, 71*, 729–745.

Vaillant, G. E. (1977). *Adaptation to life*. Boston: Little, Brown.

16

Seasons of the Heart

ELLEN BERSCHEID

Participants in the conference that led to this book were instructed to focus on "the interplay between attachment, caregiving, and sex within romantic and marital relationships." Because I was assigned to a session titled "Interfaces between Attachment Theory and Other Perspectives on Romantic Love," I assumed that the organizers wished me to represent one of those "other perspectives," namely, what has been called the "two-component theory of romantic love" presented by Elaine (Walster) Hatfield and me more than 30 years ago (Berscheid & Walster, 1974). If my assumption was correct, the organizers were disappointed. In the brief historical perspective with which I begin this chapter, I discuss the political purpose of that 1974 article, "A Little Bit about Love," to which (in my view at least) the two-component model was secondary.

Rather than the so-called "two-component model of love," the "other perspective" I shall discuss in this chapter draws on the taxonomy of love I presented in my 1985 *Handbook of Social Psychology* article on interpersonal attraction (Berscheid, 1985). Although it has been widely ignored since the day it was presented, I have found no reason to abandon my 1985 taxonomy over the past two decades. In my original presentation of that classification scheme, I briefly speculated on the "interplay" between the interpersonal affect systems I outlined—their interplay both over the lifespan of the individual and over the lifespan of a relationship. Hence, the title of this chapter: "Seasons of the Heart."

"BUT WHAT ABOUT TENDERNESS?"

My mini-historical retrospective goes back to about 25 years ago, when I was invited to participate in the annual Carnegie Mellon Symposium on Cognition, which was to address, for the first time, the interaction between cognition and affect (Berscheid, 1982). The lecture I had prepared provided a brief rendering of my emotion-in-relationship model, which focuses on the antecedents of "hot" emotion in close relationships, subsequently published in *Close Relationships* (Kelley et al., 1983/2002; Berscheid, 1983/2002). As I was walking up the path to the lecture hall where I was to deliver my talk, I noticed a gardener puttering about the many plants and bushes in the garden that fronted the building. A tall man, garbed in sandals, loose T-shirt, and baggy Japanese gardening pants, he was carefully examining the undersides of the leaves of some of the plants and pulling a few weeds here and there. Later, when it was my turn to go to the lectern, I saw the gardener again. He was sitting at the back of the dark, almost empty, auditorium, far from the symposium participants and the few others attending, all of whom were clustered in the front rows. Surmising that he was taking a break from his horticultural duties and sought the comfort of a seat in the cool lecture hall, I thought no more about it.

Much later, however, when we speakers were discussing and debating the day's offerings in an adjacent conference room, I was surprised to see the gardener casually wander into the room and sit down silently in one of the chairs lined up against the wall. After we'd finished and I was rushing out of the building to attend the dinner our hosts had arranged, I was startled when he stopped me and said, "Ellen, I really liked what you had to say today." He paused for a moment and added, "But what about tenderness?" "What about tenderness?" I replied, "Well, what *about* tenderness?" He elaborated. He said he was talking about the feeling one gets when one looks at an infant asleep in a crib. Hungry and ready to get some sleep myself, I quickly conceded that my model couldn't account for such "cool," nonarousing feelings as tenderness but that it certainly was something to think about (although *I* obviously never had). Mulling over his question as I hurried on my way, I thought, "Boy, even the gardeners at Carnegie Mellon are smart!" When I arrived at dinner, several speakers came up to me and said, "We saw Herb Simon talking to you—what did he have to say?" Thus I learned that I had mistaken psychology's first Nobel laureate for the gardener.

The point of my tale is not that there is a reason my family refers to me as "Ms. Magoo." It is that, at that time, I didn't know many people who could have answered Herb Simon's question, "But what about tenderness?" or who could have told him where that particular feeling fit into what we knew about the emotions and feelings people commonly experience in relationships. Today, however, it is easy to guess that the feeling of tenderness has something to do with "caregiving," for tenderness usually is felt for the young, weak, or vulnerable. But at that time, just 25 years ago, "caregiving" and "attachment" were foreign words to most social psychologists. At least they were to me.

ROMANTIC LOVE AND LIKING

When I went to Carnegie Mellon I had just begun to write the first chapter on interpersonal attraction to be included in *The Handbook of Social Psychology* (Lindzey & Aronson, 1985). Previous handbooks had included nothing directly on interpersonal attraction or on enduring relationships but, by the time of the third edition, social psychologists knew a lot about attraction—or "liking" for strangers in initial encounters within a laboratory setting. Virtually all attraction investigators assumed that the causal determinants of liking—or mild positive sentiment for another—were precisely the same as the causal determinants of love and other strong forms of attraction, those causal conditions simply being present in stronger magnitude in the case of strong forms of attraction, such as romantic love. This assumption, combined with the primary theoretical formulation underlying virtually all attraction research at the time—the reward–punishment perspective of the learning theories—had led to the widely accepted idea that a whole lot of rewards anticipated or received from another produced love, whereas lesser amounts produced liking.

Elaine Hatfield and I (Berscheid & Walster, 1974) had challenged that idea a few years earlier in our 1974 article. We observed that greater and greater increases in liking did not seem to culminate in romantic love as frequently as everyone seemed to assume. We argued that the causal conditions associated with romantic love were *qualitatively different* from those associated with liking. One of those differences, we said, was the role of reward and punishment, which seemed to operate in what we called a "sensible" way in the case of liking (that is, more rewards and fewer punishments from another generally resulted in liking that person more), but not in the case of romantic love. Romantic love, it seemed to us, was often characterized by what we called a "hodgepodge" of emotions, some of which—jealousy, despair, and anger, for example—were highly unpleasant. In short, our thesis was that romantic love is a different animal than liking and thus deserved to be studied on its own.

The primary purpose of the 1974 article, then, was to persuade our colleagues in the attraction arena that they were deluding themselves if they thought that by identifying the determinants of liking they were also identifying the determinants of romantic love. But how could we phrase our message diplomatically? How could we say to our colleagues, many of whom at the time were interpreting the results of their "liking" studies in romantic-love terms, "You [and we] haven't really been studying romantic love?" Elaine, who always had a clever solution for such puzzles, quickly came up with a solution: We'd rename liking "companionate love." Hence, our colleagues *were* studying love—it was just love of a different kind than romantic love. So it was that in the revision of our book *Interpersonal Attraction* (Berscheid & Walster, 1978) we included a chapter on "romantic love" and a separate chapter on "companionate love," or liking a person with whom we are interdependent. Subsequently, Walster and Walster (1978) devoted an entire book to comparing and contrasting romantic and companionate love.

Although the romantic–companionate love distinction has endured and is common today, at the time it came as a news bulletin to some. For example, one night I stayed up late to watch the *Tonight Show* because it had been advertised that Virginia Johnson (of Masters and Johnson human-sexual-response fame) would talk about love. In her interview with Johnny Carson, I was startled to hear her say that she had it on the good authority of two psychologists named Berscheid and Walster (waving our book in the air) that being romantically in love with another and liking them were two different things and had different causes. The much-married Carson was highly interested in this news and, naturally enough, wanted to know what the causes of romantic love were. Johnson quickly steered the conversation off into other matters.

Besides ourselves, Zick Rubin (1974) also was drawing attention to the difference between liking and loving and empirically developed two scales intended to capture the difference. Rubin speculated that the dimensions underlying his Love Scale were attachment, caring for the welfare of the other, and a willingness to self-disclose to the other, whereas the primary dimensions underlying his Liking Scale seemed to him to be affection and respect. After going to all the work of developing these scales, however, he was disappointed to find that, among young, heterosexual couples who scored high on another scale he'd developed—the Romanticism Scale—Liking Scale scores were as powerful predictors of their movement toward a more intense relationship as their Love Scale scores were; worse, among those who scored low on the Romanticism Scale, neither Liking scores nor Love scores predicted movement toward marriage. Rubin's report ended with a two-part question: "What are the causal, sequential links between liking and loving? Under what specific conditions does each facilitate the development of the other?" (1974, p. 400).

Social psychologists are still asking those questions. For example, Susan and Clyde Hendrick, in their chapter on "Romantic Love" in *Close Relationships: A Sourcebook* (2000), question Walster and Walster's (1978) contention, subsequently endorsed by many others, that romantic (or "passionate") love usually appears first in romantic relationships and then, if the relationship endures, gradually evolves into companionate love. In other words, the Hendricks question what they call the "either/or theory of love," which proposes that one can *either* be in a state of passionate love *or* in a state of companionate love but not in both states at the same time. The Hendricks muse that, to the contrary, "Perhaps passion does not have to die, and perhaps companionship is important from the beginnings of the relationship" (2000, p. 204). I return to their conjecture later; the point here is simply that the sequence of these varieties of affect within a single relationship is still a matter of speculation. Rubin's question of 30 years ago has yet to be answered.

Whereas the topic of romantic love was on the periphery of attraction research and of social psychology when I was embarking on my review of the interpersonal attraction literature in the early 1980s, the topic of loneliness was front and center. An important stimulus to research on loneliness had been a book, *Loneliness: The Experience of Emotional and Social Isolation*, arranged and edited by Robert S. Weiss (1973). It included an article by John Bowlby (1973), who presented some of his attachment theory ideas and emphasized that the reward–punishment perspective of the learning theories could *not* account for this type of affectional bond.

Bowlby's chapter in Weiss's book captured my attention for at least two reasons: First, Zick Rubin, who had had some training in developmental psychology, had speculated that attachment was one of the dimensions underlying romantic love (but not liking); and, second, Elaine Hatfield and I had observed that romantic love did not seem to follow reward–punishment principles. I went on to read Bowlby's 1979 book, *The Making and Breaking of Affectional Bonds*, which gave a more detailed view of his thoughts about attachment and its association with attraction and other interpersonal phenomena. Believing that Bowlby's views needed representation in the *Handbook* chapter, I scoured the literature looking for empirical studies that applied attachment theory to adult attraction. I found only one to cite: "Childhood Attachment Experience and Adult Loneliness," by Phil Shaver and Carin Rubenstein (1980).

CLASSIFYING VARIETIES OF LOVE

I regarded the *Handbook* chapter as an opportunity to put love on the radar of psychologists interested in interpersonal attraction but to do that, I believed I should make an attempt to classify the kinds of love humans typically feel for one another. At that time, there was no dearth of taxonomies of love. Most, however, had been developed by philosophers who had drawn their conclusions from their own personal experiences and observations. An example, later to be pursued empirically by Clyde and Susan Hendrick (e.g., 1986), was constructed by Lee (1973), who had published a book outlining a number of what he called "love styles." These were based on his interviews with people who had been encouraged to talk about their romantic love experiences and also on his readings of works of literature and philosophy. Lee titled his book *The Colours of Love: An Exploration of the Ways of Loving*. The "ways of loving" Lee addressed were the ways adults "loved" members of the opposite sex—or "romantic love," as it is often viewed. I, however, wanted to sketch the entire landscape of love, or positive interpersonal affect; romantic love, in my view, was only one part of that landscape.

Here, I must pause to note that the title of this volume (and the title of the conference that preceded it) confused me, undoubtedly because the term "romantic love" itself is confusing. It is often used loosely to refer to any kind of positive affect that occurs within a relationship between a man and a woman, especially a relationship that either is progressing toward or has culminated in marriage—that is, courtship or marital relationships (see Berscheid & Regan, 2005). I assumed this is the way it was used in the title of this book and the conference. However, the term "romantic love" also is used to refer to a particular *kind* of positive affect—or syndrome of emotions, feelings, attitudes, and behaviors—as opposed to other kinds of positive affect that are often observed in a relationship between a man and a woman, which is how I am using the term. I emphasize this because romantic love may be experienced in relationships with like-sex persons and in relationships in which progress toward marriage is not an objective. Moreover, adult relationships between men and women often exhibit other kinds of positive affect, and it is important to distinguish these from romantic love. Thus I found the title "Dynamics of Romantic Love: Attachment, Caregiving, and Sex" confusing because it implies that attachment, caregiving, and sex are components of romantic love. In my view, each—romantic love, attachment, caregiving, and sex—is conceptually and empirically distinguishable from the others. Although all may be observed in courtship and marital relationships, only the word "sex" refers distinctively to the romantic-love pattern of affect, as Sally Meyers and I have elaborated theoretically and supported empirically (Berscheid & Meyers, 1996; Meyers & Berscheid, 1997).

When I was attempting to construct a taxonomy of love for the 1985 *Handbook*, I believed that the taxonomist must provide *justification* for clumping some things together and for differentiating that clump of things from other clumps of things. For the behavioral scientist, it seemed to me that the most compelling reason for distinguishing seemingly like things from each other is evidence that each has different causes and different consequences. Hal Kelley subsequently elaborated this point of view with respect to theories of love in our book *Close Relationships* (Kelley et al., 1983/2002). He observed that any particular conception or theory of love has associated with it a cluster of ideas that includes four components (p. 269): first, ideas about the *historical antecedents* of the current causes of the observed phenomena; second, the *current causes* believed to be responsible at present for the observed phenomena; third, *observable manifestations*, including actions and feelings that are the characteristic indications of that kind of love; and fourth and finally, ideas about the *future course of the phenomena*, given the causes and processes currently under way.

A consideration of the types of positive affect humans may feel for other humans led me to propose that there are basically four types of positive affect systems, each of which has the same historical antecedents, namely, the human's biological heritage developed over evolutionary time but (1) different current causes, (2) different characteristic behaviors on the part of the person who experiences the affect, and also (3) different characteristics of the person who is usually the target of (or stimulus for) the affect. The four types of love I named in the *Handbook* taxonomy were the following.

Attachment Love

As originally proposed by Bowlby (e.g., 1979) and Harlow (1958), and as has now become well established, the attachment system appears to be "innate," or unlearned, and thus its *historical cause* lies in the evolutionary history of the human species and the need for infants to stay in close proximity to a protector to survive; its *immediate cause* is a threatening situation; its *characteristic behaviors* are those that promote proximity to the protector; and its interpersonal *target* is usually a familiar person who is older, stronger, and wiser than the individual. As both Bowlby and Harlow emphasized, reward–punishment principles are *not* among its causal conditions. Although Bowlby theorized that attachment is characteristic of all humans over their lifespan, this *normative* feature of attachment theory has been almost wholly ignored. As Jeff Simpson and Steven Rholes note in their introduction to their edited book, *Attachment Theory and Close Relationships* (1998), the normative component of attachment theory—"which attempts to explain modal, species-typical patterns of behavior and stages of development through which nearly all human beings pass"—has been neglected in favor of its *individual difference* component, "which attempts to explain stable, systematic deviations from the modal behavioral patterns and stages" (1998, p. 4).

Altruistic Love

My *Handbook* taxonomy named a second kind of interpersonal affect system, "altruistic love," which I defined as caring about another's welfare and taking actions to promote it regardless of whether those actions are perceived to result in future benefits to the self. Thanks to the work of Shaver and others and a greater awareness of Bowlby's attachment theory, I now realize that "altruistic love" was not the best name to give to this kind of love. Even in the early 1980s, it had many other names, including "charitable love," "brotherly love," "communal love," "agape," and Maslow's term, "B-love," or love for another's being. Today, another name—"compassionate love"—has been coined for this type of love about which researchers seem to be getting empirically serious, as evidenced by a symposium on compassionate love at the recent International Association of Relationship Research (IARR) conference at the University of Wisconsin in July 2004. As I noted in my comments there, the dictionary (e.g., *Merriam-Webster's Collegiate Dictionary*, 1993, 10th ed., p. 234) defines compassion as "sympathetic consciousness of others' distress together with a desire to alleviate it" (p. 234), a definition consistent with the findings of Bev Fehr and Sue Sprecher's systematic empirical research on people's understanding of the term (Fehr & Sprecher, 2004).

I now suspect that the interpersonal affect system underlying this kind of love is the caregiving system, identified by Bowlby and Harlow, and that it would be profitable for researchers to view it that way. The caregiving system, like the attachment system, appears to be part of the human's biological heritage. Indeed, as many have observed, the attachment system could not have evolved without the complement of a caregiving system. Like attachment, then, the *historical cause* of this kind of love—caregiving love or compassionate love or whatever you want to call it—lies in the evolutionary history of the human species. My colleague David Lykken's (1999) elaboration of caregiving love not incidentally addresses Herb Simon's question "But what about tenderness?":

> Young animals are vulnerable and relatively helpless so we, like other mammals, evolved a tendency for parents to behave in a nurturant and protective way toward their offspring. The greater probability that nurtured and protected offspring would survive to breed themselves was the cause of this evolved proclivity. But the actual mechanism that evolved to yield this useful tendency is relatively nonspecific. Like many other mammals, we seem to have an innate disposition to be protective of the helpless and vulnerable. (p. 24)

Lykken goes on to observe that "this nonspecific feeling of tenderness toward the helpless and vulnerable" (1999, p. 25) may have unanticipated consequences, such as the full range of parental emotions and nurturing impulses shown toward pet animals (and see Berscheid & Regan, 2005, pp. 154–156). Indeed, responses to distress calls not infrequently occur across species; that is, humans respond to animals' distress calls and animals often respond to ours.

In sum, whereas the *historical cause* of this type of love lies in human evolutionary history, its *current, immediate cause* is the perception that another is in distress. Its *characteristic behaviors* depend on the nature of the distress that is perceived, because the motive underlying the behavior is alleviation of the distress. The *target* of the behavior is a distressed person. If it is true that all humans are born with an unlearned caregiving system that results in responding to distress calls made by other members of the species, then, as is true of the attachment system, the causal conditions for activation of the caregiving system do *not* follow reward–punishment principles.

Social psychologists have extensively studied caregiving in adults under such rubrics as "social support" and "prosocial behavior" (see Berscheid & Collins, 2000), but many unanswered questions associated with the caregiving system remain. One of these is how early the system is activated. Caregiving in children, who less frequently have the resources to respond effectively to another's distress, has been little investigated, but there is no reason to think that distress calls are unnoticed by children or that they would not respond with distress-alleviating behavior if they could.

Romantic Love

The third interpersonal affect system I named in the *Handbook* chapter was romantic love, also frequently called "passionate love" or "erotic love." As the word "erotic" denotes, this type of love historically has been strongly associated with sexual desire. Indeed, Sally Meyers and I (Meyers & Berscheid, 1997) demonstrated that people who care for another but do *not* feel sexual desire for that person rarely describe their feelings as "romantic love." Moreover, people who *do* say they are romantically in love with another almost always also say they feel sexual desire for the other, and they also almost always say they care for, and like, the other. When they sexually desire a person but do not like or care for him or her, they are unlikely to describe their feelings as "romantic love." In other words, our results suggested that, roughly speaking:

- Romantic love = liking *with* sexual desire.
- Companionate love = liking *without* sexual desire.
- Lust = sexual desire *without* liking.

The *historical cause* of sexual desire, which appears to be a necessary but not sufficient condition for a person to describe his or her feelings toward another as "romantic love," and the sexual/reproductive system, which is its source, again lie in our evolutionary history. As Shaver and his associates discuss:

> Animals, including humans, have been constructed by evolution to place a high priority on sexual reproduction. . . . The cycle of desire and arousal

> followed by sexual behavior and orgasm can easily be viewed as an innate system with an important biological function. (Shaver, Hazan, & Bradshaw, 1988, p. 87)

The *current causes* of sexual desire have not been well established (see Regan & Berscheid, 1999), although they often include good general health and the availability of an appropriate *target*, usually a physically attractive, fertile person of the opposite sex, as evolutionary psychologists maintain. Its *characteristic behaviors*, apart from the sexual arousal–orgasm cycle, typically include planned pursuit of a person of the opposite sex with the motive to sexually mate with that person.

Friendship

The fourth, and final, variety of love I named in the *Handbook* chapter was friendship, which also often goes by other names, including "philias," "liking," "affection," "affiliation," "pragmatic love," and, as I've discussed, "companionate love." This affect system, unlike the attachment, caregiving, and sexual systems, *is* very much based on reward–punishment principles; that is, we feel positive affect for those who reward us and dislike those who punish us. Again, the *historical cause* of the behavior is our evolutionary heritage and the pain–pleasure principle that has served as the basic motivating principle underlying most psychological theories of behavior, particularly the learning theories; the *current causes* of liking, its associated *characteristic behaviors*, and its typical *targets* are listed and discussed in chapters on interpersonal attraction in social psychology textbooks.

In sum, these four seemed to me then, and seem to me now, to be human beings' biologically based and innately given positive *interpersonal affect systems*, at least at the psychological level of analysis (what the neurological level of analysis will ultimately reveal is not clear). My thesis is that each deserves to be treated separately because each has different causal conditions for activation and different consequences (i.e., associated behaviors and interpersonal targets). For example, we can be attached to persons whom we do not like or respect, are not sexually attracted to, and who, as Bowlby and other ethologists have observed, have been more a source of punishment than reward. We can, and often do, exhibit caregiving behavior toward people we do not know, do not like, are not sexually attracted to, and from whom we expect no reward; their distress activates our caregiving system and we respond. Similarly, we can be sexually attracted to unfamiliar people to whom we are not attached and do not particularly like (and whom, in fact, we know to be scoundrels); conversely, we can be sexually repulsed by people we like very much.

THE "INTERPLAY" BETWEEN TYPES OF LOVE

I have outlined in some detail the types of love I think it worthwhile to separate conceptually because one cannot consider the "interplay" among things without being clear about the nature of the things presumed to be interacting. Similarly, hypotheses about the interplay between those things cannot be investigated if each cannot be measured separately. In the *Handbook*, I suggested:

> It seems reasonable that although all forms of love may be experienced in different blends at one time in the same relationship, certain varieties may be more characteristic of some stages of a relationship than others, partially because their determinants are more likely to be in force at some stages than at others. (Berscheid, 1985, p. 437)

In other words, one set of questions about the interplay among these types of love must address how they are likely to *interact within a specific relationship*. Investigation of these questions would require samples of relationships of greater age range than those typical of unmarried college sophomores and a broader range of relationship types than courting or dating relationships. A broader range of relationship types would be necessary because some varieties of love may occur more or less often in different types of relationships and different social contexts, partly as a result of cultural beliefs that some kinds of love are more appropriate to certain types of relationships than to other types of relationships.

A second set of questions about the interplay among the four types of love must address how they are likely to *interact over the lifespan of the individual*: "Some varieties [of love] also may be more characteristic of individuals at some developmental and life cycle stages than others" (Berscheid, 1985, p. 437).

Finding the answers to the first set of questions depends somewhat on the answers to the second set of questions, because over the lifespan of a long-term relationship, both partners are aging as the relationship ages, possibly making some types of love more likely than others over time simply as a result of lifespan developmental processes.

Some Theoretical (or Possibly Semantic) Differences with Shaver and Colleagues

Shaver and his associates (1988) are among the few, if any, researchers who have attempted to address how different interpersonal affect systems may interact. Although the principal thrust of their theory was to propose that adult romantic love and infant–caregiver attachment have observable and theoretical similarities, Shaver, Hazan, and Bradshaw's (1988) theory of love goes beyond the romantic-love-equals-attachment theme to propose that "adult love is an integration of three behavioral systems (discussed by Bowlby): attachment, caregiving, and sexuality" (1988, p. 70). These theorists also hypothesize that "these three systems . . . operate differently over the course of the relationship, causing the quality of love to change accordingly" (p. 70). Although I endorse this hypothesis, my views differ from those of Shaver et al. in at least three respects.

First, three of the "behavioral systems" Shaver et al. (1988) address in their theory—attachment, caregiving, and sexuality—are generally the same as three of the "varieties of love" I include in my taxonomy. The fourth one I include—friendship—does not appear in their theory. I justified the inclusion of friendship love (or *philias*, or liking, or companionate love) as a variety of love because the tendency to move toward people and things that give pleasure and are rewarding and away from people and things that are painful and punishing is perhaps the most adaptive and fundamental of the human species' evolutionary legacies. Moreover, because it is nonspecific, the pleasure–pain principle also underlies the other three varieties of love (e.g., proximity to an attachment figure is rewarding and caregiving is pleasurable, as is sexual activity).

Second, I believe there is a difference between the phrases "romantic love" and "adult love" and, thus, that these phrases should not be used as synonyms. Whereas Shaver and his associates (1988) seem to identify "romantic love" principally with attachment, their view of romantic love also sometimes (as in the title of this book) seems to include caregiving and sexuality as well. I, on the other hand, identify "romantic love" strongly with the sexual/reproductive system—not the attachment system and not the caregiving system. Shaver et al.'s "adult love" includes the attachment system and the caregiving and sexuality systems. I agree with Shaver et al. that "adult love" (if the phrase is taken to mean love of unspecified variety within a specific relationship between two adults) may involve attachment, caregiving, and sexuality, but, as previously discussed, I *add* a fourth, companionate love (or *philias*, liking, friendship).

Third, and importantly, in the phrase "adult love is an integration of three behavioral systems," I do not know what is meant by the term "integration." I have strenuously argued that the four types of love I have named should be kept conceptually and empirically separate. How a person experiences activation of the three systems within a specific relationship is a different matter, however. Perhaps "integrated" was intended to mean "experienced together." It is true that things joined experientially tend to become integrated cognitively. If so, self-report would not be useful in examining the interplay between types of love (or behavioral systems) because people would not separate the different types of positive affect they feel for another (i.e., their melded feelings simply would be reported as "love"). If so, behavioral measures will prove more useful in investigations of the interplay between systems.

NORMATIVE PATTERNS IN TYPES OF LOVE EXPERIENCED OVER THE RELATIONSHIP'S LIFE

Despite these differences, I agree with Shaver et al. (1988) that these systems probably "operate differently over the course of the relationship" (p. 70). Although each affect system is conceptually separable from the others, it is easy to see that the partner may be the target of all of these behavioral systems at various times over the course of the individual's relationship with that person. It also seems possible that all may be active at one point in time in the relationship but that, at other times, only one or two or three may be active.

Implicit in the hypothesis that these systems operate differently over the course of the relationship is the supposition that there are *normative patterns* in the operation of these systems over the lifespan of certain types of relationships (e.g., romantic relationships). It is these normative patterns that need to be empirically determined. I should immediately note, however, that when one speaks of a normative pattern of affect over the course of a particular type of relationship, the discourse becomes somewhat tautological, because relationship "type" tends to be defined not only by the age and other characteristics of the partners and by the social context of the relationship (see Berscheid, 1994) but also by the affect system (or variety of love) currently dominant in the relationship. For example, as I have discussed, a relationship in which the partners are young adults who like each other and feel some sexual attraction for each other and whose relationship seemingly is progressing toward permanence is often described as a "romantic relationship." Similarly, a relationship in which the partners are different in age, with one partner vulnerable and weak and the other strong and nurturant, is often termed a "parental" relationship (if kinship exists) or a "mentoring" or "avuncular" relationship (if it doesn't). Thus, because the type of affect system currently dominant in the relationship is often used to classify the type of relationship it is, investigations of the course of affect over relationships of a certain type might need to be reframed as investigations of normative affect patterns over the course of relationships that vary by their initially dominant affect system.

Not a great deal is known empirically about the normative patterns of affect systems that are characteristic of different types of relationships. One reason such knowledge is sparse is that investigation of the interplay among the four types of love (or affective behavioral systems) I've described requires at minimum: (1) measures of each of the four types of love, preferably behavioral as opposed to self-report measures, permitting the construction of a "four-point profile" of the quality of love (or blend of love) present in the relationship at a given time; (2) a very large relationship population, preferably of many different relationship types (e.g., same sex–opposite sex; same age–different age; kin–nonkin, etc.), followed longitudinally.

SOME HYPOTHESES ABOUT NORMATIVE PATTERNS OF AFFECT WITHIN A "ROMANTIC RELATIONSHIP"

Although empirical evidence is lacking, many hypotheses have been advanced about the "course of love" often seen in "romantic relationships" between two adults. Again, these hypotheses concern the *normative* patterns of the appearance and disappearance of different varieties of love in a relationship between two adults (often called a "romantic" relationship when the partners are opposite-sex, experience sexual desire, and are progressing toward marriage or another quasi-permanent status, such as cohabitation).

The "Either–Or" Hypothesis

Earlier I mentioned the "either–or" hypothesis: that romantic love appears first in the relationship (and thus gives the relationship its "romantic relationship" label), companionate love appears later, and the two rarely appear together. There now is some evidence that this hypothesis is false, that, in fact, liking for another combined with sexual attraction is typical of the first stage of a "romantic relationship" between two adults. For example, Hendrick and Hendrick (1993) concluded from their study of dating couples that "there is a strong friendship component to love, even in the romantic love relationships of young adults who are merely dating" (p. 464) and that "the friendship component of romantic love does not develop later in a relationship . . . but rather is present early on and in some cases precedes the felt 'experiencing of love' " (p. 465). Supporting the Hendricks' conclusion, Meyers and Berscheid (1997) subsequently found that, if an individual said he or she was "in love" with another, that person was also highly likely to be described as a "friend" (although the reverse was not true—only rarely are people "in love" with their friends). This suggests that these two interpersonal affect systems facilitate each other—or at least do not interfere with each other—at least initially.

The Westermarck Hypothesis

Although it may seem reasonable on the face of it that all four of the systems should facilitate, or at least not inhibit, the activation of any one of the other systems over the course of the relationship (because all are varieties of love, or positive affect), some theorists have hypothesized otherwise. One of these is cultural anthropologist Arthur Wolf (1995), who conducted a lifelong investigation of the Westermarck hypothesis from Chinese archival records. Contrary to Freud (e.g., 1920/1953), who believed that an incestuous love target was the first and normative love choice of all humans, Westermarck (e.g., 1922) asserted that persons living closely together from childhood not only are likely to be sexually indifferent to each other but are likely to develop an outright aversion to sexual activity with the familiar other.

As a graduate student doing field work in China, Wolf discovered that Mother Nature had formed the conditions of a natural experiment to test Westermarck's hypothesis. At one time, there were two forms of marriage in China: one that involved early and intimate association between the future bride and groom and one that prohibited all contact between the partners prior to the marriage ceremony. In a dazzling display of scholarship, one that took him a lifetime to accomplish, Wolf painstakingly ascertained that the other characteristics of the couples and their situations were equal, at least in terms of the dependent variable, which was the spouses' sexual attraction to each other, as measured by their fertility and likelihood of divorce or separation. In the end, Wolf found support for Westermarck's hypothesis: Couples who had had early childhood association had fewer children and were more likely to separate than those who had no contact before marriage.

Of more interest to the present discussion, however, is Wolf's finding that the adverse effect on sexual attraction of early childhood association was most marked among couples brought together in the bride's first or second year. To interpret that finding, Wolf turned to Bowlby's attachment theory, which posits that these are the very years during which children form their most intense and demanding attachments. Wolf reasoned that perhaps Westermarck's aversion and Bowlby's attachment are closely related phenomena, even two sides of the same coin. A disposition to form strong emotional bonds with people who are older and wiser has survival advantages but entails the dangers of inbreeding. Thus:

> Might it not be, then, that what nature has selected for in infants and small children is a disposition one aspect of which is a strong tendency to attach socially and the other an equally strong tendency to avoid sexually? (Wolf, 1995, p. 464)

Wolf argues that the success of childhood-association marriages varied with the age at which the wife was adopted, but not the husband's age at her arrival, because the wife was usually younger than the husband and, therefore, she was the one who developed an attachment to him and, hence, an aversion to sexual relations with him (see Wolf, p. 465).

Wolf proposes, in addition, that caregiving also is a contrasexual disposition—that by evolutionary necessity both attachment and caregiving carry with them an aversion to sexual relations:

> Why doesn't the husband in a minor [childhood association] marriage ignore his wife's aversion and, if necessary, use his authority to overcome her resistance? Because having known his wife when she was still a helpless infant, and having participated in teaching her to cope, he is as averse to sexual relations with her as she is to such relations with her caretakers. (Wolf, 1995, p. 466)

Whether the giving of sustained care in an adult relationship (where there has been no childhood association) also inhibits sexual desire is not clear. The only evidence on this count I've been able to find is a "Dear Abby" piece in which a husband asks the advice columnist how he can explain to his ill wife, who is pestering him for sexual relations, that he now sees himself as her "caregiver"—not her lover. Interestingly, the only speculation that caregiving may inhibit another interpersonal affect system is found in Kunce and Shaver (1994), who wonder whether perhaps attachment and caregiving are competing systems.

It is clear that the number of questions that might be asked about the normative patterns of the activation of the four affect systems I've named over the course of a relationship are legion. Even the most elementary of these have yet to be answered. For example, how long does it take for an attachment to develop between romantic partners? Shaver and his associates (1988), in their strong identification of romantic love with attachment, seem to imply that a "romantic figure" quickly and automatically becomes an "attachment figure." However, familiarity, which appears to be an essential element in the development of attachment, takes time. In his studies of persons divorced or otherwise separated from their spouses, Weiss (1975) noted that many displayed a bewildering (at least to them) desire to reachieve proximity with their now disliked, and even hated, spouse. Weiss observed that such attachment behavior seemed most likely to be displayed if the individual had been married 2 years or longer. Moreover, as opposed to familiarity, novelty appears to be an important element in sexual attraction, which (as I've discussed) appears to be a necessary condition for an individual to describe his or her feelings as "romantic love." Thus, are attachment and sexual desire antagonists, as Wolf suspects? Furthermore, is it true that all romantic partners become attachment figures? Some evidence on this point is needed, especially because Bowlby theorized that attachment is generally felt for persons wiser, stronger, and older. Some romantic partners are dumb, weak, and young (but perhaps highly physically attractive and sexually desired). Do these partners also become attachment figures?

THE BOTTOM LINE

My thesis has been that, first, it is useful to separate the major varieties of love conceptually and empirically—not to meld two or more under a "romantic love" rubric. Second, as this suggests, it is important to differentiate between the *affect* "romantic love" and a "romantic love" *relationship*. Third, the evidence that sexual desire is necessary although not sufficient for most people to describe their feelings as romantic love is strong and should not be ignored. The sexual/reproductive system is biologically of the greatest importance to humans and other species, and, thus, it would be peculiar if it did not have special properties and influences on the operation of the other affect systems. Fourth, Wolf's hypothesis—that attachment and caregiving are contrasexual—needs investigation, especially because growing familiarity with another over time seems to facilitate attachment but diminish sexual desire (see Regan & Berscheid, 1999).

The title of this chapter was taken from John Denver's song "Seasons of the Heart," in which he laments that "A wiser man than I might know the seasons of the heart." I don't know who that "wiser man" might be. Those of us who have studied the heart must confess that we know no more than John Denver did about its seasons over the course of a relationship or over the course of a lifetime. For myself, however, I consider it an achievement that, thanks principally to the work of Phil Shaver and his many associates, we now can at least cobble together an answer to the question that haunted me for so many years: "But what about tenderness?"

REFERENCES

Berscheid, E. (1982). Attraction and emotion in interpersonal relationships. In M. S. Clark & S. T. Fiske (Eds.), *Affect and cognition* (pp. 37–54). Hillsdale, NJ: Erlbaum.

Berscheid, E. (2002). Emotion. In H. H. Kelley, E. Berscheid, A. Christensen, J. H. Harvey, T. L. Huston, G. Levinger, E. McClintock, L. A. Peplau, & D. R. Peterson, *Close relationships* (pp. 110–168). Clinton Corners, NY: Percheron Press. (Original work published 1983)

Berscheid, E. (1985). Interpersonal attraction. In G. Lindzey & E. Aronson (Eds.), *The handbook of social psychology* (3rd ed., pp. 110–168). New York: Random House.

Berscheid, E. (1994). Interpersonal relationships. *Annual Review of Psychology*, *45*, 70–129.

Berscheid, E., & Collins, W. A. (2000). Who cares? For whom and when, how, and why? *Psychological Inquiry*, *11*, 107–109.

Berscheid, E., & Meyers, S. A. (1996). A social categorical approach to a question about love. *Personal Relationships*, *3*, 19–43.

Berscheid, E., & Regan, P. (2005). *The psychology of interpersonal relationships*. New York: Prentice Hall.

Berscheid, E., & Walster, E. (1974). A little bit about love. In T. L. Huston (Ed.), *Foundations of interpersonal attraction* (pp. 355–381). New York: Academic Press.

Berscheid, E., & Walster (Hatfield), E. (1978). *Interpersonal attraction* (2nd ed.). Reading, MA: Addison Wesley.

Bowlby, J. (1973). Affectional bonds: Their nature and origin. In R. S. Weiss (Ed.), *Loneliness: The experience of emotional and social isolation* (pp. 38–52). Cambridge, MA: MIT Press.

Bowlby, J. (1979). *The making and breaking of affectional bonds*. London: Tavistock.

Denver, J. (1981). Seasons of the heart. On *The country roads collection* [CD]. New York: RCA.

Fehr, B., & Sprecher, S. (2004, July). *Compassionate love: Conceptual, relational, and behavioral issues*. Paper presented at the conference of the International Association for Relationship Research, Madison, WI.

Freud, S. (1953). *A general introduction to psychoanalysis* [J. Riviere, Trans.]. New York: Pocket Books. (Original work published 1920)

Harlow, H. F. (1958). The nature of love. *American Psychologist, 13*, 673–685.

Hendrick, C., & Hendrick, S. S. (1986). A theory and method of love. *Journal of Personality and Social Psychology, 50*, 392–402.

Hendrick, S. S., & Hendrick, C. (1993). Lovers as friends. *Journal of Social and Personal Relationships, 10*, 459–466.

Hendrick, S. S., & Hendrick, C. (2000). Romantic love. In C. Hendrick & S. S. Hendrick (Eds.), *Close relationships: A sourcebook* (pp. 203–215). Thousand Oaks, CA: Sage.

Kelley, H. H. (2002). Love and commitment. In H. H. Kelley, E. Berscheid, A. Christensen, J. H. Harvey, T. L. Huston, G. Levinger, E. McClintock, L. A. Peplau, & D. R. Peterson (Eds.), *Close relationships* (pp. 265–314). Clinton Corners, NY: Percheron Press. (Original work published 1983)

Kelley, H. H., Berscheid, E., Christensen, A., Harvey, J. H., Huston, T. L., Levinger, G., McClintock, E., Peplau, L. A., & Peterson, D. R. (2002). *Close relationships*. Clinton Corners, NY: Percheron Press. (Original work published 1983)

Kunce, L. J., & Shaver, P. R. (1994). An attachment-theoretical approach to caregiving in romantic relationships. In K. Bartholomew & D. Perlman (Eds.), *Advances in personal relationships: Vol. 5. Attachments in adulthood* (pp. 205–237). Philadelphia: Kingsley.

Lee, J. A. (1973). *Colours of love: An exploration of the ways of loving*. Toronto, Ontario, Canada: New Press.

Lindzey, G., & Aronson, E. (Eds.). (1985). *The handbook of social psychology* (3rd ed.). New York: Random House.

Lykken, D. (1999). *Happiness*. New York: Golden Books.

Meyers, S. A., & Berscheid, E. (1997). The language of love: The difference a preposition makes. *Personality and Social Psychology Bulletin, 23*, 347–362.

Regan, P. C., & Berscheid, E. (1999). *Lust: What we know about human sexual desire*. Thousand Oaks, CA: Sage.

Rubin, Z. (1974). From liking to loving: Patterns of attraction in dating relationships. In T. L. Huston (Ed.), *Foundations of interpersonal attraction* (pp. 383–402). New York: Academic Press.

Shaver, P. R., Hazan, C., & Bradshaw, D. (1988). Love as attachment: The integration of three behavioral systems. In R. J. Sternberg & M. L. Barnes (Eds.), *The psychology of love* (pp. 68–99). New Haven, CT: Yale University Press.

Shaver, P. R., & Rubenstein, C. (1980). Childhood attachment experience and adult loneliness. In L. Wheeler (Ed.), *Review of personality and social psychology* (Vol. 1, pp. 42–73). Beverly Hills, CA: Sage.

Simpson, J. A., & Rholes, W. S. (1998). Attachment in adulthood. In J. A. Simpson & W. S. Rholes (Eds.), *Attachment theory and close relationships* (pp. 3–21). New York: Guilford Press.

Walster (Hatfield), E., & Walster, G. W. (1978). *A new look at love*. Reading, MA: Addison-Wesley.

Weiss, R. S. (Ed.). (1973). *Loneliness: The experience of emotional and social isolation*. Cambridge, MA: MIT Press.

Weiss, R. S. (1975). *Marital separation*. New York: Basic Books.

Westermarck, E. (1922). *The history of human marriage* (Vol. 2, 5th ed.). New York: Allerton.

Wolf, A. P. (1995). *Sexual attraction and childhood association: A Chinese brief for Edward Westermarck*. Stanford, CA: Stanford University Press.

17

Dynamics of Romantic Love

Comments, Questions, and Future Directions

PHILLIP R. SHAVER

There is no adequate way to express my deep gratitude to the authors and editors of this stimulating and important book. When I suggested holding a conference on romantic love as a way to celebrate my 60th birthday, I had no idea my wish would be granted. Now that it *has* been granted, with results that surpass anything I had hoped for, I realize that, even if I live another 60 years, I won't be able to repay Mario Mikulincer and Gail Goodman for organizing the conference and turning it into this insightful volume in my honor. Nor can I adequately thank all of my friends, colleagues, and former students who paid their way to attend the celebration, several of whom went on to write the provocative chapters in this book. By admitting that I wanted a scientific conference for my birthday and actually receiving one, I have revealed both that I am an incurable academic and that my friends are similarly inclined. Perhaps, then, there is no better way to express my appreciation than by responding seriously to their excellent work.

In Chapter 1, Gail Goodman provides a brief account of how I became an attachment researcher. Thinking about this "psychobiography" caused me to include in this chapter another brief case study, so that readers and I can share a concrete reference point. In Chapter 2, Mario Mikulincer provides an excellent overview of the research generated over the past 20 years by Cindy Hazan's and my conceptualization of romantic love as a state motivated and organized by three behavioral systems: attachment, caregiving, and sex. Rather than recapitulate Mario's detailed and informative overview, and instead of reacting chapter by chapter to the other authors' complex and detailed descriptions of particular lines of research, which would require another volume, I will use these final pages to convey a few personal reactions, ideas, and remaining mysteries.

I begin with a brief case study, which is followed by a discussion of some of the points it raises and illustrates. I am especially interested in what we mean when we say that romantic love, or pair bonding, is based on three separate behavioral systems, so I devote several sections to implications of that claim. I then turn to the issue of individual differences in attachment, caregiving, and sex and consider ways of thinking about the fact that individual differences in the functioning of the three systems are interrelated and that priming one system has systematic effects on the others. Finally, toward the end of the chapter I consider how the attachment, or behavioral systems, approach to romantic love and couple relationships is similar to and differs from other theoretical approaches.

A REFERENCE CASE: THE FEYNMANS' ATTACHMENT RELATIONSHIP

Because this book, like most high-level scientific discourse, is quite abstract, even though it deals with some of life's most intense, engaging, and in some cases exceedingly painful and destructive experiences—sexual passion, emotional bonding, affectionate caregiving, rejection and loss, couple violence, and sexual coercion—I begin with a specific and fairly normal example of what we are theorizing about.

The Case

In the early 1940s, while working on the first atomic bomb, the Nobel Prize-winning physicist Richard Feynman wrote almost daily to his young wife, Arline Feynman. Like Richard's behavior throughout his long and eventful life, the letters (edited by Richard's daughter, Michelle Feynman, 2005) are marked by quirky brilliance, a sparkling, devilish sense of humor, intense affection, and sexual attraction. The letters as a whole are remarkable for a variety of reasons, but the most amazing letter, to my mind, is one Richard wrote at age 28, a year and a half after Arline died of tuberculosis:

> I adore you, sweetheart. I want to tell you I love you . . . I always will love you. I find it hard to understand . . . what it means to love you after you are dead—but I still want to comfort you and take care of you—and I want you to love me and take care of me. I want to have problems to discuss with you; I want to do little projects with you. . . . What should we do?
>
> When you were sick you worried because you could not give me something that you wanted to and thought I needed. You needn't have worried. Just as I told you then there was no real need because I loved you in so many ways so much. And now it is clearly even more true—you can give me nothing now yet I love you so that you stand in my way of loving anyone else—but I want [you] to stand there. You, dead, are so much better than anyone else alive.
>
> I don't understand it, for I have met many girls and very nice ones and I don't want to remain alone—but in two or three meetings they all seem ashes. You only are left to me. You are real. My darling wife, I do adore you. I love my wife. My wife is dead.
>
> P.S. Please excuse my not mailing this—but I don't know your new address. (pp. 68–69)

If anyone doubted that Bowlby's (1969/1982, 1973, 1980) theory of attachment and loss applies to adult romantic love, this letter should help change the person's mind. Richard had Arline's substance and qualities so deeply etched in his mind—in his attachment hierarchy and internal working models, to use Bowlby's terms—her vivid presence was impossible to dislodge even though Richard, who was not religious, believed he would never see her again. Arline's status as what Bowlby called Richard's "primary attachment figure" caused other attractive women, at least for a period of years, to be excluded from that role, perhaps against Richard's "better judgment." Moreover, despite his obvious brilliance in other domains, he couldn't fathom his continuing commitment to and longing for Arline. Notice that Richard was, in attachment theory terms, *attached* or emotionally bonded to Arline; he wished intensely to be near her. But he also wanted to take care of her and be taken care of by her, and he clearly grieved for her. (His daughter Michelle said in her notes on the correspondence that "This letter is well worn—much more so than others—and it appears as though he reread it often.")

Keeping Personal Experience and Everyday Observations in Mind

Whatever readers of this volume conclude about love and attachment, I hope they keep the example of Richard and Arline in mind, along with whatever experiences of intense romantic love (pair bonding, in the language of evolutionary psychology) still blaze or smolder in their own memories. Certainly I think about my own experiences when theorizing about love. My wife, Gail Goodman's, brief description of the early years of our courtship, in Chapter 1, refers to some of the memories I consult frequently, memories of a time when I failed to return to a tenured job at New York University after spending a sabbatical year at the University of Denver, where I first met Gail. Despite receiving the academic equivalent of death threats from NYU's psychology department and attorneys, I wanted to stay in Denver with Gail, and I did. I also awkwardly ended relationships with other women whom I cared about in New York so I could pursue what has proven to be a very rewarding 25-year relationship with Gail.

In my opinion, there is no theory of personality, emotions, social relationships, or psychological development that holds much more than a flickering candle to actual experience. Someday there may be, but not today. Thus it behooves us as relationship researchers to keep attachment theory, alternative theories of love (such as interdependence theory; the intimacy theory developed by Harry Reis in Chapter 15; Art and Elaine Aron's self-expansion theory, summarized in Chapter 14; and Ellen Berscheid's wise conceptual analysis in Chapter 16), and our own actual experiences of love in mind. I was delighted to see, when reading Berscheid's lovely essay (Chapter 16) that she had been moved by Nobel Prize-winner Herbert Simon's casual question, "What about tenderness?" I assume the question grew out of his keen observations of his own and other people's close relationships, not from formal work in artificial intelligence, his insightful but fairly narrow conception of emotions as interrupters of cognition, and his analyses of "satisficing" in organizational economics.

I was also pleased that the Arons raised, in Chapter 14, the issue of the Jungian "shadow," the aspect of a person or culture that is suppressed or hidden from view and complements or contradicts what is consciously emphasized. The Arons refer to the "archetype of the Divine Child," which is similar to attachment researchers' image of the perfectly secure infant who grows up to be a perfectly loving and happy adult. All of us realize, I hope, that no one is perfectly secure or perfectly "divine" and that to insist on a model of perfect security, rather than a model that acknowledges human complexity, depth, and intrapsychic conflicts and tensions, is bound to be misleading and perhaps even dangerous, because the shadow component of a mind or a culture tends to assert itself in destructive ways. By keeping our own relationships and other real relationships in mind, perhaps we will remember the complexity that even our fairly simple studies reveal: Everyone has had both more and less successful relationships and has enjoyed being loved, as well as having suffered from inevitable attachment injuries. All of us are subject to conflicting motives and impulses, the balance of which changes as a function of social context (presence or absence of partner support), external threats (wars, economic depressions, a partner's serious illness), and internal conditions (self-doubts, "compassion fatigue," and painful negative memories, dreams, or daydreams). It takes effort for anyone to balance and regulate all of the conflicting pushes, pulls, and priorities.

In the attachment field we are so accustomed to glorifying secure attachment that we rarely stop to wonder why there aren't more saints in the world, especially given that Ainsworth and her followers (e.g., Ainsworth, Blehar, Waters, & Wall, 1978; Weinfield, Sroufe, Egeland, & Carlson, 1999) labeled more than half of the middle-class children they studied "securely attached" and that researchers using the Adult Attachment Interview (AAI; e.g., Hesse, 1999; Main, 1995) have declared that more than half of middle-class American adults have a "secure state of mind with respect to attachment." Psychologists have done a great deal of research and administered megatons of psychotherapy over the past hundred or so years; yet human cruelty, damaged children, unfaithful spouses, and wars and violence have not noticeably diminished, let alone disappeared completely. Thus it is worthwhile to keep one eye on everyday experiences and the daily world news, especially experiences and stories that contradict our theories, so that we do not become deluded by theoretical oversimplifications, misleading abstractions, or wishful idealizations.

Romantic Love Engages Multiple Behavioral Systems

The fact that Richard's Feynman's love for Arline Feynman involved both attachment and caregiving (I'll get to sex in a minute) was evident when he said, "I still want to comfort you and take care of you—and I want you to love me and take care of me." That was not mere rhetoric. He actually *had* taken care of Arline while she was ill, very tenderly, and even though she was living mainly in a tuberculosis sanitarium at the time, she did a great deal, in letters and in the considerable time they spent together, to take care of Richard's emotional, sexual, and other needs. In a letter to Arline written months before she died, Richard said: "Without you I would be empty and weak like I was before I knew you" (Feynman, 2005, p. 48). They both shared their everyday experiences, frustrations, and new discoveries, including discoveries about their own feelings—in ways that fit well with Reis's insightful discussion of intimacy in Chapter 15 of this volume.

One thing to notice about Richard's wish to care for Arline, as expressed in the letter I quoted, is that this aspect or form of love (i.e., caregiving) is not only what Berscheid (Chapter 16) calls an "affect," or a feeling. It is also not, as I believe she would agree, an attitude. In my opinion, the psychology of emotions and its extension into the field of close relationships made a mistake when it conceptualized emotions, including forms of love, primarily as "affects," feelings, or attitudes—that is, as subjective states that might be located in an abstract mental space defined by the dimensions of valence and arousal. (For an excellent contemporary example of this approach, with which I disagree despite admiring the author's scope, see Barrett, 2006a, 2006b.)

We can see some of the difficulties inherent in the "affect" or "feeling" conceptualization of love in the following passages (here combined for brevity) from Berscheid's chapter in this volume:

> The title of this volume (and the title of the conference that preceded it) confused me, undoubtedly because the term "romantic love" itself is confusing. It is often used loosely to refer to any kind of positive affect that occurs within a relationship between a man and a woman, especially a relationship that either is progressing toward or has culminated in marriage. . . . However, the term "romantic love" also is used to refer to a particular *kind* of positive affect—or syndrome of emotions, feelings, attitudes, and behaviors—as opposed to other kinds of positive affect that are often observed in a relationship between a man and a woman, which is how I am using the term. (p. 409)

Except for the single word "behaviors" that sneaked in at the end of the inserted, dashed phrase, the passage is all about feelings or affects. (The fact that the term "romantic love" confounds a kind of relationship, a couple relationship that includes sex or at least sexual interests, with a kind of "affect" related to one of several different behavioral systems, only one of which is sexual, is important, and I will return to it later.)

An advantage of conceptualizing romantic love in terms of innate, motivated, dynamic, and generally functional behavioral systems is that focusing our attention on such systems forces us to think about *motives*, *actions*, and *action tendencies* rather than just feelings. Aron and Aron (Chapter 14) make a related observation:

> We hypothesized . . . that passionate love is best conceptualized as a goal-oriented motivational state in which the individual is experiencing an intense desire to merge with the partner. That is, we conceive of passionate love as the experience that corresponds to the intense desire to expand the self by including another person in the self. Thus passionate love is not a distinct emotion in its own right (such as sadness or happiness) but rather can evoke a variety of emotions according to whether and how the desire is fulfilled or frustrated. (p. 364)

None of us, I assume, would deny that feelings are important (see Shaver, Morgan, & Wu, 1996, for an example of my own efforts to characterize feelings of love), but I think it is crucial that we tie them theoretically to motives and goals—or, in the language of attachment theory, to innate behavioral systems. The attachment system causes a lonely or distressed person to seek physical and psychological proximity to a comforting protector or supporter; that is, it *moves* the person, both figuratively and literally, in the direction of a real or imagined attachment figure. If the person's goal of seeking proximity is frustrated or rebuffed, he or she is likely to protest, cry, become aggressive, and so on. (Bowlby's books, such as the second and third volumes of his *Attachment and Loss* trilogy, published in 1973 and 1980, had subtitles including the words anxiety, anger, sadness, and depression.) The caregiving system influences a person to feel troubled by another person's vulnerability, distress, or need, and it *moves* a compassionate, caring person toward a needy other in ways that can be observed in behavior and detected in the motor cortex of the brain during "compassion meditation" (e.g., Lutz, Greischar, Rowlings, Ricard, & Davidson, 2004). The sexual system does more than cause feelings or affects; it *moves* a person to engage in sexual activities. Both the desires involved and experienced when a behavioral system is activated and the emotions evoked by successfully attaining or failing to attain the behavioral systems' set goals (as Bowlby called them) are "affective" (felt), but the feelings are not the only parts of the process that have psychological significance.

One of the most important advances in emotion theory in the past few decades, and one to which I tried to make at least a small contribution (e.g., Reis & Shaver, 1988; Schwartz & Shaver, 1987; Shaver et al., 1996; Shaver, Schwartz, Kirson, & O'Connor, 1987), was to place *goals* and *action tendencies* rather than feelings or affects at the center of the emotion process (e.g., Frijda, 1986; Oatley & Jenkins, 1996). Chapter 7 of this volume, by Nancy Collins, AnaMarie Guichard, Máire Ford, and Brooke Feeney, does a marvelous job of showing that caring involves a motivated set of actions and action tendencies, not a mere feeling (although I'm not denying that caring feelings are extremely important; they help us realize, make sense of, and remember our motives and motivational inclinations). If caregiving tendencies did not express themselves in behavior, the caregiving system postulated by Bowlby would never have evolved.

Richard and Arline Feynman did not write a great deal about sex, at least not in the letters published by Richard's daughter (from a subsequent marriage), but the two lovers had been devoted and amorous high school sweethearts who went on to spend many weekends together while Richard was in college and graduate school. Even after they married and her health was declining, Arline wrote to Richard: "I'm so excited and happy and bursting with joy—I think, eat, and sleep 'you'—our life, our love, our marriage. . . . I love you sweetheart—body and soul—I long to be near you again . . . you're a wonderful husband and lover. Come to me soon—I need you and want you" (Feynman, 2005, p. 24). In another letter, after feeling that she might be pregnant, she wrote, "I could rave about you endlessly dear, everything about you seems so extra-special and nice to me—your legs are strong and muscular . . . then there is the baby talk you use sometimes when you love me . . . I adore you" (p. 27). During the final year of her life, despite being weak and frequently in pain, Arline wrote, "It's good to know that even if medicine fails, there is always your smile, and your hand—it's effective dearest" (p. 34).

Maybe I'm a dirty old man (as Gail Goodman explains in Chapter 1, I have definitely begun to think of myself as old), but I can imagine only one activity that Arline might have been referring to when praising Richard's healing hand. Like the attachment and caregiving systems, the sexual system motivates actions, not just feelings.

STILL, WHAT ABOUT THE *FEELING* OF "LOVE"? WHAT DOES IT MEAN TO SAY "I LOVE YOU"?

A big challenge, once we place romantic love and pair bonding in a behavioral systems framework, is to figure out how best to integrate the separate systems and to do so in a way that acknowledges the feeling aspect and the everyday language of love. Certainly, Richard and Arline's letters revealed and expressed strong feelings, and the lovers often used the term "love" for their feelings, although, viewed in terms of behavioral systems theory, they sometimes seemed to be talking about wanting to see each other and be physically close, wanting to be taken care of, wanting to take care of the other, and wanting to "make love" to each other. In accord with my wish not to get lost in abstractions, I wouldn't want to endorse a cybernetic model of behavioral systems that left out experiences, feelings, words, and values. (As a colleague recently asked in an e-mail message, "If we're talking about mechanical behavioral systems rather than human emotions, couldn't two robots be 'in love' and 'pair bonded'?" [Louise Sundararajan, personal communication, 2005]).

Bowlby, the originator of the behavioral system perspective, clearly believed that the operation of the attachment system is closely associated with what we, in ordinary language, call "love":

> Many of the most intense of all human emotions arise during the formation, the maintenance, the disruption and the renewal of affectional bonds—which for that reason are sometimes called emotional bonds. In terms of subjective experience, the formation of a bond is described as falling in love, maintaining a bond as loving someone, and losing a partner as grieving over someone. Similarly, the threat of loss arouses anxiety and actual loss causes sorrow, whilst both situations are likely to arouse anger. Finally, the unchallenged maintenance of a bond is experienced as a source of security, and the renewal as a source of joy. (1979, p. 69)

All of these emotions are evident in the letters exchanged by Richard and Arline Feynman, and one can easily see in their correspondence the kinds of challenges and misunderstandings—usually amounting to unintended breaches of trust or violations of expectations about giving and receiving care—that sometimes cause negative attachment-related emotions to erupt (as demonstrated by other couples in the studies described by Jeff Simpson, Lorne Campbell, and Yanna Weisberg in Chapter 9 of this volume). The Feynmans' interactions, extending over many years, also corresponded well with Collins et al.'s (Chapter 7) laboratory experiments on the dynamic interrelation of one partner's attachment needs and the other partner's caregiving efforts.

As explained subsequently, the term "love" is broad enough in everyday language to be associated with an attachment, or "affectional," bond to a caring other, the "care" associated with the caregiving behavioral system, and the sexual attraction and satisfaction associated with the sexual system. That is, the ordinary-language term "love" is used for all of the feelings associated with all three of the behavioral systems that Hazan and I (Hazan & Shaver, 1987) thought were involved in romantic pair-bond or couple relationships, especially the positive feelings, but also many of the negative ones. The idea that "love hurts" has been expressed in countless love songs over the centuries. (See Aron and Aron, Chapter 14, for examples of the diverse emotions associated with love).

This means, as Ekman (1992) explained when deciding that love is not a basic emotion, that the term "love" is used for just about any notable emotion generated in "romantic love" relationships. Ekman called these relationships "plots," meaning that they involve more than one person, usually in particular kinds of roles relevant to a particular emotion term. According to Ekman, many different discrete emotions arise in such scenarios (jealousy is another example of a "plot"—one that by definition involves three social roles), so there cannot be only a single emotion term that accurately applies to them, and—of great interest to Ekman when he was deciding which emotions are and which are not "basic"—there is no single, easily identifiable facial expression associated with a love plot or a jealousy plot.

As scientists, when we contemplate the workings of the attachment, caregiving, and sexual systems, we move beyond thinking about consciously available feelings in one person's subjective consciousness to a set of partly unconscious motivational processes that cause people to approach, touch, and interact with each other in order to receive protection and comfort, to offer protection or provide support, or to engage in sexual activities. When all three of the behavioral systems are organized around a particular person, we have what I mean by "romantic love" (which, when it occurs in only one member of a dyad, can be one-sided and may qualify for the term "infatuation"). When both the attachment, caregiving, and sexual systems of both members of a dyad are organized around each other, we have what I would call a "romantic relationship." What matters in these cases is not any particular emotion but the ways in which several behavioral systems and kinds of emotion (including but not limited to the ones mentioned in the passage I quoted from Bowlby) are organized around successive interactions, and eventually a relationship, with a particular person. I think Berscheid and I come close to agreeing about this, although I admit that the language and the various constructs involved are devilishly difficult to pin down precisely.

What about Exploration and Affiliation?

Several of the chapter authors mention explicitly or imply that Hazan and I (Hazan & Shaver, 1987; Shaver, Hazan, & Bradshaw, 1988) were too restrictive in characterizing romantic love in terms of only three of the behavioral systems discussed by Bowlby (1969/1982). In particular, we left out the exploration and affiliation systems. This is an important point, because the natural link between Bowlby's theory and self-expansion theory as outlined by Aron and Aron in Chapter 14 is the exploration system. Bowlby used the term "exploration" to refer to the human infant's very evident curiosity, playfulness, and intense interest in developing personal efficacy and competence (e.g., standing up, walking, making interesting events happen over and over again). Bowlby and Ainsworth placed enormous emphasis on the role of secure attachment in promoting exploration, learning, and personal growth. They might well have called these processes "self-expansion."

Exploration is also important to Collins et al. in Chapter 7, because caregiving in an adult relationship often amounts to supporting a partner emotionally and in other ways while he or she attempts to solve personally important problems, achieve desirable goals at work, and so on. Exploration and self-expansion are also obviously important to Reis's discussion of intimacy in Chapter 15. What makes intimacy so exciting and rewarding when it goes well is that a person is helped by a partner to see more deeply and unambivalently into him- or herself and to have previously confusing, hidden, or disapproved aspects of the self understood and, in many cases, genuinely sympathized with or approved of. When this goes on in both directions in a relationship, the two partners come to feel "larger," freer, less conflicted and distorted, and more complete. The result is "self-expanding," without a doubt, and not only because one "includes the other in the self," in the Arons' terms, but also because more of the self has become visible, understood, and accepted by the other and the self.

I have less to say about affiliation per se, but Berscheid (Chapter 16) is surely correct that friendship, or companionship, between loving partners is a significant part of love. Simply doing things together, being playful together, and having fun of all kinds together (e.g., leisure activities, home improvement projects, vacationing) are important, as Richard Feynman indicated when he said, "I want to do little projects with you. . . . What should we do?" Also important is the sense of security and identity couple members enjoy based on a shared history.

Thinking about these additional behavioral systems helps me realize that "love," or "romantic love" (meaning the set of forces that draw members of a couple together and cause them to care about each other), is a broad, overarching term used for all of the forces, including sexual attraction and involvement, that cause members of a couple to care for and about each other as specific individuals. "I love him" is a way of saying, "I have a lot of my behavioral systems wrapped firmly around him, and the image of him, in ways that make it very difficult for me to think about trading him in for anyone else." I still think this makes attachment a very central part of the process of this kind of love, along with caring and sex, but it might be appropriate to include exploration and affiliation as well. They both contribute to the emotional force of love, to the selection of one partner rather than another, and to the likelihood that what begins as self-expansion and infatuation will evolve into a lasting attachment.

Appraisal and Bestowal

Another, related way to think about "romantic love" is to notice that anyone with whom I establish a "pair bond" in a mutual, multi-behavioral-system way has a very special *value* to me. *Feeling* that value, and *feeling* myself assigning it to one particular person, especially if it places her ahead of all others in my personal pantheon, or attachment hierarchy, is an important part of what I mean by "loving" that person. And if the sexual behavioral system is involved (in line with the emphasis Berscheid places on that system when using the term "romantic"), then the love is likely to qualify as "romantic."

In Singer's (1984) comprehensive historical study of the philosophy of love, he concluded that the term "love" refers to two related but distinct ways of valuing a person: *appraisal* and *bestowal*. Interestingly, without articulating a theory of the underlying processes, he noticed that when one person "loves" another in the romantic sense, the lover "appraises" the beloved individual as being more valuable (at least to the lover) than other people and as more valuable than most other people believe the lover to be. This kind of appraisal is relatively easy to explain in terms of what the lover "does for me," and in that respect it is somewhat like becoming attached to someone because he or she provides a safe haven and secure base. Harlow (1959), in his famous studies of rhesus monkey infants' attachments to a cloth surrogate mother, called this process "love." According to Singer, the other kind of human valuation, which he calls "bestowal," goes beyond and is more mysterious than appraisal. He claims that bestowal involves both creative imagination and generosity and is therefore a form of "giving":

> Only in relation to our bestowal does another person enjoy the kind of value that love creates. . . . The bestowing of value shows itself . . . in caring about the needs and interests of the beloved, by wishing to benefit or

> protect her, by delighting in her achievements, by encouraging her independence while also accepting and sustaining her dependency, by respecting her individuality, by giving her pleasure, by taking pleasures with her, by feeling glad when she is present and sad when she is not, by sharing ideas and emotions with her, by sympathizing with her weaknesses and depending upon her strength, by developing common pursuits, by allowing her to become second nature to him—"her smiles, her frowns, her ups, her downs" [to quote a once-popular song]—by wanting children who may perpetuate their love. (pp. 6–7)

Although Singer never says so (he is definitely not an attachment theorist), I think the bestowal process is mainly a product of the caregiving system. Consider how much it helps parents to view their children as special, as cute or beautiful, as potential geniuses, as exceptionally funny, and so on. Often, this allows parents to see and foster the genuine potential in their children that other people do not care enough to notice. For many adults, perhaps including parents themselves, it is as funny to notice this biased parental bestowal of value on a particular child as it to see a romantic Jack go gaga over Jill. But for a child, the parent's special care and bestowal of high value is a godsend. It is what allows the potential to become manifest in reality.

For some reason, the bestowal process has been underemphasized in psychology. This may have something to do with the long immersion of American psychology (and Anglo-American culture generally) in utilitarianism, market economics, and rewards and punishments. It is fairly easy for us to ask and answer the question "What's in it for me (or Jack)?" in terms of rewards and punishments. It is more difficult to say why one person would bestow special value on another through a generous act of imagination. But if my hunch is correct, caregiving, sensitive responsiveness, and bestowal are more important to a lasting romantic "pair bond" relationship than attachment and sex are, even though attachment and sex often contribute to it or follow from it (see Diamond, Chapter 11, this volume, for intriguing examples of two-way influence).

Although as scientists we may be inclined to view bestowal skeptically or cynically, looking back at Richard Feynman's letter to his dead wife, I think you'll see the bestowal process in full swing, and at least for me it is difficult to smirk about it in that case. Richard really did bestow Arline with precious, and for a while totally irreplaceable, qualities, which made it easy for him to take care of her and difficult for him to "turn her in for a new model" when she died. Why? Although I obviously cannot say for sure, I find it useful to conceptualize Richard as having activated his caregiving system with respect to Arline, even though that may not have been his original reason for being attracted to her. Singer (1984), like Berscheid (1988), realized that the initial attraction in a romantic relationship is often sexual, but he thought romantic love was more than sexual attraction or infatuation:

> If a woman is *simply* a means to sexual satisfaction, a man may be said to want her, but not to love her. For his sexual desire to become a part of love, it must function as a way of responding to the character and special properties of this particular woman. Desire wants what it wants for the sake of some private gratification, whereas love demands an interest in that vague complexity we call another person. No wonder lovers sound like metaphysicians, and scientists are more comfortable in the study of desire. For love is an attitude with no clear objective. Through it one human being affirms the significance of another, much as a painter highlights a figure by defining it in a sharpened outline. But the beloved is not a painted figure. She is not static: she is fluid, changing, indefinable—*alive*. The lover is attending to a *person*. And who can say what that is? (p. 8)

I agree with, and even marvel at, most of what Singer says in that passage, except when he says "love is an attitude with no clear objective." When viewed from the perspective of the caregiving system, noticing, appreciating, and bestowing admirable qualities on a particular other person is part of what allows one of us human adults to see more deeply into another (see Diamond, Chapter 11, and Reis, Chapter 15, this volume, for examples), to understand and share each other's goals and perspectives (Aron & Aron, Chapter 14), to take care of one another (Collins et al., Chapter 7), to commit to a relationship partner, to engage in a long-term, mutually supportive relationship with the partner, and often, to wish to have and take care of children with him or her (see Brumbaugh & Fraley, Chapter 4, this volume). In the same way that the motivational goal of the attachment system is the self's protection, security, expansion, and development, the goal of the caregiving system is the other person's protection, security, expansion, and development (Mikulincer, Chapter 2, this volume). Contrary to cynical psychologies, I believe that it feels as good to achieve the latter kinds of goals as it does to achieve the former kinds, which is one reason for being hopeful and optimistic about the human species despite its many weaknesses, self-destructive tendencies, and failings.

There may be a sense in which both kinds of rewards, those from the attachment side and those from the caregiving side, become part of an amplifying cycle, for reasons discussed by Aron and Aron in Chapter 14 and Reis in Chapter 15. As already mentioned, the Arons contend that one of the exciting aspects of a romantic relationship is the rapid self-expansion such a relationship provides to both partners. They can expand their knowledge, identities, emotional repertoires, skills, and capacities by experiencing, understanding, valuing, and incorporating their partner's qualities and perspectives into themselves. This sounds somewhat "selfish" and egotistical at first, partly because of the term *self*-expansion, but if you consider the example of a parent feeling excited, edified, and rewarded by intimate, loving interactions with his (in my case) child, you will notice that the parent's self-expansion comes partly from seeing the world anew through the child's eyes, noticing the profound impact a parent has on a child's feelings and development, appreciating the child's rapidly expanding skills, and empathizing with the child's distress. In other words, it can be "self-expanding" to take care of another person's needs sensitively and responsively.

Reis (Chapter 15) explains well, in what is for me a remarkable "expansion" of the theory of intimacy he and I sketched in 1988 (Reis & Shaver, 1988), how two people's sensitivity and responsiveness to each other can enlarge and illuminate *both* people's worlds. When two people see and "feel" deeply into each other, and consequently experience, understand, and express more of themselves, they *both* "expand"—and not in a *folie à deux* manner. As each person grows, becomes more secure, risks "exploring" more of self, partner, and world (to call again on Bowlby's notion of an exploration behavioral system), and reflects positive feelings back onto the partner, both people's attachment and caregiving systems are gratified, renewed, and reinforced. Although this kind of intimacy definitely happens in sexual relationships and can be facilitated by mutually rewarding sexual experiences, the mutual self-expansion that occurs often includes much more than sex.

The double-barreled valuing process—appraisal plus bestowal—is interesting in part because we have all noticed, I'm sure, that when a person falls in love, his or her friends are often perplexed by the extreme value placed on the beloved. Jack's friends find it a little silly, stupid, or crazy, perhaps even embarrassing, that Jack perceives Jill to be so uniquely and incredibly wonderful. To them, although she may be quite all right, she is certainly "nothing special." Murray, Holmes, and Griffin (1996) call this peculiar form of valuation a "positive illusion," but I prefer Singer's term "bestowal" because it avoids the cynicism inherent in the term "illusion." Besides, as Reis explains in Chapter 15, recent research shows that a "positive illusion" has measurably good effects on a partner by virtue of being associated with the bestower's very real sensitive and responsive care. It may be misleading to conceptualize the bestower's perceptions of the "bestowee's" potential as illusory if the bestowee goes on to realize the potential in ways that everyone can see. We might be more accurate to call the bestowal "beneficial discernment" rather than illusion.

PUTTING THE THREE BEHAVIORAL SYSTEMS TOGETHER

The evidence reviewed in this volume indicates that the three behavioral systems emphasized by Hazan and me (Hazan & Shaver, 1987) in our theorizing about romantic love—attachment, caregiving, and sex—are systematically interrelated, and in more ways than by simply receiving the blanket designation "love" in everyday discourse. Why is this the case?

As a starting point, notice that secure people (understood here as those who score relatively low on both the attachment insecurity dimensions of anxiety and avoidance; see Mikulincer, Chapter 2, this volume) find it relatively easy to get psychologically close to others and, when threatened or stressed, to call on memories of supportive experiences with attachment figures. They are also sensitive and responsive caregivers who allow their relationship partners to cope with challenges autonomously if the partners are inclined to do so but offer well timed and appropriately structured comfort and assistance if that is what is needed (e.g., Collins et al., Chapter 7). In other words, attachment security is related to sensitive and responsive caregiving.

Similarly, people with a secure attachment orientation view sex as a mutually enjoyable way to foster intimacy and affection in the context of a stable relationship (see Cooper et al., Chapter 10, and Gillath & Schachner, Chapter 13, this volume). Secure people are not usually sexually anxious, out to prove themselves sexually, or inclined to cynically manipulate or "use" their sexual partners. We do not know much yet about the interplay between the caregiving and sexual systems, but Gillath's preliminary experimental studies (discussed in Chapter 13), in which participants were subliminally primed with photographs of naked members of the opposite sex, indicate that priming the sexual system moves people, on average, toward greater self-disclosure and more constructive handling of conflicts—tendencies usually associated with attachment security and supportive caregiving. I can imagine that priming people with a sense of caring might also alter the nature of the sexual inclinations, at least slightly—for example, by causing them to be more partner- than self-oriented.

How can we best conceptualize the relations among the behavioral systems? Bowlby and Ainsworth began their theorizing by portraying attachment security as a "secure base for exploration," which suggested that the attachment system was primary, came first in development, and formed either a solid or a shaky foundation for the other behavioral systems. Following Bowlby and Ainsworth's lead, my coauthors and I have, over the years, tended to treat the attachment-system aspect of romantic love as primary. One reason for doing this is that attachment behavior and attachment styles, or orientations, show up early in infant development, whereas caregiving (e.g., as first indicated, for example, by empathy in 3-year-olds; Kestenbaum, Farber, & Sroufe, 1989) appears next, and sex—at least genital sexuality—appears later. With this developmental progression in mind, we looked initially for predictive links between measures of adult attachment style and measures of caregiving (e.g., Kunce & Shaver, 1994; also Collins et al., Chapter 7, and Mikulincer, Shaver, & Slav, Chapter 8, this volume) and sex (e.g., Cooper, Shaver, & Collins, 1998; Davis, Shaver, & Vernon, 2004; Schachner & Shaver, 2004; Tracy, Shaver, Albino, & Cooper, 2003; and Levy, Kelly, & Jack, Chapter 6,

Cooper et al., Chapter 10, Davis, Chapter 12, and Gillath & Schachner, Chapter 13, this volume).

More recently, however, we have learned that we can experimentally prime any one of the behavioral systems and see causal effects on the others. In other words, at least in adults, the behavioral systems are intertwined, such that activation of one has effects on the others and that individual differences in one tend to be correlated with individual differences in the others. There are, as already mentioned, two ways to think about this. First, we can view the attachment system as appearing first in development because its function, assuring protection (i.e., survival), is biologically crucial. Once a child has a functioning attachment system and has begun to adapt it to the local caregiving environment (i.e., once a fairly stable attachment style has developed), the child's caregiving system comes on line to deal with sibling and peer relationships and to be molded by moral socialization and enculturation. Given that children with different attachment styles act in and experience social relationships somewhat differently, the operating parameters of the caregiving system may be shaped in certain predictable directions. Also important are imitation and modeling of primary caregivers, which create similarities in caregiving between parents and children and between a child's attachment system (shaped by the parents) and his or her caregiving system (modeled on those of the parents).

We know empirically that caregivers' behavior initially causes similarities between caregivers' and children's attachment styles (e.g., de Wolff & van IJzendoorn, 1997; van IJzendoorn, 1995). Parental attachment and caregiving anxieties encourage offspring attachment anxiety, and parental attachment and caregiving avoidance encourage offspring attachment avoidance (perhaps partly for genetic reasons, as discussed later, but probably not primarily for those reasons). The anxious or avoidant child is likely to become an anxious or avoidant caregiver by two routes besides genetic similarity—by reacting systematically to the parent's caregiving regime and by copying the caregiver's behavior through a modeling process.

Once the attachment and caregiving systems have developed in tandem and accommodated to each other, they are available to influence presexual peer relationships and then adolescent and adult sexual relationships. Hence, when we study sexual motives and behavior in college and adult samples, the operating parameters of the sexual system are predictable to some extent from the operating parameters of the attachment and caregiving systems. But also, given that priming the sexual system with pictures of naked members of the opposite sex has effects on the attachment and caregiving systems (see Gillath & Schachner, Chapter 13), it seems likely that once pregenital romantic and fully sexual romantic relationships begin, sexual experiences feed back on the operating parameters of the attachment and caregiving systems. (This remains to be studied.)

A second way to think about the empirically documented interrelations among the attachment, caregiving, and sexual systems is to view all of them as being affected by pervasive individual differences in temperament or personality. I have conducted several studies to see whether global attachment styles, or attachment-style dimensions, are completely redundant with one or more of the "Big Five" personality traits: openness to experience, conscientiousness, extroversion, agreeableness, and neuroticism (McCrae & Costa, 1996). They definitely are not. In two of our studies (Noftle & Shaver, in press; Shaver & Brennan, 1992), we compared attachment-style scales with measures of the "Big Five" traits to see which sets of variables best predicted relationship quality and outcomes. Using different measures of attachment style and different measures of the "Big Five" traits, we found that attachment measures consistently outperformed personality trait measures, using both contemporaneous and longitudinal research designs.

Moreover, in several of our laboratory experiments on both conscious and unconscious mental processes related to attachment style (e.g., Mikulincer, Gillath, & Shaver, 2002; Mikulincer, Shaver, & Slav, Chapter 8, this volume), we controlled for neuroticism, general anxiety, self-esteem, or interpersonal trust and still obtained predicted effects of attachment anxiety and avoidance. Simpson, Davis, and other authors of chapters in the present volume have included similar statistical controls in their studies and obtained similar results: Attachment effects are never fully, and usually not even partially, explained by alternative personality constructs. In a recent study using functional magnetic resonance imaging, we (Gillath, Bunge, Shaver, Wendelken, & Mikulincer, 2005) found different patterns of brain activation associated with neuroticism and attachment anxiety.

Still, the correlation between neuroticism and attachment anxiety is often substantial (around .40 or .45), and the correlation between avoidant attachment and agreeableness or extraversion is often statistically significant, although not large. Graziano and Tobin (2002) have shown that agreeableness is positively related to compassion and altruism in some of the same ways that avoidant attachment is negatively related to those same prosocial states, but it seems unlikely, given the relatively modest correlation between avoidance and agreeableness, that the attachment effects are redundant with the agreeableness effects. Moreover, there is nothing in the conceptualization of the "Big Five" traits that would have led to the huge research program generated over the past 20 years by adult attachment theory. Thus attachment theory and its associated measures are scientifically fruitful, whether or not we think of attachment styles as personality traits.

Whatever kinds of qualities they measure, attachment-style measures might be influenced by genes. In the case of the "Big Five" personality traits, about half of the individual-difference variance is attributable to genetic factors (Bouchard & Loehlin, 2001). To date, only a handful of behavior genetic studies of infant attachment patterns have been published. Four of these studies (Bokhorst et al., 2003; Bakersman-Kranenberg, van IJzendoorn,

Bokhorst, & Schuengel, 2004; O'Connor & Croft, 2001; Ricciuti, 1992) turned up little evidence of heritability but garnered some evidence for effects of shared environment on attachment patterns (as would be expected if twins' common caregiving environment mattered). In some cases, however, the sample sizes were small or the attachment-style measures differed substantially from the "gold standard" Strange Situation test (Ainsworth et al., 1978), so the absence of evidence for genetic influences may still not be compelling. In one study (Finkel & Matheny, 2000), the heritability of attachment security, based on a nonstandard measure of security, was estimated to be 25%, and there was no substantial effect of shared environment. But the attachment measure used in that study was more similar than usual to measures of infant temperament, perhaps thereby skewing the results in the direction of genetic determination.

At the adult level, Brussoni, Jang, Livesley, and MacBeth (2000) estimated that 43%, 25%, and 37%, respectively, of the variability in fearful, preoccupied, and secure attachment (assessed with Griffin and Bartholomew's, 1994, self-report measures) was attributable to genes, but the four attachment measures were intercorrelated, so the results might all reflect a single genetic influence. Variability in dismissing attachment, however, was not at all attributable to genes in that study. Crawford et al. (2005) used proxy versions of the Experience in Close Relationships (ECR) attachment anxiety and avoidance scales (Brennan, Clark, & Shaver, 1998) and found that roughly 40% of the variance in anxious attachment was attributable to genetic factors but that none of the variance in avoidant attachment was due to genes. Interestingly, in that study about 33% of the variance in avoidance was attributable to shared environment.

These preliminary studies are interesting and thought provoking even if they are not yet totally clear in their implications. It seems possible that similarities and differences in what is tapped by the Strange Situation, the AAI, and self-report measures such as the ECR attachment scales can eventually be illuminated by determining the extent to which they have similar or different genetic determinants. Because the ECR self-report attachment scales share variance with "Big Five" neuroticism and are similar in assessment method, they may be more affected than AAI classifications (Hesse, 1999) by genes.

My goal in touching on the matter of genetic influences is not to prejudge or resolve it, because no one can resolve it at present, but to encourage readers to remain open to whatever the evidence eventually dictates. The large and very systematic network of research findings obtained to date by adult attachment researchers will continue to be quite meaningful and significant, both scientifically and clinically, no matter how behavior genetic studies turn out. Nevertheless, it behooves us to include measures of personality and temperament variables in our studies, to take genes into account by pursuing twin studies or doing actual genetic assessments, and to keep in mind that some of the effects we attribute to attachment history may be due in part to genes or to interactions between genes and attachment history. Eventually, and perhaps not too far in the future, we will be able to examine actual genetic profiles associated with different patterns of scores on attachment, caregiving, and sexual motivation measures. Gillath is beginning to explore the possibilities in my lab at the moment.

To summarize this section, there are systematic links between the attachment, caregiving, and sexual systems and between individual differences in the parameters of the three systems (all of which might be characterized in terms of "hyperactivation" and "deactivation," as Mikulincer does in Chapter 2 of this volume). We don't know yet whether these links are due to inherent properties of the behavioral systems (e.g., to shared brain mechanisms or to the way they unfold and overlap in development), to the roles played by parental attachment figures in shaping the three systems' parameters, to common influences of central personality traits, or to genes. This uncertainty leaves the field wide open for a variety of future studies.

FURTHER QUESTIONS

Throughout the book, chapter authors have raised important additional questions and challenges for attachment research or for a behavioral systems approach to romantic love. In this section I address some of them.

What Is Adult Attachment?

In Chapter 3, Hazan, Campa, and Gur-Yalsh ask how we can recognize and confidently assess adult attachment. Investigators of infant attachment generally bypass this question by assuming that a child's primary caregiver, often the child's mother, is likely to be *a* primary if not *the* primary attachment figure. In studies of college students and their romantic partners, we often assume, or at least hope, that most relationships that have lasted beyond a certain point (say, several months) are either genuine attachments or at worst what Bowlby, discussing young infants, called "attachments in the making." This practice is sometimes questioned, even though the results of studies based on it have generally yielded clear and theory-compatible results.

In their discussion of the problems inherent in delineating adult attachment, Hazan et al. refer to four defining classes of behavior discussed by Bowlby (1969/1982): *proximity maintenance, safe haven, separation distress*, and *secure base*. They say "these features of attachment and the dynamic functioning of the attachment system are most readily observable in the behavior of 12-month-olds in relation to their primary caregivers (typically mothers)" (p. 49). In the case of adults, they say we are surest that adult romantic pair bonds qualify as attachments when we see one partner grieve following the death or loss of the other.

Although I agree with these statements, and in fact chose the example of Richard Feynman's letter to his dead wife partly because it was written while he was grieving, I think one can also see Richard and Arline's attachment to each other in their other letters and behavior (as recounted and reflected in their correspondence well before Arline died). They repeatedly chose to stay together even when there were forces pulling them apart, such as separations entailed by his work or her illness and his parents' concern that it was unwise to marry someone who was becoming increasingly ill. The two lovers traversed great distances to be together, and when that was impossible, they communicated frequently by other means.

Also, although not shown in the letters I quoted, it was evident in others that Arline's and Richard's feelings were buoyed up or brought down depending on the condition and receptiveness of their partner. The two lovers were part of a dynamic dyadic system (as characterized well by Bartholomew and Allison in Chapter 5, Collins et al. in Chapter 7, Mikulincer et al. in Chapter 8, Simpson et al. in Chapter 9, and Reis in Chapter 15), and I doubt that a day went by when they were unaware of each other's existence and of the importance to each of the other's well-being. Moreover, when they were separated, they longed to get back together and looked forward to seeing and touching each other again.

Thus, although I understand what worries Hazan et al. about having to rely on any particular imperfect indicator of adult attachment, such as behaviors in a single real or artificial situation, self-reports, or physiological reactions in an experimental setting, I believe we can do a decent job of detecting attachment if we combine several such indicators. In the studies in which I have been involved, we have measured attachment by asking to whom a person would turn if he or she needed one or more of the comforts provided by attachment figures (using the WHOTO scale designed by Hazan and Zeifman, 1994, and subsequently adapted by other researchers, including Bartholomew and Fraley), by seeing whose names become more readily available cognitively following subliminal threats (e.g., Mikulincer et al., 2002), by seeing whose names, when encountered subliminally or activated in association with conscious memories of that person's loving kindness, increase a person's activation of other behavioral systems, such as caregiving (e.g., Gillath, Shaver, & Mikulincer, 2005; Mikulincer, Shaver, Gillath, & Nitzberg, 2005).

Because letters seem to be a revealing way to assess adult attachment in the case of Richard and Arline Feynman, we might also use methods and materials such as love letters, e-mail correspondence, experience sampling, daily diaries, and so on to supplement behavioral observations and more general self-reports or self-descriptions. That these methods have great value has already been demonstrated in diary studies by Collins and Feeney (2005), Pietromonaco and Feldman Barrett (1997), Tidwell, Reis, and Shaver (1996), and some of the other authors of this volume (e.g., Mikulincer et al., Chapter 8; Simpson et al., Chapter 9).

A valuable supplementary approach might be to study existing correspondence between relationship partners. An example that has fascinated Mikulincer and me is the published correspondence between Gauguin, Van Gogh, and their friends and relatives (see Druick & Zegers, 2001, a book designed for a joint exhibit of the two artists' work). Although I assume these artists were not romantic or sexual partners in a literal sense (see Diamond, Chapter 11, this volume, for a pioneering study of the complexity of same-sex attraction and attachment), their relationship had many of the qualities of such a relationship. Gauguin, who left not only his wife and children but also Van Gogh when he moved to Tahiti, was clearly avoidant; and Van Gogh, who fell apart psychologically and famously cut off his ear when Gauguin left their collaborative relationship, was clearly anxious and preoccupied. Van Gogh did everything he possibly could to lure Gauguin into a collaborative relationship and to keep him from jettisoning it, and all the while Gauguin was writing to friends complaining about Van Gogh's annoying leech-like neediness and dependency.

Despite hoping, with Hazan et al., that we can do a better job of operationally identifying adult attachment, it would be a mistake, at least in some research contexts, to draw too sharp a line between attachment and nonattachment relationships. Besides the still undeveloped example of Gauguin and Van Gogh (and related studies of attachment and affiliation by Furman, 1999, and Mikulincer & Selinger, 2001), we might consider studies by Rom and Mikulincer (2003), who built on pioneering work by Smith, Murphy, and Coats (1999) to show that people can be "attached" to groups in which they work and that individual differences in attachment style, measured similarly to the way we measure them in the context of romantic relationships, predict how people feel and behave in the groups to which they are "attached." Moreover, group cohesion, which is related to the degree to which people feel integrated into and sensitively and responsively treated by a particular group, interacts with attachment style to predict work performance (even in the military, which might seem like an odd place to look for "love," although it is surely a context in which threats and fears and the wish for protection are rampant). In a similar vein, Kirkpatrick (2004) conducted several studies of "attachment to God" and summarized other researchers' studies of attachment and religion. Many of the individual differences in attachment style documented in the domain of romantic relationships reappear in relation to God and other religious figures, such as the Virgin Mary and the Buddha.

This should not be surprising, because we know that part of what underlies individual differences in attachment style is what Bowlby called "internal working models," cognitive–affective structures that come into play when a person feels threatened or is moved to perceive another person, group, or imaginary personage as a possible protector, safe haven, or secure base. Just as the mental structures or working models that originally applied to one's mother can be extended to actual and potential romantic partners (e.g., Zayas & Shoda, 2005), the models (expectations, assumptions, and lists of virtues or scary attributes) that apply to parents and romantic partners can be extended or transferred (Andersen & Chen, 2002) to group leaders, the Buddha, religious mentors, and so on. One of the simplest and most common Buddhist prayers is "I take *refuge* in the Buddha, the Dharma [the Buddha's teachings], and the Sangha [the community of fellow Buddhist practitioners]." This is a way of saying, "The living religious tradition to which I am attached, which includes vivid images of both legendary and currently living exemplary loving and protective individuals, serves me as a safe haven and secure base."

Hazan and colleagues (Chapter 3) say that "what distinguishes our attachment figures from everyone else is that, in a very literal sense, they reside inside of us" (a notion that fits well with Aron and Aron's ideas in Chapter 14 about "inclusion of the other in the self"):

> Their effects on us do not require their physical presence. We carry around mental images of them that we invoke when we need comforting. We go about our daily business more confidently because we know they are cheering us on and ready to help if needed. Our emotional reactions are tempered by anticipating their embrace or reassuring words. Our physiological homeostasis is sustained beyond immediate interactions because our physiological systems have been conditioned to them. (Hazan et al., p. 65, this volume)

I agree completely. But notice that these statements could apply to any person, symbolic figure, religious entity, group, or even culture to which a person becomes attached.

Mikulincer and I (Mikulincer & Shaver, 2004) have demonstrated in a preliminary way that when people are threatened or worn down by failure, they can call on symbolic residues of past good attachment relationships both to ease their current distress and to bolster their sense of themselves as strong, worthy, self-sustaining people who share some of their attachment figures' admirable qualities. I assume this can be done with Jesus and the Buddha almost as well as it can be done with Mom or "Putzie" (Richard Feynman's "baby talk" term of endearment for his wife Arline). Moreover, Mikulincer, Florian, and Hirschberger (2003) showed that attachment relationships can serve some of the "terror management" functions previously attributed only to self-esteem enhancement and adherence to a cultural worldview. My colleagues and I (Hart, Shaver, & Goldenberg, 2005) recently followed up this work and found that threatening one of the three main security-maintaining strategies (attachment, self-esteem, or worldview) evoked defensive responses in the others, suggesting a common underlying security-maintenance system. Both religions and political ideologies seem well designed to bolster this tripartite security system.

This is a huge and important topic, well beyond the scope of this chapter, but I hope by merely mentioning it to convey why I wouldn't want the effort to pin down a specific definition of attachment to keep us from exploring how some of our insights regarding attachment might extend into other social and psychological domains. In the same way that Bowlby (1969/1982) created attachment theory from very diverse ideas and research findings in psychoanalysis, ethology, cybernetics, cognitive and developmental psychology, and community psychiatry, we or our intellectual offspring can bring together new ideas, issues, and findings to create an intellectual framework and body of knowledge that reaches beyond today's attachment theory.

Perhaps this is an appropriate place to make a different but related point. There is a natural tension among psychological researchers when one theory or approach to research threatens to invade the territory staked out by another or when one subfield's interpretation and use of a seminal theoretical text, such as Bowlby's (1969/1982) first volume in the *Attachment and Loss* trilogy, differs from another subfield's interpretation or use of it. Relationship theorists who are not "attached" to attachment theory are quick to demand that "attachment" be defined more restrictively so that attachment researchers do not invade the territory of closeness researchers, interdependence researchers, group researchers, and so on. Moreover, attachment researchers who use observational or interview assessments of attachment style (e.g., the AAI; Hesse, 1999) are sometimes resistant to findings obtained with self-report questionnaires and social-cognition research paradigms (see, for example, the exchange between Shaver & Mikulincer, 2002a, 2002b, and Waters, Crowell, Elliott, Corcoran, & Treboux, 2002). Similarly, most of us self-report attachment researchers tend to ignore the AAI literature (although Bartholomew, Furman, and Simpson are important exceptions).

In my opinion, a healthy response to this kind of territory marking is to leave the boundaries loose for the time being, not because they should necessarily remain loose forever but because we are making interesting discoveries on all sides of all the fences I have just obliquely referred to and because we might not have made these discoveries if we had subdivided the intellectual territory prematurely and built more solid fences around the subterritories. The attitude I am recommending requires tolerance of ambiguity and openness to uncertainty and exploration, which we know are facilitated by security and impeded by insecurity and defensiveness. Fortunately, these intellectual tensions occur within a shared professional arena in which, to a great extent, we can attain greater courage and security simply by granting it to each other. The openness demonstrated by the authors of this book, especially the Arons, Reis, and Berscheid, who were chosen to represent alternative or complementary perspectives, provides an admirable set of examples.

My own preference for openness, broad scope, and perhaps even open-minded, temporary fuzziness affects my reading of Brumbaugh and Fraley's ambitious chapter (Chapter 4). They do a heroic job of reviewing gargantuan literatures on biological, cultural, and individual-difference determinants of mating and marriage patterns. In their biological analyses they find modest support for three hypotheses regarding the extension of infant–parent attachment capacities into the realm of adolescent and adult romantic love and mating: the paternal-care hypothesis, the developmental-immaturity or neoteny hypothesis, and the concealed-ovulation hypothesis. None of these hypotheses explains a great deal of the cross-species variance in mating systems, however, and I suspect the reason is twofold: (1) The nature of attachments in adulthood need not be completely explicable in terms of adaptive modules of the brain designed by evolution specifically for adult functions. It seems possible that modules or systems "designed" originally for infant–caregiver attachment simply continue to exist and are used as well in the adult pair-bonding context; and (2) whatever the biological processes involved in adult attachment turn out to be, they interact to such an extent with other emotional and cognitive processes that they are not likely to have a simple, tightly delimited, modular function of the kind imagined by evolutionary psychologists. (For a provocative critical review of the search for such modules in contemporary evolutionary psychology, see Buller, 2005.)

An instructive example of another system with the same kind of complexity is human language. Centuries of speculation have gone into trying to determine "*the* function" of human language, but I doubt that it has just one function. Once human language came into existence for whatever primary function or functions it originally served, it became the vehicle for myriad mental and communicative processes that almost certainly do not correspond to a single biological function. Moreover, human language seems to be a case in which there really are no clear phylogenetic antecedents, at least not ones that look anything like human language. There are not such antecedents even among our closest primate cousins (who, you may have noticed, have not said or published much lately).

Another example of an important human activity that involves attachment circuitry but probably not circuitry specifically evolved for its own purpose is religion (Kirkpatrick, 2004). Many scientists have tried to imagine what evolutionary function or functions religion might have had, but Kirkpatrick (2004) argues persuasively that religion is a multidimensional, multicomponent phenomenon that takes advantage of several different evolved behavioral systems without, most likely, being due at all to the evolution of a specific "religion module" in the brain. (For a somewhat different but generally compatible and very interesting analysis, see Rue, 2005.)

If many of the processes and functions associated with attachment can be observed in leader–follower, student–teacher, and devotee–God relationships, it doesn't make sense to restrict our consideration of them solely to their child–parent or reproductive relationship contexts. If my intuitions about this matter are correct, we should keep trying to discover how each of the behavioral systems works and what role it plays, separately and in collaboration with other psychological processes, in various social phenomena. It seems possible, for example, that the caregiving system comes into play most directly when a person serves as a parent, less directly but still powerfully when a person cares for a romantic partner, less directly but still notably when the person exhibits compassion and provides altruistic assistance to suffering members of an extended family or tribal or ethnic group, and even less directly when the person shows compassion and kindness to needy strangers (Gillath, Shaver, & Mikulincer, 2005; Mikulincer et al., 2005). The question of whether the caregiving behavioral system evolved specifically for its use in adult romantic or pair-bond relationships or was shaped in additional ways because of genetic payoffs for caregiving in relationships with village members and strangers should remain open.

My unrestricted, wait-and-see attitude extends to the case of recent efforts to determine whether people have a single attachment style in their relationships with parents, siblings, close friends, and various romantic partners (in cases in which there is more than one partner across time). Much of this research is still unpublished, but my impression from hearing about it at conferences and reviewing manuscripts submitted to journals is that the different attachment styles, as measured, are usually substantially correlated despite not being identical across all relationships. Undoubtedly, a person's relationship motives, worries, and behaviors are not the same across all relationships. Many studies show that both partners' attachment styles (and, I assume, caregiving and sexual styles as well, if those were measured) have effects on the relationship and on both partners' measurable feelings about it. For this to be the case (i.e., for there to be joint causality), the partners must affect each other's perceptions, satisfactions, and dissatisfactions. Given that some of these affected states involve trust and distrust, security and insecurity, commitment and infidelity, and many other such issues, the partners' responses to attachment measures should also be affected. This cross-relationship variability must not be so great, however, that it makes "global attachment style" a misleading or meaningless concept, because in many studies (reviewed by Mikulincer & Shaver, 2003, and Shaver & Mikulincer, 2005) we have found that people's scores on global attachment measures predict complex reactions to laboratory and real-world situations. Thus, although it is not unimportant to measure relationship-specific attachment styles, it would be a mistake to ignore a person's general attachment or caregiving or sexual tendencies while pursuing only differences between relationships.

Relations between Attachment Theory and Other Theories and Perspectives

Several chapters in this volume demonstrate that adopting an attachment theoretical approach to adolescent and adult couple relationships provides a useful perspective on, or a striking alternative to, other theoretical approaches. For example, in Chapter 5, Bartholomew and Allison question the reigning feminist perspective on partner violence and abuse and show that both partners' attachment histories and styles contribute to two important dyadic behavior patterns in abusive relationships: pursuing–distancing and pursuing–pursuing. The first pattern tends to occur, the authors say, "in couples with incompatible attachment needs (i.e., closeness vs. distance) . . . [and is generally observed] when individuals with preoccupied tendencies [are] partnered with more avoidant (fearful or dismissing) individuals" (p. 116). In this kind of interaction, either partner is capable of becoming violent, regardless of gender. The pursuing–pursuing pattern tends to occur in couples in which both partners are anxious or preoccupied. Such joint causality has been observed as well in much nonattachment research, in which mutual violence and abuse is predicted by both partners being high on measures of neuroticism or negative affectivity (e.g., Moffitt, Robins, & Caspi, 2001; Robins, Caspi, & Moffitt, 2000, 2002).

Interestingly, Bartholomew and Allison also say that interpersonal problems in abusive relationships are partly a matter of poor caregiving: "When both partners showed preoccupied tendencies, they tended to compete for support and attention from each other. Moreover, neither partner was able to recognize or meet his or her partner's needs, leading to mutual frustration and, at times, aggression" (p. 116). The authors go on to say that future research is likely to reveal that both partners in violent and abusive relationships suffer from "deficits in the ability to effectively ask for care, . . . perceive and appropriately respond to a partner's need for care, and . . . accept and benefit from partner care. . . . In relationships in which a partner's attachment needs are chronically frustrated, caregiving may indirectly fulfill attachment needs and may even serve to inhibit the activation of the attachment system" (p. 118). This is similar to using sexual behavior to serve attachment needs, as described in Chapter 12 by Davis and Chapter 13 by Gillath and Schachner.

In Chapter 6, Levy, Kelly, and Jack compare attachment theory with Buss's (1999; Buss, Larsen, & Westen, 1996) evolutionary theory of mating, two alternative ways to explain gender differences in sexual and emotional jealousy. As Levy et al. explain, "Buss et al. . . . found that men tend to view sexual infidelity as more distressful than women do, and women tend to view emotional infidelity as more distressful. They also found that men displayed greater physiological distress than did women while imagining a mate's sexual infidelity" (p. 130). These kinds of data have been viewed by Buss and his colleagues as evidence that men are worried about paternity certainty whereas women, who are pretty certain their children are their own, are worried lest their male partners commit their resources to other women and those women's offspring. Instead, Levy et al. thought the sex differences in kinds of jealousy might be explained by the fact that men are more likely than women to have a dismissingly avoidant attachment style (e.g., Shaver et al., 1996), and because this style has been associated with sexual promiscuity, lack of interest in psychological intimacy (e.g., Davis et al., 2004; Schachner & Shaver, 2002, 2004), and projection of one's own negative traits onto others (Mikulincer & Horesh, 1999)—possibly including attributing sexual infidelity to them—dismissing men might be more sexually than emotionally jealous. If so, this could explain the gender difference in types of jealousy without relying on Buss's theory.

Levy et al. found, in a large-sample study, that dismissing women were roughly 4 times as likely as secure women to say that sexual jealousy was more distressing than emotional jealousy and that dismissing men were nearly 50 times as likely as secure men to say that sexual jealousy was more troubling. Secure individuals of both genders were more likely to find emotional infidelity more distressing than sexual infidelity. Thus, although there were still notable gender differences in kinds of jealous reactions to partner infidelity, there were also important attachment-style differences moderating the gender differences. As the authors point out, the attachment perspective on jealousy suggests social and clinical interventions to reduce male sexual jealousy, which can sometimes escalate to violence or even murder, which the nonattachment version of evolutionary psychology does not.

Some of the studies described in Chapter 13, by Gillath and Schachner, show that, indeed, augmenting people's sense of security can incline them more toward a stable, long-term relationship, which shows that altering the attachment system can have effects on the sexual system. These results supplement previous studies by our research group (e.g., Gillath, Shaver, Mikulincer, Nitzberg, et al., 2005; Mikulincer et al., 2005) showing that augmenting a person's sense of attachment security causes the person to become more compassionate and altruistic. They also fit with results reported by Mikulincer et al. in Chapter 8 of this volume, which indicate that attachment security fosters gratitude and forgiveness, two prosocial orientations that should contribute to stability and quality of a long-term couple relationship. Combined with Davis's very comprehensive analysis of the process of sexual coercion (Chapter 12), these various clues from attachment research suggest possible methods of intervention to reduce relationship dysfunction and sexual violence.

Are Attachment and Sexual Attraction Incompatible?

In Chapter 16, Berscheid provocatively suggests, based on two kinds of evidence, that attachment and sexual attraction might be incompatible. First, sexual attraction and enthusiasm tend to wane over the course of long marriages, even though the partners remain quite attached to each other (Regan & Berscheid, 1999). Second, Wolf (1995) showed, in a fascinating study of an unusual marriage system once practiced in certain areas of Taiwan, that couples who were betrothed and brought up together as young children tended not to have good or long-lasting sexual and marital relationships in adulthood. (The couples were formed by parents when the partners-to-be, especially the girls, were quite young.)

I won't dispute the first kind of evidence, because it would require a lengthy analysis and because it does not, in any case, imply that it is the attachment per se that causes or contributes to the decline in sexual excitement. The second kind of evidence deserves attention, however, especially because most readers of this chapter will not have read Wolf's work, as I had not before Berscheid brought it to my attention in her chapter.

There turn out to be many complexities involved in the special cases of child betrothal discussed by Wolf (1995). First, the child brides-to-be were voluntarily given away by their own parents and placed in adoptive homes, where they were often treated very badly. Here are typical comments from two such brides quoted by Wolf: (1) "When I think of my childhood, I wonder why my fate was so bad. My foster mother beat me too often and too hard. I was always trembling with fear" (p. 61). (2) "They adopt someone else's daughter to do their work. I used to get so angry with my parents because they gave me away. . . . If they hadn't given me away, I probably would have had a very happy life. . . . I felt, 'No one pays attention to me, because I am an adopted daughter' " (p. 63).

Needless to say, there could be many reasons why such women's marriages were not as successful or satisfying, on average, as those of other women raised more normally, without this having anything to do with being attached to their husband-to-be. The live-in future brides often felt heartlessly rejected by their own parents and cruelly mistreated by their future husband's family, including the future husband himself. Wolf (1995) also mentions that couples of this kind tended to get married 2 years earlier, on average, than comparison couples, which in itself might have made their relationships less likely to succeed.

Most important and surprising to me, however, was Wolf's repeated and insistent claim that he was definitely *not* claiming that *adult* attachment interferes with *adult* sexual attraction or marital satisfaction. On p. 16, for example, he says, "That husband and wife commonly form enduring attachments is entirely irrelevant." The reason is that his main idea was that child husbands- and brides-to-be become familiar with each other before they have sexual motives, which then makes it difficult to view their adoptive sibling as a sex partner later on. He would not have advanced a similar hypothesis about a teenage girl adopted into a family with a teenage boy, nor did he believe in any way, shape, or form that adult spouses who were attached could not be sexually attracted to each other. Thus, although it is very important for us to look empirically at how the three behavioral systems under discussion in this book interact with and affect each other, there is no reason at present to predict that sex and attachment or sex and caregiving or caregiving and attachment cannot coexist and function in a mutually coordinated fashion.

CONCLUDING COMMENTS

I will end simply by saying, again, thanks so much to everyone involved in celebrating my watershed birthday and creating this stimulating, informative, and forward-looking book. I don't generally agree with cheery psychologists and gerontologists who say that old age is the best phase of life. But I would certainly agree that a 60th birthday celebration staged by bright, inventive colleagues, students, and friends can be delightful. I am utterly amazed by what has grown up from the tentative little theoretical acorn that Cindy Hazan and I planted in the *Journal of Personality and Social Psychology* almost 20 years ago, and I am grateful to everyone who helped it become a large and sturdy oak tree, even the people who corrected its dangerous lean with guy wires, trimmed its wayward branches, and assaulted it with bug spray from time to time. As I have tried to indicate here, the theory has benefited and will continue to benefit from criticisms and amendments offered by observant scientists with new data and alternative perspectives. I look forward to future birthdays, further discussions and debates, and new research methods and findings and to watching, for many more years, what develops from our mutual intellectual and social endeavors.

REFERENCES

Ainsworth, M. D. S., Blehar, M. C., Waters, E., & Wall, S. (1978). *Patterns of attachment: A psychological study of the Strange Situation.* Hillsdale, NJ: Erlbaum.

Andersen, S. M., & Chen, S. (2002). The relational self: An interpersonal social-cognitive theory. *Psychological Review, 109*, 619–645.

Bakermans-Kranenburg, M. J., van IJzendoorn, M. H., Bokhorst, C. L., & Schuengel, C. (2004). The importance of shared environment in infant–father attachment: A behavioral genetic study of the attachment Q-sort. *Journal of Family Psychology, 18*, 545–549.

Barrett, L. F. (2006a). Are emotions natural kinds? *Perspectives in Psychological Science, 1*, 28–58.

Barrett, L. F. (2006b). Solving the emotion paradox: Categorization and the experience of emotion. *Personality and Social Psychology Review, 10*, 20–46.

Berscheid, E. (1988). Some comments on love's anatomy: Or, whatever happened to old-fashioned lust? In R. J. Sternberg & M. L. Barnes (Eds.), *The psychology of love* (pp. 359–374). New Haven, CT: Yale University Press.

Bokhorst, C. L., Bakermans-Kranenburg, M. J., Fearon, P., van IJzendoorn, M. H., Fonagy, P., Schuengel, C., et al. (2003). The importance of shared environment in mother–infant attachment security: A behavioral genetic study. *Child Development, 74*, 1769–1782.

Bouchard, T. J., & Loehlin, J. C. (2001). Genes, evolution, and personality. *Behavior Genetics, 31*, 243–273.

Bowlby, J. (1973). *Attachment and loss: Vol. 2. Separation: Anxiety and anger.* New York: Basic Books.

Bowlby, J. (1979). *The making and breaking of affectional bonds*. London: Tavistock.

Bowlby, J. (1980). *Attachment and loss: Vol. 3. Loss: Sadness and depression.* New York: Basic Books.

Bowlby, J. (1982). *Attachment and loss: Vol. 1. Attachment* (2nd ed.). New York: Basic Books. (Original work published 1969)

Brennan, K. A., Clark, C. L., & Shaver, P. R. (1998). Self-report measurement of adult romantic attachment: An integrative overview. In J. A. Simpson & W. S. Rholes (Eds.), *Attachment theory and close relationships* (pp. 46–76). New York: Guilford Press.

Brussoni, M. J., Jang, K. L., Livesley, W. J., & MacBeth, T. M. (2000). Genetic and environmental influences on adult attachment styles. *Personal Relationships, 7*, 283–289.

Buller, D. J. (2005). *Adapting minds: Evolutionary psychology and the persistent quest for human nature*. Cambridge, MA: MIT Press.

Buss, D. M. (1999). *Evolutionary psychology: The new science of the mind.* Boston: Allyn & Bacon.

Buss, D. M., Larsen, R. J., & Westen, D. (1996). Sex differences in jealousy: Not gone, not forgotten, and not explained by alternative hypotheses. *Psychological Science, 7*, 373–375.

Collins, N. L., & Feeney, B. C. (2005). *Attachment processes in daily interaction: Feeling supported and feeling secure*. Unpublished manuscript, University of California, Santa Barbara.

Cooper, M. L., Shaver, P. R., & Collins, N. L. (1998). Attachment styles, emotion regulation, and adjustment in adolescence. *Journal of Personality and Social Psychology, 74*, 1380–1397.

Crawford, T. N., Jang, K. L., Livesley, W. J., Shaver, P. R., Cohen, P., & Ganiban, J. (2005). *The overlap between self-reported attachment insecurity and personality disorders in adults: Genetic and environmental influences*. Submitted for publication.

Davis, D., Shaver, P. R., & Vernon, M. L. (2004). Attachment style and subjective motivations for sex. *Personality and Social Psychology Bulletin, 30*, 1076–1090.

de Wolff, M., & van IJzendoorn, M. H. (1997). Sensitivity and attachment: A meta-analysis on parental antecedents of infant attachment. *Child Development, 68*, 571–591.

Druick, D. W., & Zegers, P. K. (2001). *Van Gogh and Gauguin: The studio of the south*. Chicago: Art Institute of Chicago.

Ekman, P. (1992). An argument for basic emotions. *Cognition and Emotion*, 6, 169–200.

Feynman, M. (Ed.). (2005). *Perfectly reasonable deviations from the beaten track: The letters of Richard P. Feynman*. New York: Basic Books.

Finkel, D., & Matheny, A. P. (2000). Genetic and environmental influences on a measure of infant attachment security. *Twin Research*, *3*, 242–250.

Frijda, N. H. (1986). *The emotions*. Cambridge, UK: Cambridge University Press.

Furman, W. (1999). Friends and lovers: The role of peer relationships in adolescent romantic relationships. In W. A. Collins & B. Laursen (Eds.), *Minnesota symposia on child psychology: Vol. 30. Relationships as developmental contexts* (pp. 133–154). Mahwah, NJ: Erlbaum.

Gillath, O., Bunge, S. A., Shaver, P. R., Wendelken, C., & Mikulincer, M. (2005). Attachment-style differences and ability to suppress negative thoughts: Exploring the neural correlates. *Neuroimage, 28*, 835–847.

Gillath, O., Shaver, P. R., & Mikulincer, M. (2005). An attachment-theoretical approach to compassion and altruism. In P. Gilbert (Ed.), *Compassion: Conceptualizations, research, and use in psychotherapy* (pp. 121–147). London: Brunner-Routledge.

Gillath, O., Shaver, P. R., Mikulincer, M., Nitzberg, R. E., Erez, A., & van IJzendoorn, M. H. (2005). Attachment, caregiving, and volunteering: Placing volunteerism in an attachment-theoretical framework. *Personal Relationships*, *12*, 425–446.

Graziano, W. G., & Tobin, R. M. (2002). Agreeableness: Dimension of personality or social desirability artifact? *Journal of Personality*, *70*, 695–727.

Griffin, D. W., & Bartholomew, K. (1994). The metaphysics of measurement: The case of adult attachment. In K. Bartholomew & D. Perlman (Eds.), *Advances in personal relationships: Vol. 5. Attachment processes in adulthood* (pp. 17–52). London: Kingsley.

Harlow, H. F. (1959). Love in infant monkeys. *Scientific American*, *200*, 68–86.

Hart, J. J., Shaver, P. R., & Goldenberg, J. L. (2005). Attachment, self-esteem, worldviews, and terror management: Evidence for a tripartite security system. *Journal of Personality and Social Psychology*, *88*, 999–1013.

Hazan, C., & Shaver, P. R. (1987). Romantic love conceptualized as an attachment process. *Journal of Personality and Social Psychology*, *52*, 511–524.

Hazan, C., & Zeifman, D. (1994). Sex and the psychological tether. In K. Bartholomew & D. Perlman (Eds.), *Advances in personal relationships: Vol. 5. Attachment processes in adulthood* (pp. 151–177) London: Kingsley.

Hesse, E. (1999). The Adult Attachment Interview: Historical and current perspectives. In J. Cassidy & P. R. Shaver (Eds.), *Handbook of attachment: Theory, research, and clinical applications* (pp. 395–433. New York: Guilford Press.

Kestenbaum, R., Farber, E. A., & Sroufe, L. A. (1989, Summer). Individual differences in empathy among preschoolers: Relation to attachment history. *New Directions for Child Development*, *44*, 51–64.

Kirkpatrick, L. A. (2004). *Attachment, evolution, and the psychology of religion*. New York: Guilford Press.

Kunce, L. J., & Shaver, P. R. (1994). An attachment-theoretical approach to caregiving in romantic relationships. In K. Bartholomew & D. Perlman (Eds.), *Advances in personal relationships: Vol. 5. Attachment processes in adulthood* (pp. 205–237). London, England: Kingsley.

Lutz, A., Greischar, L. L., Rowlings, N. B., Ricard, M., & Davidson, R. J. (2004). Long-term meditators self-induce high amplitude gamma synchrony during mental practice. *Proceedings of the National Academy of Sciences, 101*, 16369–16373.

Main, M. (1995). Attachment: Overview, with implications for clinical work. In S. Goldberg, R. Muir, & J. Kerr (Eds.), *Attachment theory: Social, developmental, and clinical perspectives* (pp. 407–474). Hillsdale, NJ: Analytic Press.

McCrae, R. R., & Costa, P. T., Jr. (1996). Toward a new generation of personality theories: Theoretical contexts for the five-factor model. In J. S. Wiggins (Ed.), *The five-factor model of personality: Theoretical perspectives* (pp. 51–87). New York: Guilford Press.

Mikulincer, M., Florian, V., & Hirschberger, G. (2003). The existential function of close relationships: Introducing death into the science of love. *Personality and Social Psychology Review, 7*, 20–40.

Mikulincer, M., Gillath, O., & Shaver, P. R. (2002). Activation of the attachment system in adulthood: Threat-related primes increase the accessibility of mental representations of attachment figures. *Journal of Personality and Social Psychology, 83*, 881–895.

Mikulincer, M., & Horesh, N. (1999). Adult attachment style and the perception of others: The role of projective mechanisms. *Journal of Personality and Social Psychology, 76*, 1022–1034.

Mikulincer, M., & Selinger, M. (2001). The interplay between attachment and affiliation systems in adolescents' same-sex friendships: The role of attachment style. *Journal of Social and Personal Relationships, 18*, 81–106.

Mikulincer, M., & Shaver, P. R. (2003). The attachment behavioral system in adulthood: Activation, psychodynamics, and interpersonal processes. In M. P. Zanna (Ed.), *Advances in experimental social psychology* (Vol. 35, pp. 53–152). New York: Academic Press.

Mikulincer, M., & Shaver, P. R. (2004). Security-based self-representations in adulthood: Contents and processes. In W. S. Rholes & J. A. Simpson (Eds.), *Adult attachment: Theory, research, and clinical implications* (pp. 159–195). New York: Guilford Press.

Mikulincer, M., Shaver, P. R., Gillath, O., & Nitzberg, R. E. (2005). Attachment, caregiving, and altruism: Boosting attachment security increases compassion and helping. *Journal of Personality and Social Psychology, 89*, 817–839.

Moffitt, T. E., Robins, R. W., & Caspi, A. (2001). A couples analysis of partner abuse with implications for abuse-prevention policy. *Criminology and Public Policy, 1*, 5–36.

Murray, S. L., Holmes, J. G., & Griffin, D. W. (1996). The benefits of positive illusions: Idealization and the construction of satisfaction in close relationships. *Journal of Personality and Social Psychology, 70*, 79–98.

Noftle, E. E., & Shaver, P. R. (in press). Attachment dimensions and the Big Five personality traits as predictors of close relationship outcomes. *Journal of Research in Personality.*

Oatley, K., & Jenkins, J. M. (1996). *Understanding emotions.* Cambridge, MA: Blackwell.

O'Connor, T. G., & Croft, C. M. (2001). A twin study of attachment in preschool children. *Child Development, 72,* 1501–1511.

Pietromonaco, P. R., & Feldman Barrett, L. (1997). Working models of attachment and daily social interactions. *Journal of Personality and Social Psychology, 73,* 1409–1423.

Regan, P. C., & Berscheid, E. (1999). *Lust: What we know about human sexual desire.* Thousand Oaks, CA: Sage.

Reis, H. T., & Shaver, P. R. (1988). Intimacy as an interpersonal process. In S. Duck (Ed.), *Handbook of research in personal relationships* (pp. 367–389). London: Wiley.

Ricciuti, A. E. (1992). Child–mother attachment: A twin study. *Dissertation Abstracts International, 54,* 3364. (UMI No. 9324873).

Robins, R. W., Caspi, A., & Moffitt, T. E. (2000). Two personalities, one relationship: Both partners' personality traits shape the quality of their relationship. *Journal of Personality and Social Psychology, 79,* 251–259.

Robins, R. W., Caspi, A., & Moffitt, T. E. (2002). It's not just who you're with, it's who you are: Personality and relationship experiences across multiple relationships. *Journal of Personality, 70,* 925–964.

Rom, E., & Mikulincer, M. (2003). Attachment theory and group processes: The association between attachment style and group-related representations, goals, memories, and functioning. *Journal of Personality and Social Psychology, 84,* 1220–1235.

Rue, L. (2005). *Religion is not about God: How spiritual traditions nurture our biological nature and what to expect when they fail.* New Brunswick, NJ: Rutgers University Press.

Schachner, D. A., & Shaver, P. R. (2002). Attachment style and human mate poaching. *New Review of Social Psychology, 1,* 122–129.

Schachner, D. A., & Shaver, P. R. (2004). Attachment dimensions and motives for sex. *Personal Relationships, 11,* 179–195.

Schwartz, J., & Shaver, P. R. (1987). Emotions and emotion knowledge in interpersonal relations. In W. Jones & D. Perlman (Eds.), *Advances in personal relationships* (Vol. 1, pp. 197–241). Greenwich, CT: JAI Press.

Shaver, P. R., & Brennan, K. A. (1992). Attachment styles and the "big five" personality traits: Their connections with each other and with romantic relationship outcomes. *Personality and Social Psychology Bulletin, 18,* 536–545.

Shaver, P. R., Hazan, C., & Bradshaw, D. (1988). Love as attachment: The integration of three behavioral systems. In R. J. Sternberg & M. Barnes (Eds.), *The psychology of love* (pp. 68–99). New Haven, CT: Yale University Press.

Shaver, P. R., & Mikulincer, M. (2002a). Attachment-related psychodynamics. *Attachment and Human Development, 4,* 133–161.

Shaver, P. R., & Mikulincer, M. (2002b). Dialogue on adult attachment: Diversity and integration. *Attachment and Human Development, 4,* 243–257.

Shaver, P. R., & Mikulincer, M. (2005). Attachment theory and research: Resurrection of the psychodynamic approach to personality. *Journal of Research in Personality, 39,* 22–45.

Shaver, P. R., Morgan, H. J., & Wu, S. (1996). Is love a "basic" emotion? *Personal Relationships, 3,* 81–96.

Shaver, P. R., Schwartz, J., Kirson, D., & O'Connor, C. (1987). Emotion knowledge: Further exploration of a prototype approach. *Journal of Personality and Social Psychology, 52*, 1061–1086.

Singer, I. (1984). *The nature of love: Vol. 1. Plato to Luther* (2nd ed.). Chicago: University of Chicago Press.

Smith, E. R., Murphy, J., & Coats, S. (1999). Attachment to groups: Theory and measurement. *Journal of Personality and Social Psychology, 77*, 94–110.

Tidwell , M. C. O., Reis, H. T., & Shaver, P. R. (1996). Attachment, attractiveness, and social interaction: A diary study. *Journal of Personality and Social Psychology, 71*, 729–745.

Tracy, J. L., Shaver, P. R., Albino, A. W., & Cooper, M. L. (2003). Attachment styles and adolescent sexuality. In P. Florsheim (Ed.), *Adolescent romance and sexual behavior: Theory, research, and practical implications* (pp. 137–159). Mahwah, NJ: Erlbaum.

van IJzendoorn, M. H. (1995). Adult attachment representations, parental responsiveness, and infant attachment: A meta-analysis on the predictive validity of the Adult Attachment Interview. *Psychological Bulletin, 117*, 387–403.

Waters, E., Crowell, J., Elliott, M., Corcoran, D., & Treboux, D. (2002). Bowlby's secure base theory and the social/personality psychology of attachment styles: Work(s) in progress. *Attachment and Human Development*, 4, 230–242.

Weinfield, N. S., Sroufe, L. A., Egeland, B., & Carlson, E. A. (1999). The nature of individual differences in infant–caregiver attachment. In J. Cassidy & P. R. Shaver (Eds.), *Handbook of attachment: Theory, research, and clinical applications* (pp. 68–88). New York: Guilford Press.

Wolf, A. P. (1995). *Sexual attraction and childhood association: A Chinese brief for Edward Westermarck*. Stanford, CA: Stanford University Press.

Zayas, V., & Shoda, Y. (2005). Do automatic reactions elicited by thoughts of romantic partner, mother, and self relate to adult romantic attachment? *Personality and Social Psychology Bulletin, 31*, 1011–1025.

Index

N

O

P